Black Holes of Smooth Muscle Physiology

Myogenic Automaticity and Vascular Basal Tone

nova
Medicine & Health
New York

Vascular Research Developments Series

The VSITE Review
Young Kim, MD
ISBN: 978-1-53619-934-5
eBook ISBN: 978-1-68507-030-4

Peripheral Artery Disease: From Risk Factors to Management
Jeremy D. Parks (Editor)
ISBN: 978-1-53619-968-0
eBook ISBN: 978-1-53619-986-4

More information about this series can be found at
https://novapublishers.com/product-category/series/vascular-research-developments/

Anatoly Soloviev

Black Holes of Smooth Muscle Physiology

Myogenic Automaticity and Vascular Basal Tone

nova
Medicine & Health
New York

DOI: https://doi.org/10.52305/SDST7340

Library of Congress Cataloging-in-Publication Data

ISBN: 979-8-89530-703-8 (Hardcover)
ISBN: 979-8-89530-764-9 (eBook)

Published by Nova Science Publishers, Inc. † New York

Contents

Foreword

The term 'vascular tone' refers to blood vessels existing in a state of partial constriction. Arterial vascular tone is particularly important, having two vital physiological functions: to maintain arterial blood pressure essential for an adequate arterio-venous pressure-gradient and thus blood flow throughout the body; and to modulate blood flow to the various tissues and organs in concert with their metabolic requirements. Ultimately, vascular tone is subject to the degree of vascular smooth muscle cell contraction. The biology of vascular smooth muscle contraction and relaxation has been an area of intense study for over a century, from Bayliss's observations on the effects of pressure changes on bat-wing arteries to modern investigations of miRNA, molecular microscopy and the whole variety of 'omics'. Agents modulating vascular tone are amongst the most widely prescribed drugs in the world. Yet, disorders of vascular tone persist, from primary hypertension to coronary and cerebral vasospasm to the recently identified '-NOCA' diseases (Ischemia, Angina or Myocardial Infarction with Non-Occluded Coronary Arteries).

At the outset of this engrossing and comprehensive new book, Anatoly Soloviev argues that failure to understand the fundamental mechanisms controlling basal vascular smooth muscle tone - a "black hole" at the centre of vascular physiology - is impeding development of effective therapeutic strategies against diseases, or indeed syndromes involving abnormal vessel constriction. The book sets out to explore the hole and fill it with some engrossing, cogently argued theories. Ideas and evidence are communicated in the author unique style combining physiology and biophysics with other scientific disciplines, history, literate quotations and admirable acknowledgement of his Ukranian, Russian and eastern European forebears and colleagues.

Chapters 3 and 4 discuss vascular smooth muscle cells as physiological oscillators, exhibiting rhythmic cycles of contraction and relaxation analogous with gastrointestinal and uterine smooth muscle. As an example of this oscillatory activity, Chapter 3 describes the biophysics of the arterial myogenic response, an intrinsic contractile or relaxation reaction of the smooth muscle cells to altered longitudinal stretch or tension, driven by corresponding changes in arterial intralumenal pressure. Myogenic responsiveness of vascular smooth muscle cells and arteries is later developed as a key idea of the book.

This discussion is then expanded into the meat of the book's key issue, vascular smooth muscle tone and the function of resistance arteries in blood flow autoregulation, the phenomenon of maintained local blood flow satisfying tissue or organ metabolic requirements in the face of varying system-wide forces. Chapters 5-8 detail some theories advanced to explain the phenomenon and describe some supporting examples in engaging and entertaining detail, with some enlightening historical insights. The theories include the aforementioned myogenic or Ostroumov-Bayliss response of intralumenal pressure-driven vasoconstriction; the metabolic theory whereby cells produce paracrine vasoactive substances in accord with their metabolic activity; and changes in perivascular fluid pressure resulting from pressure-induced modulation of capillary filtration. This last idea is described as "exotic," but the authors make a detailed argument supporting its potential role in reactive hyperemia of skeletal muscle, a classic example of blood flow autoregulation traditionally explained from a myogenic or metabolic standpoint.

Chapter 9 delves into the black hole more deeply, further exploring the idea of myogenic responsiveness as a key controller of basal vascular smooth muscle cell contraction. The term myogenic derives from our understanding of a muscle-dependent response independent of neuro-humoral or other extracellular signalling factors. Starting from Bjorn Folkow's 1964 description of vascular smooth muscle cells as "mechanoreceptors with a built-in contractile system," the chapter is both expansive in comparing vascular myogenic tone with other examples of fundamental oscillatory control systems modulated by a variety of inputs, and detailed in discussing possible molecular mechanisms of vascular smooth muscle myogenic activity. Some interesting ideas are explored, including whether myogenically active vascular smooth muscle cells represent a subpopulation within the vessel wall, electrically coupled to other non-myogenic cells, leading to the possibility of vascular 'pacemaker' cells equivalent to the gastrointestinal interstitial cells of Cajal. Vasomotion - rhythmic cycles of contraction and dilation of resistance arteries, oscillations with modifiable frequencies– is also discussed as a physiological manifestation of myogenic responsiveness.

Chapter 10 explores a thesis dear to the authors' hearts, that metabolic autoregulation - contraction or relaxation of vascular smooth muscle caused by the tissue's metabolic requirements - is mediated by the vascular smooth muscle cells' response to changes in oxygen supply through glycolysis. Following an elegant preliminary argument both for and against the hypothesis, data is shown demonstrating that contractile force of the cell is inhibited in hypoxia through effects on Ca2+ entry and intracellular Ca2+ release. Glycolysis, an oscillatory cell process, is proposed as an underlying mechanism linking cellular [O_2] to ATP production, glycolytic ATP primarily devoted to the activity of plasmalemmal Na^+/K^+-ATP-dependent pump – and from there, oscillations in cell membrane potential, Ca2+-entry and contraction. Several different lines of argument are developed in support of the idea, a very interesting one with some still unexplained components, as noted by the author.

The impact of other vascular cells on basal vascular smooth muscle and arterial tone is explored in Chapter 11. These include factors associated with the vessel's adventitial layer, including immunomodulatory cells and factors released by perivascular adipose tissue. Vascular endothelial cells and their multiple vasoactive agents and structures are also discussed, including the potential impact of endothelial dysfunction on hypercontractility of the overlying smooth muscle. Chapters 12 and 13 discuss dynamics of the two key ions in vascular smooth muscle contraction, Ca^{2+} and K^+, with a concise discussion of the various channels, pumps and other mechanisms involved in modulating their intracellular concentrations. It was gratifying to see the large-conductance Ca^{2+}-activated K^+-channel (known variously as BKCa, KCa1.1 and Maxi-K) given prominence. Also included here is a gratifying, lengthy discussion on the potential roles of transient receptor potential ion channels (TRP), a large family of voltage-independent, non-selective cation channels serving a variety of cellular roles still being explored. The authors are smart to focus on these channels, and to introduce the idea of TRP subtypes being intimately involved in heterogeneity of vascular tone control. The idea that vascular smooth muscle cells in arteries or blood vessels in differing tissues and organs would express differing control systems linked to tissue function is a very important one. Several examples are described here.

Chapters 14 and 15 take seeming digressions from the central thesis in exploring, respectively, the role of water channels (aquaporins) and electromagnetic fields in vascular smooth muscle cell function. The former are placed cleverly in context given the authors' interest in trans-mural and indeed trans-membrane pressures as mechanical stimuli controlling vascular tone.

The discussion on electromagnetic fields involves mitochondrial and microtubule activity and links these to the authors' interest in coupled oscillators. There is a remarkable discussion on the use of gold nano-particles to modulate vascular ion channel activity through interaction with cellular electromagnetic fields. Chapter 16 briefly discusses the role of reaction oxygen species in modulation of vascular tone - as with TRP channels, this is an evolving area with much remaining to be explored. Nevertheless, the authors make a smart link back to the effect of superoxide and hydrogen peroxide on Na+/K+-ATPase activity in the context of their main theses.

Chapter 17 is arguably the most fascinating and absorbing section of the book. It fundamentally describes the effects of ionizing radiation on vascular smooth muscle cell contraction, arterial resistance and blood pressure, based on the authors' experiences after the Chernobyl disaster in 1986. The primary inhibiting effect of ionizing radiation on vascular BKCa expression and function is described and supported by evidence, together with effects on other ion channels and potential mechanistic roles for ROS and protein kinase C. Amazing reading. Chapter 18 is a brief summary on the potential for miRNA to modulate vascular tone. As with some of the immediately preceding chapters, the role of miRNA in vascular smooth muscle physiology is a developing field with much remaining to be discovered.

In Chapter 19 and the conclusion, the author looks ahead from their key idea that myogenic responsiveness - their Ostroumov-Bayliss response, first described in 1902 – is the fundamental controller of basal vascular smooth muscle tone; if not filling the black hole, at least shrinking it substantially. The chapter addresses one of the fundamental unanswered questions of myogenic responses; what is the cellular tension- or stretch-sensor coupling the mechanical stimulus to contraction? Some of the proposed mechanisms are discussed, including mechano-sensitive ion channels including TRP, G-protein coupled receptors, and indeed G-proteins themselves and integrins. The possibility of non-traditional cellular contractile mechanisms activated by these sensors is also explored. Once again, the diversity of potential tension-sensors and associated contractile mechanisms should emphasize the key idea of vascular heterogeneity. It is entirely possible and indeed encouraging, from a therapeutic point of view, that there is no single, fundamental mechanism establishing basal vascular tone, and indeed such mechanisms are variable throughout the body. Cerebral arteries establish basal tone through a signalling pathway different from the arteries in the coronary circulation, different again from renal arteries, etc.

Overall, this book is terrifically detailed, with an engaging tone and interesting perspectives on the idea of basal vascular smooth muscle tone. The ideas are informed by extensive experience in the field and solid, detailed experimental evidence. Congratulations to Tony and his comrades on their achievement, and enjoy his book!

Tim Murphy, BSc (Hons), PhD.
UNSW Sydney, Australia,
February 2025.
President, ANZMS Senior Lecturer,
School of Biomedical Sciences,
Faculty of Medicine,
The University of New South Wales,
Sydney, Australia

Acknowledgments

My sincere gratitude to all my teachers, who at different times and in different ways (by their personal example or advice) helped and supported me in my scientific way. I am grateful to all those who are now alive and well, and to those who are no longer with us, but who have always remained dear to my heart. These are Yury M. Smirnov, Igor I. Grechishkin, Grigory P. Conradi, Vladimir M. Khayutin, Moisey I. Gurevich, Semen A. Bershtein, Platon G. Kostyuk, David A. Brown, Thomas B. Bolton, Per Hellstrand, Alison M. Gurney, Richard Gryglewsky, Bjorn Folkov, John Shepherd, Robert Furchgott and Paul Vanhoutte. And, of course, my deep gratitude to my collaborators and colleagues, without whose participation this book would never have appeared – Sergey M. Tishkin, Irina V. Ivanova, Igor V. Kizub, Sergey V. Kyrychenko, Alexander V. Parshikov, Vadym G. Sydorenko, Tatiana V. Novochatska, Igor L. Monchak, Dariia O. Dryn, Maria I. Melnyk. Many thanks to Professor A. V. Zholos for his professional advice regarding the role of calcium "window current" and various TRP channels in vascular function.

Chapter 1

Introduction

"What we call the beginning is often the end.
And to make an end is to make a beginning.
The end is where we start from."
T. S. Eliot

The existence of local regulation of blood flow has been known since the time of Claude Bernard. It became clear that the blood supply to various organs depends on the level of their functional activity and metabolism. Unfortunately, at that time, physiologists could only measure blood pressure, but not parameters of linear or volumetric blood flow. Of course, blood pressure is an important parameter. However, it should be remembered that this is an integral value, depending both on the work of the heart and on the state of the vascular bed as a whole. That is, at that time it was technically possible to study mainly systemic blood flow. It is clear that where systemic hemodynamics is studied, and the main indicator is arterial pressure, their central, nervous regulation comes first.

The situation changed radically when it became possible to measure blood flow in tissues and the contractile and electrical characteristics of isolated smooth muscles and cells *in vitro*. It is quite clear that by this time, a huge number of questions had accumulated in the physiology of blood circulation, and the main one, of course, was the question of the nature of vascular tone. I have dealt with this problem for 50 long years, and my current feelings are ambivalent. On the one hand, there have been and are successes in our field of research, sometimes even very tangible ones. On the other hand, there is a feeling of futility of effort. The problem multiplies before our eyes, divides, breaks up into parts, and, most importantly, does not come into hand in its entirety.

Why did the term "black holes" appear in the title of our book? A black hole, as you know, is a region of space-time, the gravitational attraction of which is so strong that even objects moving at the speed of light, including quanta of light itself, cannot leave it. Astrophysicists think so. For everyone else, the abyss is that which has no bottom. The Great Russian scientist and poet of the past, Mikhail Lomonosov, wrote about the cosmos... "The abyss has opened, full of stars that have no number, and the abyss has no bottom." A living cell is a microcosm within us, and its main secrets remain hidden to us until now, as well as the main secrets of the universe.

Undoubtedly, doing science is not only a way to earn a living, but also an exciting journey through the world of mysteries. Only now, more and more, there is a feeling that in our profession it is very often impossible to achieve a specific goal and unequivocally solve the problem. As soon as you successfully solve one part of the problem, a dozen new ones immediately appear. Each new solution creates a maze of new possibilities. In other words, the closer you get to something, the further it moves away from you. Thomas Eliot was right when he wrote that where something ends, something must begin. The end is where the beginning is.

It is a common thing for a scientist when at the end of research to have a feeling that everything that has been done disappears somewhere, but there is still no solution to the problem. It is as if you are digging a deep hole, trying to get to the bottom of something, and suddenly you notice that more and more new branches appear in the earthen passage you dug, and all the soil you throw out by some miracle disappears somewhere.

One can, of course, console oneself by investing one's small brick in the general building of some grandiose concept that will someday radically change people's ideas about the functioning of living things. But in this process of cognition, there must be some key nodes, when a certain mechanism of regulation of physiological functions becomes clear completely and irrevocably. At such nodal points, the existing presentation paradigm must at least partially change (Kuhn, 1962).

In any branch of science, there are directions, the study of which lasts for decades without visible real progress. In medicine, this is, for example, the treatment of arterial hypertension (AH). Many discoveries have been made, and even more new drugs have been created. Undoubtedly, the quality of life of patients suffering from this disease has improved. But for some reason, the mortality rate is decreasing very little. This means that we are doing something wrong. This means that we do not know something important for the effective treatment of this disease. Namely, we do not fully understand the nature of vascular tone and its architectonics. An effective drug cannot be created if the pharmacological target is not precisely defined.

Unfortunately, in the last 20-30 years, studies of the mechanisms of regulation of regional blood flow and basal tone in the physiology of blood circulation have not been a priority. Researchers prefer to solve specific problems, mainly related to conducting preclinical studies of potential drugs. I am well aware of this type of research, when its participants solve their narrowly specialized tasks set before them by sponsors, often without even having an idea of the main goal of the research.

One reason for this state of affairs is that such studies often require the use of anesthetized animals. For quite understandable and well-known reasons, this creates many additional problems. Of course, the factor mentioned above of the seeming futility of research on such a global problem as basal vascular tone also played its role. In addition, pharmaceutical companies pay much more for their work than universities. However, I think it would be a big strategic mistake to accept this state of affairs.

Chapter 2

Two Main Problems of Modern Pharmaco-Therapy

Why do we attach so much importance to the problem of basal tone? The reason is simple. It lies in the insufficiently high efficiency of modern pharmacotherapy for vascular diseases. This is a serious problem since the effectiveness of disease treatment of the cardiovascular system has not changed over the past 40-50 years, amounting to less than 60% at best (that is subject to all the principles of evidence-based medicine). For example, despite the availability of a huge arsenal of drugs, mortality from the consequences of arterial hypertension (AH), at best, does not decline. This disease is easy to diagnose but unfortunately difficult to treat.

Patients have to take medicines for hypertension for life since when they are canceled, the disease with all its symptoms inevitably returns. Most drugs currently play the role of a kind of "pharmacological crutches." Take away the crutches and the person will fall. If you end the pharmacological support, all the symptoms do not just return, but they reappear in an enhanced form - such is a somewhat pharmacological rebound. This way, you will have to use the services of a pharmacy and a doctor for the rest of your life. This is not a cure; it is an imitation of a cure, not more.

Deviation 1. *It seems that we live in a time of substitution and confusion of concepts. Not only in politics but also in science. What meaning do we put into the term treatment, therapy (Greek θεραπεία - treatment, recovery)? Most often, this is understood as a process, the purpose of which is to alleviate, remove or eliminate the symptoms and manifestations of a particular disease, pathological condition, or other impairment of life, normalize disturbed life processes, and restore health.*

It turns out that the result of this process is not the elimination of the very cause of the disease, but only the minimization of its manifestations, i.e., symptoms. If so, it becomes clear why, despite intensive research and the availability of a huge number of new antihypertensive drugs, hypertension, for example, and its complications continue to dominate among the leading causes of death in the working population. Despite the declared successes in treatment, mortality and disability rates in AH practically do not decrease.

As already mentioned, this disease is easy to diagnose but difficult to treat. With the abolition of drugs, AH, as a rule, returns. You will have to be treated for all your life, i.e., the meaning of treatment comes down to the banal elimination of symptoms and improving the quality of life, which in itself is not so bad (if you also do not pay attention to the side effects of drugs). Not bad, if the task of cure is not set. I emphasize, not only to treat but also to cure! It turns out that at present, the process of treatment is more important for us - pharmaceutical companies produce drugs, patients buy, symptoms go away, profits grow - everything seems to be fine.

Among specialists dealing with the problems of hypertension, everyone is well aware of the so-called "rule of halves," which was introduced into circulation in 1960 in the USA. Its essence is that half of patients with hypertension do not know that they are sick. Half of those who know about their disease are not treated. Only half of the patients achieve satisfactory results. You can rephrase this statement in such a way that half of those who are treated do it wrong. If this rule is true, then a simple calculation shows that at best, just over 12% (according to maximum estimates of up to 25%) of patients with AH receive the correct treatment. The figure is depressingly low, even if we imagine that it is actually 2-3 times higher. Moreover, "correct" in this case means only that they are treated following modern ideas about the etiology and pathogenesis of AH, i.e., receive inhibitors of the sympathetic nervous system, diuretics, calcium antagonists, beta-blockers, blockers of the synthesis of angiotensin-converting enzyme (ACE) and its receptors, etc. In other words, the "correctness" of treatment directly depends on how "correctly" certain links of AH pathogenesis are identified.

The appearance of each group of drugs from the above gave rise to new hopes in due time, but periods of euphoria quickly gave way to pessimistic moods. Without going into details, we note that, like many years ago, the effectiveness of the treatment of hypertension continues to be insufficient. There is reason to believe that the main reason for this lies, apparently, in the multiplicity and complexity of the mechanisms leading to an increase in blood pressure, and the lack of knowledge about the key links in its pathogenesis.

Indeed, pathophysiology has long known that many organs and systems are involved in the mechanisms of high blood pressure: dysfunction of the heart, resistive and capacitive vessels, cortical and medulla of the adrenal glands, the juxtaglomerular apparatus of the kidneys, the autonomic nervous system, etc. A multi-circuit and multi-level system of regulation and stabilization of blood pressure includes many subsystems that ensure the optimal mode of operation of the heart and the value of peripheral vascular resistance, at which the work performed by the myocardium is minimal. This system consists of many humoral and neural circuits that regulate the functions of the heart and blood vessels, and, despite its inherent reliability, is quite easily vulnerable precisely because of its great complexity. It may seem that the search for a single main mechanism responsible for the development of hypertension and the maintenance of a high level of systemic arterial pressure is unpromising. If so, then the time of the predicted "victory" over AH is pushed back into the infinitely distant future. This would be too pessimistic a forecast.

The nature of the physiological regulation of functions is such that the mechanisms of management and control of the functional systems of a living organism are often duplicated many times over (Barcroft, 1934). Barcroft wrote that duplication occurs so often that it is hardly accidental. It obviously constitutes a well-known property of function architecture and makes it all the more impressive in that it is implemented in such different ways. Barcroft wondered why, in this case, the heart itself was not duplicated. In this regard, it is appropriate to mention Michael Joiner's ideas on redundancy in physiology (Joyner, 2013). He wrote "... redundant mechanisms operate to govern the behavior of complex systems." This idea is similar to the idea of redundant safety systems in the design or management of complex human activities like building planes, care of patients in the operating room or intensive care units, or perhaps underground mining. If one safety system fails, then complementary or backup systems are there to ensure that the plane continues to fly, the patient survives, and/or the mine does not collapse.

Examples parallel to the safety story abound in physiology. Perhaps the most widely used example is blood pressure regulation, where a host of local and neural factors integrate the actions of the cardiovascular system and kidney to keep blood pressure within a narrow range, even when one or more elements of the system is less than fully functional.

Indeed, the heart obviously does not have a full-fledged doubler, but there is an extensive vascular system with built-in mechanisms of autoregulation. Moreover, it is thanks to them that the heart can do its job of providing adequate perfusion of organs and tissues. The variety of forms of regulation of the function (in this case, the level of blood pressure) in turn creates the preconditions for damage to various parts of various regulatory mechanisms involved in the regulation of blood pressure. In other words, the more responsible the task performed by the system and the greater the number of regulatory mechanisms involved in maintaining a particular parameter, the greater the likelihood of their damage during the pathological process. It is obvious that the currently available set of drugs, firstly, not etiologically targeted, and, secondly, does not allow influencing all critically important links.

Consider this statement on the example of calcium channel blockers (calcium antagonists). There is no doubt that their use for the treatment of AH has significantly improved the prognosis and quality of life of patients. The use of calcium antagonists convincingly substantiated experimentally, since the entry of extracellular calcium through the voltage-gated calcium channels (VGCCs) of the L-type in the plasma membrane of VSMCs is significantly increased in both experimental animals and humans (Hermsmeyer, 1993). In addition, the number of calcium channels themselves per unit area of the plasma membrane surface is also increased under hypertension (Chatelain et al. 1984). All this creates the prerequisites for excessive calcium entry into the muscle cell and the development of its hypercontraction. However, unfortunately, the blockade of the inward calcium current does not always lead to a stable decrease in the level of vascular tone to the predicted values.

The reason is simple. Calcium channels work in tandem with potassium ion channels. A decrease in the activity of potassium channels leads to depolarization of cell membranes and promotes the entry of calcium into the cell. Therefore, it may be necessary first to normalize potassium conductivity or the work of the sodium-potassium ATPase, which largely determines the level of membrane potential in smooth muscle cells.

The point is also that although vascular tone is indeed to a large extent a function of the intracellular concentration of calcium ions ($[Ca^{2+}]_i$), this mechanism is not the only and decisive one in the regulation of vascular tone. It has now been proven that vascular tone can vary within a fairly wide range against the background of unchanged $[Ca^{2+}]_i$. This happens due to shifts in the so-called affinity (sensitivity) of the contractile proteins of a smooth muscle cell to calcium ions (more on this will be discussed below).

Let us assume that the main cause of hypertension is an excess supply of calcium ions to smooth muscle cells. However, this does not mean that blockade of the inward calcium current will be the only correct treatment. It is more important to know what led to an increase in calcium entry into the cell, i.e., need to know why it happened.

For instance, Goulopoulou and Web (Goulopoulou & Webb, 2014) hypothesized that in the pre-hypertensive state, necrotic cell injury during hypoxic and ischemic events leads to the local release of damage-associated molecular patterns (DAMPs). DAMPs activate the so-called Toll-like receptors (TLRs) in the arterial smooth muscle cell leading to disturbed Ca^{2+} signaling. This altered Ca^{2+} pattern leads to increased vasoconstriction and reduced vasodilation contributing to overt hypertension. Although we have not yet identified specific pharmacological targets for the treatment of hypertension, this is a move in the right direction.

The quality of life of patients with hypertension has undoubtedly improved now, but whether the quality of treatment has improved radically is a moot point. There are many antihypertensive drugs. However, paradoxically, with all the positive and negative (side) manifestations of their action, according to generalized data in both in Europe and US media in recent years, simple diuretic drugs are one of the best in terms of price-quality ratio (Baguet et al. 2007). The analysis showed that the weighted mean reduction in SBP over 8-12 weeks was greatest with diuretics, particularly indapamide 1.5 mg/day (mean change from baseline, - 22.2 mm Hg), which reduced systolic blood pressure more than any of the other drugs evaluated (at any dose considered). The weighted mean reduction in diastolic blood pressure was generally similar across all antihypertensive drug classes, ranging from -11.4 mm Hg with the beta-blocker atenolol and calcium channel antagonists to -10.3 mm Hg with angiotensin II receptor antagonists.

It was not a surprising discovery since thiazide diuretics are recommended as one of the first medicines to treat high blood pressure. Although diuretics are no longer considered the preferred agent for the treatment of hypertension in adults and children, they remain acceptable first-line options. Diuretics effectively decrease blood pressure in hypertensive patients, and in adults with hypertension, they reduce the risk of adverse cardiovascular outcomes. Yes, they differ only in their specific action and do not relieve the disease itself but effectively reduce blood pressure (at least in the initial stages of the disease) because they help the kidneys remove excess fluid and salt compounds.

Thus, the load on the heart is reduced, which in turn leads to a decrease in blood pressure. Its mechanism of action is similar to bloodletting, which is the oldest method of treating this disease since in both cases the volume of circulating blood decreases. Numerous studies have shown that diuretics effectively and at the same time safely affect the body and, in some cases, successfully relieve hypertension. The drugs of this group are especially widely used for the treatment of elderly patients, who are contraindicated in many modern antihypertensive drugs. Diuretics can be used effectively in heart failure and osteoporosis, diseases also common in older patients (Moser, 2005).

There is reason to believe that in some cases they are better than many other drugs for high blood pressure help in the treatment of hypertension in patients with metabolic disorders. It is known that people with high blood pressure and metabolic disorders are more at risk of developing cardiovascular diseases such as ischemic disease, heart rhythm disorders, cerebrovascular accidents, etc. In other studies, (Baguet et al. 2007; Fretheim et al. 2012) patients divided into groups received one of the following drugs: diuretic chlorthalidone, calcium channel blocker amlodipine, alpha-blocker doxazosin, ACE inhibitor lisinopril.

Most patients were followed up for an average of about 5 years, but in the group of patients treated with alpha blockers, trials were completed after a median of 3 years, due to an increase in cardiovascular complications. Among the patients examined, almost half had evidence of metabolic syndrome, which was defined as high blood pressure in combination with at least two of the following: diabetes mellitus or prediabetes, a body mass index (BMI) of at least 30, high triglyceride levels, or low lipoprotein levels high density ("good" cholesterol). Patients with metabolic syndrome who took diuretics had a lower incidence of cardiac abnormalities than those who took the other three drugs. Patients taking an ACE inhibitor had an increased risk of developing a dry, tickly cough, feeling dizzy or lightheaded, especially when you stand up or sit up quickly, headaches, blurred vision diarrhea, etc. Alpha blockers may improve total cholesterol. However, some research suggests that long-term use of some alpha blockers may cause some unwanted effects. Bradycardia and hypotension are two adverse effects that may commonly occur. Fatigue, dizziness, nausea, and constipation are also widely reported. Some patients report sexual dysfunction and erectile dysfunction. Less commonly, bronchospasm presents in patients on beta-blockers. (Side effects can be reported to the FDA online at www.fda.gov/safety or call 1-800-FDA-1088 (1-800-332-1088).

More recent studies (Fretheim et al. 2012) have shown that data obtained were mixed, with few significant differences and no class of drugs emerging as superior for more than one outcome. An important finding for overall mortality, based on moderate- to high-quality evidence, was that beta-blockers (atenolol) were inferior to angiotensin receptor blockers (relative risk (RR) 1.14; 95% confidence interval (CI) 1.02–1.28). ACE inhibitors were inferior to calcium channel blockers for the risk of stroke (RR 1.19, 1.03–1.38) but superior for the risk of heart failure (RR 0.82, 0.69–0.94), both based on moderate-quality evidence. Diuretics reduced the risk of myocardial infarction compared with beta-blockers (RR 0.82; 0.68–0.98) and reduced the risk of heart failure compared with calcium blockers (RR 0.73; 0.62–0.84), beta-blockers (RR 0.73; 0.54–0.96), and alpha-blockers (RR 0.51; 0.40–0.64). Interestingly, the risk of diabetes increased with diuretics compared with ACE inhibitors (RR 1.43; 1.12 -- 1.83) and calcium blockers RR 1.27; 1.05 -- 1.57). The authors concluded that beta-blockers (atenolol) and alpha-blockers might not be first-choice drugs because they were the only drug classes that did not have significant advantages over others on any measure.

To a certain extent, these data are an indicator of the crisis of modern pharmacotherapy of AH. It is also possible that we underestimate the role of water metabolism disorders in the pathogenesis of AH. We will return to this question below.

Thus, for the time being, we have focused on eliminating the symptoms of arterial disease, i.e., the visible part of the iceberg. Why are we doing this? Because it cannot be otherwise, since we do not know how the main link in the pathogenesis of high blood pressure is formed - we do not accept the role of basal vascular tone in this process.

How often do you, our reader, repair your car yourself? Most likely, you can wipe it with a rag on the outside. You entrust serious work to a specialist, a person who knows how this car works. In our case, the problem is that no one knows how the basal tone is formed. And how do you treat what you do not know? We act, “treating” the symptoms that lie on the surface, that is, we reduce the pressure inside the vessels and, therefore, reduce the risk of complications of hypertension. But we do not eliminate the cause of the increase in pressure. This can and should be done in different ways, i.e., at different levels of the most complex hierarchical structure of the vascular tone regulation system, which is based on basal tone.

Thus, contrary to television advertising, a modern drug does not always hit the target exactly. We just don’t know exactly what needs to be treated. There are two main reasons for this sad state of affairs in the pharmacotherapy of hypertension: genetic polymorphism (this problem is solved quite simply, but not cheaply) and, most importantly, the lack of reliable information about correctly identified pharmacological targets, i.e., cellular and subcellular structures, which are the main triggers of the pathological process. In other words, contrary to television advertising, modern medicine is not always exactly on target. We just don’t know how to treat it. We act like that archer who first shoots and then draws a target circle around the arrow. Such is self-deception.

A natural question arises - do we always correctly understand the "language of nature" (in this case, the symptoms of the disease), and if so, do we correctly translate it into terms that we understand? Judging by the results of practical medicine, the answer is no. To some extent, infections have been defeated, and surgeons rejoice at their successes, but the joy of their victories is overshadowed by the lack of real success among therapists and the emergence of new, no less terrible diseases.

We understand that not all physicians and pharmacologists will like what I write, but, nevertheless, I deliberately sharpen the problem before us - the need for a proper study of the nature of basal VSM tone.

Deviation 2. *What is a disease? The antonym of this word is the word health - i.e., the state of any living organism in which it as a whole and all its organs are able to perform their functions properly. If it is allowed to joke about this, then the absence of illness, i.e., health is the state of a person when there is still the strength not to go to the doctor.*

The disease is usually defined as a violation of the normal functioning, working capacity, and life expectancy of the body and its ability to adapt to constantly changing conditions of the external and internal environment, which occurs in response to the action of pathogenic factors with the simultaneous activation of protective - compensatory-adaptive reactions and mechanisms. The disease is a state of the body, expressed in a violation of its normal life, life expectancy, and the ability to maintain its homeostasis. This is a consequence of the limited energy and functionality of the living system in relation to pathogenic factors.

The definition, frankly, is even more vague and uncertain than the definition of health.

So, what is disease? The punishment of the gods, as the ancients believed. A condition in which the correct mixing of the main elements and fluids of the human body is disturbed (Galen), the conflict between the internal environment of a person and the influence of external pathogenic factors (Alkomen, Croton, later Sydenham)? Alternatively, disease comes from outside with microbes (Pasteur). In 1851, Claude Bernard wrote - "... the health of a person and his morbid condition basically do not have much difference, as they thought about it in the old days and as some of our modern doctors think."

Health and disease should not be understood as two opposite poles or as two belligerents. These are outdated and obsolete views. In fact, the difference between these two states, health and disease, is very small. We are talking about excess or deficiency, disproportion, disharmony of normal phenomena in the body. That is the essence of the disease state. In the history of medicine, there is not a single confirmed case of a disease that leads to the appearance of some fundamentally new states of the body that would completely change the situation or lead to the emergence of new specific substances.

In other words, the idea is that illness is, in fact, nothing more than a deviation from normal physiological activity. The famous French scientist and surgeon Rene Leriche concluded that the disease "is not a simple morphological change in tissues, although it is due to them and that it is often recognized by their appearance. It cannot be said that the disease is an abnormal condition caused by a deviation of physiological activity caused by morphologically determined pathological changes in tissues. It is also impossible to say that the disease is a function of a person, i.e., the patient himself, since the patient may not know that he is sick. Perhaps the disease is a collection of symptoms. However, for the patient, illness is one thing, and for the doctor, it is often quite another.

Any disease begins with imperceptible violations of the local functional balance (first phase). The renowned oncologist Sir Conneway wrote that we are becoming more and more convinced that our body for most of our lives is preparing for cancer. This preparation arises in connection with frequent malnutrition, hormonal dysfunctions, various excesses, intoxications, infections and parasitic infestations, as well as repeated injuries that are detected during x-ray examination or post-mortem autopsy.

When the final stage of the disease begins, the patient himself already feels it. Since it is natural for a person to feel that he is the center of the universe, he often has the false impression that everything that happens revolves around him. When a person falls ill, he thinks that nature and his body will organize protection for him from the threat hanging over him. He has the impression that he was a battlefield between some evil forces and the protective instinct of the body.

We often make a disease prognosis based on the so-called body's defenses, but at the same time, we proceed from our own desires and fears, replacing the real thing with what it seems. In fact, our tissues simply "ignore" us. They live their own lives, along the line indicated by their heredity, and are not at all "interested" in the goals that people set for themselves, that is, they live their own independent plant life. It is time for us to get rid of the childish notions that sometimes dominate medical science and study pathology as if we were not personally interested in the issue under study, that is, to consider the problem objectively.

The problem of genetic polymorphism can currently be solved quite simply (modern science allows this), but this will require huge additional government investments in medicine. So far, for various reasons, this does not seem realistic in many countries. So, our main task is to determine the main pharmacological target of the pathological process as accurately as possible.

Therefore, we must focus on pharmacological targets. The emergence of targeted drugs will become possible only after the identification of the target and a detailed study of the mechanisms of interaction of a potential drug with this pharmacological target. Sir James Black, a prominent Scottish physician and pharmacologist who developed propranolol and cimetidine and who was awarded the Nobel Prize in Physiology or Medicine in 1988, together with Elion and Hitchings, "for their discoveries of important principles for drug treatment" defined his drug discovery pathway as follows:

1. Identify the clinical problem.
2. Characterize the underlying biological processes.
3. Establish the regulatory molecules and receptors involved.
4. Design compounds, which antagonize this process by acting through the same receptor pathway (McGregor, 2010).

The target can be determined only in the process of a detailed study of the pathogenesis of the disease at the cellular and molecular level. Only in this way will we be able to realize the dream of Paul Ehrlich about the "magic bullet" in the future and move on to low-dose targeted pharmacotherapy. In the meantime, "shoot" at the target, and then draw a circle, indicating the place of impact as the center.

Why is it important to accurately identify the target molecule? Therefore, only in this case is the guarantee of delivery of the "letter to the addressee" and a decrease in the number and severity of side effects guaranteed. I repeat once again, only in this way, having studied the interaction of the drug with a correctly identified target molecule, it will be possible to talk about low-dose targeted therapy.

Of course, basal tone, by itself, cannot serve as a real pharmacological target. Moreover, we still poorly understand what it is. Here are the individual cellular and molecular structures responsible for its formation; they can be targets. What are these structures and mechanisms?

Potential pharmacological targets of a cell can be: receptors (and their associated ion channels), ion channels and cell membrane pumps, mitochondria (including mitochondrial pores and mitochondrial ion channels), the contractile apparatus of muscle cells, the sarcoplasmic reticulum, for example, a ligand, inositol 1,4,5-trisphosphate (IP_3) - controlled calcium channels of the reticulum, enzymatic cellular systems, genes (a practical example is gene therapy for AH, the introduction of copies of genes responsible for vasodilation or the use of so-called antisense RNA to suppress the translation or transcription of genes that are responsible for the production of vasoconstrictors).

The big problem is that the "pharmacological target" is as inexhaustible as the "atom." As soon as the researcher establishes that the target is, for example, an ATP-dependent potassium channel or a high-conductivity calcium-dependent potassium channel, how will the question arise of which subunit of this is the target, etc.? In a number of scientific disciplines, without knowing which effective treatment of diseases is impossible, in the first place, of course, is physiology and pathophysiology. The reason for this is simple - effective treatment in the vast majority of cases is impossible without knowledge of the pathogenesis of the disease.

It is interesting to note that the word PHYSIOLOGY, written in Chinese, consists of 3 hieroglyphs - life, logic, and teaching, i.e., can be translated as STUDYING THE LOGIC OF LIFE. At one time, academician Pavlov astutely wrote that the physiology of the future would be the physiology of the cell. We are already living in this time, and some of us are engaged in this particular cellular physiology.

It has long been known that any living organism is a community of various cells. The human body, for example, is made up of about 100 trillion of its own cells plus an incalculable number (quadrillions?!) of bacteria that inhabit the digestive tract. Cells, being a structural and functional component of tissues and organs, are in contact with tissue fluid, lymph, and blood plasma, and, obviously, therefore, each cell is surrounded (protected) by a plasma membrane - a shell 7-10 nm thick, which is formed by a double molecular layer, consisting mainly of phospholipids and proteins integrated into them. Many protein structures are embedded in the plasma membrane. There are receptors in the cell membrane that perceive external chemical signals and provide a "communication" of the cell with neighboring cells, both close and distant. Active and passive transport complexes are also built into the membrane, through which the cell exchanges matter with the environment. In particular, among them there are so-called. ion channels, pores formed by transmembrane proteins, through which ions passively diffuse towards a lower concentration. Typically, these pores allow only certain ions to pass through, such as potassium, sodium, calcium, and chloride. Some of the ion channels are associated with their own receptors.

Thus, in living systems, a conjugated transfer of matter and information across cell membranes constantly occurs: for example, a fat-soluble (lipophilic) signaling molecule of nitrogen monoxide (NO) passes through the cell membrane and activates an intracellular "receptor" (soluble guanylate cyclase), which, in turn, causes relaxation of blood vessels and increased blood flow. Another signaling molecule, acetylcholine, by binding to G-protein coupled muscarinic receptors, leads to the release of NO from endothelial cells (EC) and relaxation of underlying VSMCs or promotes contraction, if acetylcholine acts directly on smooth muscle (in the case when the endothelial lining was damaged). Signal transmission can also occur through receptors that activate one or another intracellular mediator (angiotensin, cAMP, cGMP, IP_3, DAG):

How does this extremely important system of regulation work, and why do we still know it so poorly? The main reason for our lack of awareness in this area is the extreme complexity of the regulatory systems under study. Imagine a system consisting of only 10 elements, but each element of which can influence each of the 90 interelement connections. The number of states in which such a system can be is equal to 290! A huge number is unthinkable, and this is in the presence of only 10 elements in the system. And this is true for a system consisting of only 10 elements. We have to deal with systems that are immeasurably more complex.

The creation of target-specific "magic bullets" has been a therapeutic goal since Ehrlich and a pragmatic criterion in drug design for many years. It should be noted that in recent years, when creating new drugs, the paradigm of target centricity has ceased to be the main and even more so the only model. A detailed analysis of regulatory signaling pathways indicates that many molecules are capable of interacting with several different targets (Keiser et al. 2009). As one of the founders of this direction aptly put it, old drugs can and should teach new tricks (Nosengo, 2016).

Clearly, so-called drug repositioning is a complement to the discovery of new molecules, not an alternative. More of both is needed. Modern medicine understands that each disease is actually a complex of several different diseases.

Chapter 3

The Main Features of Living Systems

So, we are dealing with very complex probabilistic systems that can self-organize. In biology, for a long time, the erroneous point of view dominated that living systems are characterized by inner balance. In fact, "a living cell is a complex organized system that is thermodynamically infinitely incredible and can be in this state only as long as free energy can be used to maintain this organization" (A. Hill, 1929).

After another 6 years, Bauer (1935) formulated the "principle of stable imbalance" of the thermodynamic organization of all living things. In his opinion, living systems are characterized by: 1) the presence of free energy, which discharges spontaneously without external influence (autorhythmic activity in smooth muscle cells!); 2) the ability to respond to external stimulation, restoring disturbed gradients (i.e., the possession of irritability and excitability); 3) accumulation of free energy due to work against factors leading to an equilibrium state.

In other words, "all and only living systems are never in equilibrium and perform constant work due to their free energy against the equilibrium required by the laws of physics and chemistry under existing external conditions" (Müller & Igamberdiev, 2024).

Self-Oscillatory Processes in Nonlinear Living Systems

Chemists are well aware of the so-called Belousov-Zhabotinsky reaction - a class of chemical reactions occurring in an oscillatory mode, in which some reaction parameters (color, concentration of components, temperature, etc.) change periodically, forming a complex spatial-temporal structure of the reaction medium. Currently, this name combines a whole class of related chemical systems that are similar in mechanism but differ in the catalysts used (Ce^{3+}, Mn^{2+} and Fe^{2+}, Ru^{2+} complexes), organic reducing agents (malonic acid, bromomalonic acid, citric acid, malic acid, etc.) and oxidizing agents (bromates, iodates, etc.).

Deviation 3. *The discovery of self-oscillatory processes in living systems is associated with the name of Boris Belousov, who conducted research on the Krebs cycle, trying to find its inorganic counterpart. Thanks to one of the experiments in 1951, he discovered self-oscillations in the oxidation of citric acid with potassium bromate in an acidic medium in the presence of a catalyst,* Ce^{3+} *(cerium ions). The course of the reaction varied with time, which was manifested by a periodic change in the color of the solution from colorless (*Ce^{3+}*) to yellow (*Ce^{4+}*) and back. Belousov's article on this topic was rejected twice in the editorial offices of domestic Russian journals, but subsequently, it became one of the most cited articles in this area, and the reaction was called the Belousov reaction. This reaction was further investigated when Professor Simon Shnol suggested to his graduate student, Anatoly Zhabotinsky, to investigate the mechanism of the reaction. Belousov declined an invitation to conduct joint research, although he seemed satisfied that his work would be continued. Jabotinsky's group carried out detailed studies of the reaction, including its various variants, and developed the first mathematical model. A.M. Zhabotinsky «Concentration auto-oscillations» presented the main results in this matter in 1974 (Tomita & Kitahara, 1975).*

Now it is clear that the main characteristics of any self-oscillatory process are the following:

1. Self-oscillatory processes are established due to the phenomena occurring within the system itself.
2. The amplitude of self-oscillations depends only on the properties of the system itself.
3. Self-oscillatory processes in a system are possible only when it is sufficiently far from the equilibrium point.
4. The reason for the self-oscillation of processes is the presence of a large number of interacting elements and feedback between them.
5. Self-oscillatory processes are always stable while the resulting deviations always fade. In living systems, self-oscillations often occur, which can be a potential substrate for automation.

In the physiology of the heart, the concept of a pacemaker is long known, and it has been studied much better than the autorhythmic activity of smooth muscles. It is firmly established that normal cardiac function depends on adequate timing of excitation and contraction at an appropriate pacemaker rate. A good, healthy heart works almost like a Swiss chronometer. This complex task is successfully solved due to the highly specialized electrical properties of various elements of the heart system, including the sinoatrial node, atria, atrioventricular node, the Purkinje conduction system, and the ventricles. In addition, different regions of the heart are supplied with different combinations of ion channels, pumps, and exchangers, resulting in different action potential waveforms and durations.

The pacemaker activity of a cell can be defined as its ability to spontaneously and cyclically generate an electrical signal. To do this, the membrane potential of the sinoatrial node cell must slowly depolarize to a threshold, which is a certain level required to generate an action potential. This pacemaker depolarization is the result of a small inward current passing through the cell membrane and is a key feature of cardiac automatism. This depolarization occurs during diastole at the end of the action potential and is responsible for triggering the next action potential. It is very important to understand that without diastolic depolarization, the heart simply cannot contract spontaneously. The decisive condition for rhythmic automatism is the presence of inward (inward) currents at diastolic potential and the fine dynamic integration of the functioning of sarcolemma ion channels, transporters, and Ca^{2+} cyclic proteins (Weisbrod et al. 2016a). This work is, of course, about cardiac pacemakers. Nevertheless, there is reason to believe that the main principles of the functioning of triggers in different living systems differ little from each other.

Thus, Weisbord et al. (2016) analyzed the main models of the cardiac oscillator functioning in detail. Below I will allow myself to quote a few fragments from this very useful and important review (Figure 1). The first of them is the model of the membrane clock or potential clock. This model includes a combination of different ion channel activities during diastolic depolarization. One of the most important candidates is the "funny current" or "I_f," discovered in 1979 and responsible for the acceleration of the heart rate when stimulated by norepinephrine (Brown & Difrancesco, 1980; Brown et al. 1979). Initially erroneously described as a "potassium" current, this "pacemaker current" was actually a nonspecific cationic current produced by hyperpolarization-activated and cyclic nucleotide-gated channels (HCN channels), which structurally resemble the K^+ channel superfamily. Despite having a potassium selectivity, its filter motif, and an overall structure resembling potassium channel, HCN channels are also permeable to Na^+ ions and, to a much lesser extent, to Ca^{2+} ions. Under physiological stress, the influx of Na^+ through the HCN channels is greater than the outward of K^+.

Functionally, the I_f current is distinguished by unique electrophysiological properties. While all other existing voltage-gated cationic currents are activated by depolarization, HCN channels open in response to membrane hyperpolarization. This difference explains the reason why the atypical current has been called the "funny current." Physiologically, at the end of an action potential, membrane hyperpolarization activates HCN channels, which slowly generate an inwardly directed depolarizing current until it reaches a threshold and then generates a new action potential.

In general, if this channel did not exist, it would have to be invented. Like Maxwell's demon, which allows physicists to "plug" successfully the holes of their ignorance. Of course, this channel is an almost ideal candidate for the role of a trigger activity generator in living systems.

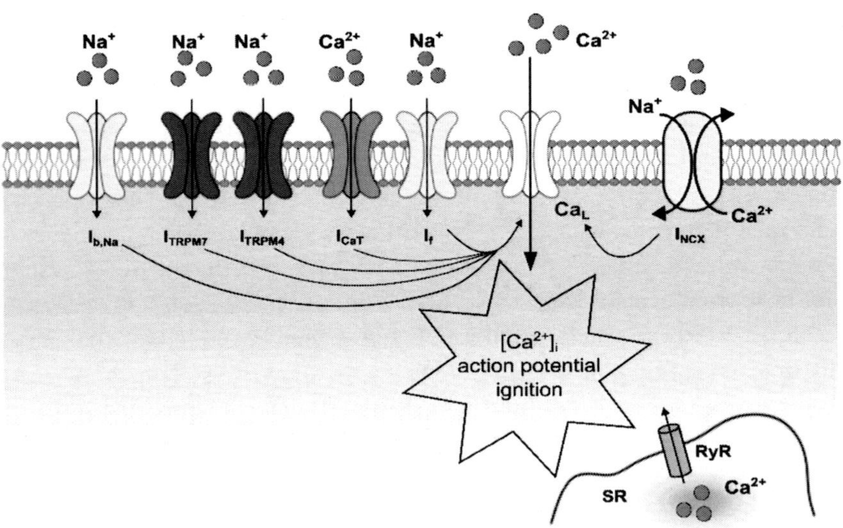

Figure 1. At first, the scheme of "membrane clock" and "calcium clock" models were presented by Weisbord et al. (Weisbrod et al. 2016b). This integrative model includes the different ion channels and coupled channel-receptor units that are tightly involved in this process of Ca2+ spark generation. Different currents such as If, the sustained sodium-dependent inward background current (Ib), Na+, T-type C2+ channel (Cav3.1 and Cav3.2), TRPM4 and TRPM7 inward currents are all good candidates that may be responsible for the diastolic depolarization, alone or in different combinations. Diastolic spontaneous calcium release increases the cytoplasmic calcium concentrations and activates NCX-1 in the forward mode. The inward NCX current depolarizes the membrane until the threshold is achieved.

Discovered some 40 years ago, the If current has since been known as the "pacemaker" current due to its role in the initiation and modulation of the heartbeat and of neuronal excitability. However, this is not all, the "funny" current keeps entertaining the researchers; indeed, several data discovering novel and uncanonical roles of f/HCN channel are quickly accumulating. The data obtained indicate the expression and cellular functions of HCN/f channels in a variety of systems/organs, particularly in sour taste transduction, hormone secretion, activation of astrocytes and microglia, inhibition of osteoclastogenesis, renal ammonium excretion, and peristalsis in the gastrointestinal and urinary systems. That is, they are also present in smooth muscles (Majgaard et al. 2022).

Where else are they available? Myometrial smooth muscle displays an intrinsic pacemaker activity, which drives uterine contractions, and several factors, including hormones, stretch, and paracrine molecules, can modulate this activity. Uterine contractions occur both in the non-pregnant state (during the menstrual cycle) and during gestation, and according to different physiological or pathophysiological conditions they vary in frequency, duration, amplitude, and direction of propagation (Aguilar & Mitchell, 2010).

To date, the mechanism behind the pacemaker activity of the uterus is still largely unknown (by the way, as in other types of smooth muscles), and neither an anatomical pacemaker region nor the presence of widely distributed pacemaker cells, has been identified properly. However, based on the evidence that small isolated myometrial strips show spontaneous rhythmic contractions, it is likely that some myocytes are endowed with an intrinsic pacemaker activity (Wray & Prendergast, 2019).

The involvement of the If current in myometrial automaticity was suggested in the 1990s when the current was measured in freshly isolated single longitudinal and circular smooth muscle cells isolated from pregnant rat uterus (Okabe et al. 1999). The I_f density was larger in circular than in longitudinal myometrial cells and this finding well correlates with the evidence that spontaneous action potentials were frequently observed in circular but not in longitudinal myocytes.

This observation led to the hypothesis that the slow activation of the If current at resting membrane potential might cause a slow depolarization, driving the membrane potential to the threshold for action potential firing. In agreement with this conjecture, Okabe et al. (1999) observed that under voltage-clamp conditions, inward currents (I_h) were activated by long hyperpolarizing pulses below -60 mV in circular but not in longitudinal muscle cells. Application of extracellular but not intracellular Cs^+ reduced the amplitude of I_h in a concentration-dependent manner (an IC_{50} of 0.15 mM). Additional data indicated that inhibition by ZD7288 (100-200 μM) decreased the force amplitude of spontaneous and oxytocin-induced contractions of longitudinal uterine strips isolated from in-term pregnant rats (Gur et al. 2021). Unexpectedly, in addition to decreasing the force amplitude, ZD7288 also increased the frequency of contractions. The interpretation of these results is not straightforward since ZD7288 was used at high concentrations and therefore non-specific effects on other ion channels are likely contributing.

Another type of smooth muscle where this type of current was detected is corpus cavernosum. Recently, Gur and colleagues (Gur et al. 2021) verified the hypothesis that HCN channels may also be functionally expressed in the smooth muscle of the corpus cavernosum. Their study indeed identified the presence of HCN3 and HCN4 proteins in smooth muscle cells of the human penile corpus cavernosum and showed that ivabradine (100 nM - 1 mM) was able to induce a concentration-dependent relaxation of tissue strips of the human corpus cavernosum previously contracted by phenylephrine. This effect was independent of the nitric oxide (NO)/soluble guanylyl cyclase pathway since it was maintained in the presence of both nonspecific nitric oxide synthase (NAME) and soluble guanylyl cyclase (ODQ) inhibitors. Gur and co-workers thus proposed that the direct inhibition of HCN channels in penile tissue may contribute to the beneficial effects of ivabradine on erectile dysfunction (ED) and that HCN block may be a useful treatment for patients who have cardiovascular risk factors and ED. In addition, they also reported evidence that ivabradine may affect other ion channels such as L-type Ca^{2+} and K^+ channels.

In addition, the last case is gastrointestinal smooth muscle cells. The I_f current was identified in isolated longitudinal smooth muscle cells of rabbit Jejunum (Benham et al. 1987) and in circular smooth muscle cells of guinea pig ileal muscle (Yanagida et al. 2000). Obviously, the presence of the current suggests a possible involvement in the slow depolarization observed in response to hyperpolarizing current stimuli, possibly caused by various inhibitory neurotransmitters and hormones.

Here is such an encouraging and useful review presented by Benzoni et al. regarding the widespread expression and diverse functional roles of HCN/If channels (Benzoni et al. 2021).

Although hyperpolarization-activated cation (HCN) ion channels are well established to underlie cardiac pacemaker activity, their role in smooth muscle organs remains relatively controversial. These channels are clearly expressed in tissues where HCN channel conductance is required for peristalsis. For instance, in renal pelvic smooth muscle (RPSM) pacemaker tissues. Recently, Yang et al. (2023) confirmed that HCN ion channels play a broad, evolutionarily conserved pacemaker role in both cardiac and smooth muscle organs and have implications for channelopathies as putative etiologies of smooth muscle disorders (Yang et al. 2023). They postulated that translational studies in human and swine demonstrate HCN channels are conserved in the multi-calyceal RPSM and that HCN channels underlie pacemaker activity that drives peristalsis.

Let us hope that soon there will be something interesting in the same respect for VSMs.

The second model of the cardiac oscillator is the calcium clock model. Calcium is known to play a central role in the E-C coupling in "working" cardiomyocytes. In fact, during this physiological process, the depolarization of the sarcolemma generates an inward calcium current through the activation of the L-type Ca^{2+} channels, which is responsible for triggering a calcium-induced calcium release (CICR), a synchronous calcic wave, from the ryanodine (RyR) and IP_3 receptors of the sarcoplasmic reticulum (SR). The subsequent $[Ca^{2+}]_i$ increase is a key feature of a proper actin-myosin interaction and cardiomyocyte contraction. In addition to the calcium wave, which results from a synchronous release through the SR receptors, spontaneous local calcium sparks have been observed in both working myocardium and Purkinje fiber cells. These spontaneous Ca^{2+} oscillations occur locally in a submembrane region of the cell and propagate rapidly. These phenomena are also observed in atrial pacemaker cells. In fact, with the help of calcium imaging techniques, Ca^{2+} chelating fluorophores, and electrophysiology, Ca^{2+} transients were visualized during the diastolic slope and preceded the large entry of calcium through the calcium channels.

Alternative pharmacological approaches with SR blockers revealed modifications in the rate and the shape of the action potential from guinea pig sinoatrial cells. Evidence for a functional interaction between the ryanodine receptor (RyR)-mediated Ca^{2+} release and the cardiac isoform of the NCX-1 Na^+ /Ca^{2+} exchanger gave rise to an alternative theory, "the calcium clock," in which diastolic spontaneous Ca^{2+} release activates the Na^+/Ca^{2+} NCX-1 exchanger in its forward mode. In these conditions, the net electrogenic inward current resulting from the entrance of 3 Na^+ and the extrusion of 1 Ca^{2+} depolarizes the membrane of the cell toward the threshold and generates an action potential (Weisbrod et al. 2016a)

The calcium-activated potassium channel family exhibits the unique characteristics of a transducer between the ubiquitous cytoplasmic calcium signals and the electrical variations of the cell membrane. Among the diverse types of channels that exhibit these properties, the calcium-activated potassium channel family (K_{Ca}) is heterogeneous. According to their unitary conductance, they have been classified into three subfamilies: BK, IK and SK, which are "large," "intermediate" and "small" conductance channels, respectively (Vergara et al. 1998).

The BK_{Ca} channels ($K_{Ca}1.1$), or "large conductance Ca^{2+}-activated potassium channels," were first identified in 1979 by Heyer and Lux in the pacemaker neurons of the snail (Heyer & Lux, 1976) and cloned 15 years later. This subfamily of channels differs from the IK and SK channels in their structure and biophysical properties. In addition to the well-known six transmembrane domains present in each subunit of voltage-gated potassium channels, an S0 membrane segment in the N-terminus and a cytoplasmic hydrophobic C-terminus containing a "calcium bowl" extend the α-subunit. Four β-subunits have been reported to be associated with the main structure of the protein. BK channels exhibit a large unitary conductance (≈ 250 pS) and are modulated by increased cytoplasmic calcium concentrations and membrane depolarization (Jiang et al. 1999). They are abundant in the central nervous system and smooth muscle cells (Nelson et al. 1995).

The protective roles of BK_{Ca} channels, such as spike frequency adaptation, explain their increased expression in excitable cells. Pharmacologically, they are sensitive to charybdotoxin, paxilline and iberiotoxin. The small conductance calcium-activated potassium channels SK1 (KCa2.1), SK2 (KCa 2.2) and SK3 ($K_{Ca}2.3$) are encoded by three different genes, KCNN1, KCNN2, and KCNN3, respectively. Structurally, they are very similar to the voltage-gated potassium channel superfamily. These channels do not have an EF-hand domain motif, and their activity is only calcium-dependent. All of the SK channels exhibit similar steady-state activation curves for Ca^{2+} (half activation of approximately 300–700 nmol/L, which is a relatively low affinity). Electrically, SK channels contrast with Ohmic currents and display a strong inward rectification at positive voltages. The mechanism is still not clear but easy to explain by an intracellular Mg^{2+} or Ca^{2+} voltage-dependent block. The three subtypes differ in their tissue expression patterns and their pharmacological sensitivities to the bee venom toxin, apamin.

Thus, oscillations in $[Ca^{2+}]_i$ c are known as a universal signaling mechanism in all eukaryotic cells. These oscillations can be triggered either by fluctuations in membrane potential, leading to the repetitive opening and closing of voltage-gated Ca^{2+} channels, or, more commonly, through activation of cell-surface receptors that can increase the levels of intracellular

IP_3. It is important that an oscillatory calcium signal provides numerous signaling advantages over a sustained increase in $[Ca^{2+}]_i$. It is clear that increasing $[Ca^{2+}]_i$ to high levels only transiently, allows to avoid the toxic effects that arise from a maintained Ca^{2+} signal.

The second advantage, oscillatory signals support long-lasting cellular responses because they circumvent the desensitization of Ca^{2+}-dependent responses that can occur during a prolonged Ca^{2+} signal. Additionally, oscillations in $[Ca^{2+}]_i$ increase the ability of low levels of stimulation to activate responses. One or two large Ca^{2+} spikes can be detected more easily than a sustained increase in $[Ca^{2+}]_i$ of the same average amplitude over the same length of time, increasing the signal-to-noise ratio. Finally, oscillatory Ca^{2+} signals impart information in both their amplitude and frequency and thus provide a mechanism for selective recruitment of downstream targets (Parekh, 2011).

Symposium report of McHale and his co-workers (2006) devoted to the origin of spontaneous rhythmicity in smooth muscles concluded that spontaneous activity in the gastrointestinal tract originates, not in smooth muscle cells themselves, but in specialized pacemaker cells, interstitial Cajal cells (ICC) or ICC-like cells (McHale et al. 2006). This may also be true in many other smooth muscle types, but detailed experiments would be required to confirm it properly. Their own studies of spontaneous electrical events in the interstitial cells of the rabbit urethra would suggest that the former is generated by the oscillatory release of calcium from intracellular stores. The 'prime oscillator' would appear to be the ryanodine-sensitive store rather than the IP_3-sensitive store since blockade of the former with tetracaine or with ryanodine stopped oscillations completely whereas inhibition of the action or production of IP_3 did not. The influx of calcium across the plasma membrane (probably via the sodium/calcium exchanger) triggers calcium release from the ryanodine-sensitive store, which causes further release from nearby IP_3-sensitive stores. This sets up a regenerative wave raising calcium concentration near the calcium-activated chloride channels to a level sufficiently high to activate them. The efflux of chloride ions through these provides the depolarizing current underlying the pacemaker potential. This, in turn, will depolarize the membrane sufficiently to activate the T- and L-type voltage-operated channels.

Chapter 4

Myogenic Automaticity in Smooth Muscles as an Example of Autooscillations in Nonlinear Living Systems

Living systems are always open, thermodynamic systems that constantly exchange matter, energy, and information with the environment (the exchange of matter, energy, and information also occurs between parts (subsystems) of the system). Negative entropy (increase in orderliness) and the ability to self-organize are also characteristic of living systems. Dynamic processes in biological systems, their self-organization, stability, and transitions from a stationary state to a non-stationary state are provided by various mechanisms of self-regulation. Self-regulation is the intrinsic property of biological systems to maintain the parameters of automatical activity of the processes taking place at a given level. Biologists call this homeostasis, although it would be more correct to speak about homeokinesis since everything is so-called constants (parameters) of the organism that are "floating," i.e., dynamic constants.

All living systems of the organic world are organized hierarchically and are represented by a large number of levels of structural and functional organization, such as, for example, the system of blood pressure regulation. Each level has its specific mechanisms of self-regulation, based, as a rule, on the principle of feedback, when the deviation of some parameter from the required level leads to the "inclusion" of functions that eliminate the imbalance, returning this parameter to the desired level. In the case of negative feedback, the sign of the change is opposite to the sign of the initial deviation, and with positive feedback, the sign of the change coincides with the sign of deviation; while the system goes from one stationary state and into another. This happens, for example, in a disease when a so-called vicious circle is formed. This property allows biological systems to be in different stationary states and, on the one hand, to function in certain respects regardless of the environment, and on the other, to adapt to the environment under appropriate conditions. In addition to stationary, biological systems, as already indicated above, also have self-oscillatory states, when the values of parameters fluctuate in time with a certain amplitude. Such states are the basis of periodic biological processes, biological rhythms, biological clocks, etc.

Most systems of the Universe are open in nature, which means that stability and equilibrium do not dominate in the Universe, but instability and non-equilibrium do. It is because of this that the Universe is capable of development, evolution, and self-organization. Stable and equilibrium systems are not capable of self-organization; they are the dead ends of evolution. From here, my negative relation is the term "stabilization of membranes" often found in our literature. Stabilization, the absence of gradients means nothing more than cell death.

Due to the selectivity to external environmental influences, nonequilibrium systems perceive differences in the external environment and "take them into account" in their functioning. At the same time, some weak effects may have a greater impact on the evolution of the system than the effects, although stronger, but not adequate to thc system's own trends. In other words, the principle of superposition does not apply to nonlinear systems: there are situations where the effect of the combined action of causes A and B has nothing to do with the results of the effects of A and B separately. This is obviously the main difference between nonlinear systems in which undamped oscillations may occur, i.e., the autorhythmic activity that interests us.

Processes in nonlinear systems are often of a threshold nature - with a smooth change in external conditions, the behavior of the system changes abruptly (recall, for example, the development of an action potential when the critical level of depolarization is reached). In other words, in states far from equilibrium, very weak disturbances can be amplified to giant waves that destroy the existing structure and contribute to its radical qualitative change (positive feedback, or, as doctors say, the "vicious circle" of the disease, i.e., self-accelerating and self-accelerating pathological process). For each system, there is some optimal "nonlinearity corridor" that promotes structure formation. Very strong nonlinearity, as well as very weak nonlinearity, is incompatible with the formation of local structures. However, within the limits of only the optimal "corridor," the amplification of nonlinearity increases the number of ways of formation and the forms of local structures, as well as the number of options for the evolution of the system and its routes to the future.

It is non-linear systems, being non-equilibrium and open, themselves create and maintain heterogeneities in the medium. In such conditions, positive feedback relations can sometimes be created between the system and the environment, i.e., the system influences its environment in such a way that conditions are generated in the environment, which in turn determines changes in the system itself. The consequences of this kind of interaction between an open system and its environment can be the most unexpected and unusual, including the development of pathological conditions (again a vicious circle).

What properties should a functional system have in order for oscillations to occur in it? First of all, it is the presence of feedback, i.e., processes leading to the fact that the result of the functioning of a system affects the parameters on which the functioning of this system depends. In other words, a signal proportional to its output signal (or, in the general case, being a function of this signal) is fed to the input of the system.

Thus, a distinction is made between positive and negative feedback. Negative feedback changes the input signal in such a way as to counteract the change in the output signal. This makes the system more resistant to random parameter changes. Positive feedback, on the other hand, amplifies the change in the output signal. Systems with strong positive feedback tend to be unstable, and undamped oscillations can occur in them. That is, in such a system, a so-called vicious circle may arise when the pathological process spontaneously accelerates. Nevertheless, biological systems are usually a combination of positive and negative feedback.

On the phase plane, self-oscillations are usually depicted as a closed isolated trajectory - a limit circle. To a mathematically unprepared reader, a circle is a limit cycle. There are stable and unstable limit cycles. A limit cycle is called stable if there is such a region on the phase plane containing this limit cycle, a neighborhood ε, that all phase trajectories starting in the neighborhood ε asymptotically approach the limit cycle at $t \to \infty$. If, on the contrary, in any arbitrarily small neighborhood ε of the limit cycle, there is at least one phase trajectory that does not approach the limit cycle at $t \to \infty$, then such a limit cycle is called unstable.

Limit cycles are possible only in a system whose right-hand sides are represented by non-linear functions. Translated into a commonly understood language, this means that self-oscillations and autowaves, multistability, and non-equilibrium steady-state distributions can exist only in nonlinear systems.

Thus, among a wide class of dynamic systems (DS) that implement oscillation modes, there are systems capable of performing undamped oscillations that have many special properties and are called self-oscillatory by Andronov (Andronov, 1966). Andronov for autonomous DS on the plane introduced the definition of self-oscillatory systems in the following way:

$$x = F(x, \mu), x \in R2, \tag{1}$$

having a stable T - periodic solution $x(t) \equiv x(t+T)$.

The DS will be self-oscillatory in the sense of Andronov if the following two conditions are satisfied:

1. The solution x(t) is stable with respect to small changes in the system itself (i.e., to changes in the evolution operator F);
2. The solution x(t) in the limit $t \to \infty$ does not depend on the choice of initial conditions (at least within some region of the phase space). A closed trajectory on the phase plane as an image of a periodic solution x(t) that satisfies the above conditions is called, as already indicated earlier, a limit cycle.

The definition of a self-oscillating system, which can be found in many books and textbooks, requires the fulfillment of the second condition (independence from the initial data). However, Andronov added to this definition the requirement that the DS be rough (condition 1), which has a very deep meaning. In modern DS theory, this condition was evaluated as structural stability and topological equivalence of the DS.

Any self-oscillatory DS is non-linear and dissipative. These two conditions provide the self-oscillatory regime in the sense of independence from the initial conditions. Changes in the initial conditions uniquely lead to a change in the initial energy, which eventually takes on a certain value in the regime of steady self-oscillations. This is possible only for dissipative systems. Secondly, the change in the initial energy in the direction of increase or decrease is controlled by the system itself, and therefore, the properties of the DS must be different for its various states. Only non-linear DS possess such properties.

Deviation 4. *A dissipative system (or a dissipative structure, from Latin dissipatio - "I disperse, destroy") is an open system that operates far from thermodynamic equilibrium. In other words, this is a stable state that occurs in a non-equilibrium medium under the condition of dissipation (dissipation) of energy that comes from outside. A dissipative system is sometimes also called a stationary open system or a non-equilibrium open system.*

In the modern theory of oscillations, the concept of self-oscillations is significantly expanded in comparison with Andronov's definition. First, it can be generalized to DSs of dimension N>2. Second, it applies not only to systems with periodic solutions but also to DSs with quasi-periodic and chaotic solutions. We can give the following general definition for a self-oscillating system - autonomous DS is called self-oscillatory if its solution is represented in the phase space as an attractor with a finite or infinite basin of attraction. An attractor can be periodic (limit cycle), quasi-periodic (n-dimensional torus), or chaotic (strange attractor). The DS m999ust be coarse, which means that the topological structure of the solution is insensitive to small changes in the evolution operator. The introduced concept of an attractor and its basin of attraction essentially means the second requirement of Andronov's definition: a change in the initial conditions within the basin of attraction does not change the properties of the steady-state solution, which depends solely on the properties of the DS.

Self-organizing systems are usually very complex open systems that are characterized by a huge number of degrees of freedom. However, not all degrees of freedom of the system are equally important for its functioning. Over time, the system allocates a small number of leading, defining degrees of freedom, to which the others "adapt." So, by the way, neonatal cardiomyocytes behave in culture - they adapt to the frequency of reduction of more active "neighbors" in the culture medium. Such basic degrees of freedom of the system are called attractors. Attractors characterize the directions in which an open nonlinear medium can evolve. In other words, attractors are those structures towards which self-organization processes take place in nonlinear media. For a visual illustration, the concept of an attractor is often used, the image of the cone "funnel," which draws in the trajectory of the evolution of a nonlinear system.

Rhythmic cell activity plays an important role in the regulation of vital functions. In contractile systems, such as the heart and smooth muscles, regular oscillations of the membrane potential are responsible for maintaining the pumping function and the proper level of tonic tension that provides motility or tissue perfusion. The existence of two main types of cell oscillators is assumed - firstly, these are cytoplasmic oscillators - glycolytic, mitochondrial, and possibly associated with intracellular $[Ca^{2+}]_i$ oscillations. Secondly - membrane oscillators are based on cyclical changes in membrane potential. These changes in membrane potential can be associated with the cyclic operation of Na^+/K^+ pumps or with changes in the ionic conductivity of the plasma membrane. The main problem of identification is the same, which starts and supports the cyclic operation of ion pumps? How are changes in ionic conductivity, leading to depolarization of the cell membrane, replaced by processes that promote repolarization?

For ionic Na^+/K^+ pumps, there is an explanation related to providing them with energy from the glycolytic oscillator. The trigger for switching the two main ionic conductivities (potassium and sodium), which determine the level of membrane potential and, accordingly, the outward and inward current, can serve as the level of intracellular calcium concentration. Calcium ions, like sodium ions, determine the amount of inward current, while potassium ions form the outward current. The opening of potassium channels leads to hyperpolarization of the membrane, and when they are closed, the membrane depolarizes and starts to let in calcium ions. When the level of depolarization reaches a certain value, the potassium channels open again, and the process repeats cyclically. In reality, this process, of course, is much more complicated, since a great many have already been identified as channels (potassium, calcium, chloride, sodium) and their kinetics, as well as their activation and inactivation parameters differ significantly. However, the overall picture is approximately the same as described above.

Chapter 5

Vascular Tone and Its Regulation

The term vascular tone is usually understood as a state of prolonged excitation of smooth muscles, which manifests itself in the corresponding intensity of their contractile activity and is not accompanied by the development of visible fatigue. The latter does not mean that the level of vascular tonic tension (as well as other types of smooth muscles, SM) is a constant value and does not change with time. It is influenced by numerous factors that can increase or decrease the contractile strength/activity of vascular SM cells. Since the nature of the processes that cause and maintain this activity has not been fully elucidated, the tone of the vascular wall is usually presented as a result mainly due to the integration of contractions of a large number of smooth muscle cells, including those with their own authoritarian activity.

It should also be recalled that the regulation of blood flow and intraluminal pressure in accordance with the metabolic and other needs of the body is provided by a complex of central remote (neurogenic) and local (humoral and myogenic) regulatory mechanisms, the last of which is inherent in tissues. In other words, two main regulatory circuits control the level of blood flow. Denervation of one or another vascular site leads to a rapidly developing relaxation of the vessels and in the pressure drop in the zone of denervation. It is interesting that after 20-40 minutes the normal blood supply to the tissues, as usual, is completely restored (Soloviev, 1973) even in the absence of external neurogenic control. The network local regulation mechanisms are able to provide adequate adaptive vascular bed responses in response to changes in blood flow and metabolism even in the absence of external neurogenic control.

However, one objection could significantly shake the concept of the existence of peripheral tone. It lies in the possibility of the existence of the so-called active vasodilation, i.e., vasodilation with increased activity of the vasodilatory nerves, and not due to the weakening or cessation of excitation of the vasoconstrictor nerves. In this case, the expansion of previously denervated vessels may not be explained by a decrease in vascular tone at all. True, for this, vasodilation must be active in the full sense of the word, i.e., carried out due to the active contraction of special muscles of the vascular wall, an increase in the tonic tension of which would lead to an increase in the diameter of the vessels. Apart from the longitudinal layer of smooth muscles of the portal vein and some abdominal veins, nothing comes to mind.

Thus, the main purpose of this book is to analyze the architectonics of integral vascular tone and mainly to shed light on the intrinsic mechanism (nature) of basal (resting) vascular tone formation (triggering) and its maintenance in health and disease.

Blood Flow Autoregulation

The autoregulation (i.e., self-regulation or myogenic regulation) of the blood flow represents a tendency to preserve its value in organ vessels despite changes in the inflow or outflow of blood. Of course, this does not mean at all that with significant and abrupt changes in blood pressure (for example, with drops of up to 100 and more mm Hg), the organ blood flow will remain constant. The essence of autoregulation is that changes in blood pressure always cause less change in blood flow than it could be in a passive-elastic, for example, rubber tube (Figure. 2). This means that the vessel actively responds to changes in intravascular pressure.

Myogenic autoregulation of blood flow is most pronounced and effective in the vessels of the kidneys and brain. Pressure changes in these vessels almost do not cause changes in blood flow. Somewhat less it is pronounced in the intestinal vessels, moderately effective in the myocardium, relatively little effective in skeletal muscle vessels, and very weakly expressed in the lung tissues. Obviously, these differences are due to differences in the level of basal tone in these vascular zones. It is possible also that this is due both to the specifics of functioning and to the varying degree of the need to maintain an optimal level of blood supply in these organs to ensure the vital activity of the organism as a whole.

As a model for the movement of blood through the vessels, in the first approximation, we can consider the following equation, which describes the flow of fluid through the pipe:

$$Q = \frac{P1-P2}{8\eta L} \cdot \pi R^4, \qquad (2)$$

where Q is the volumetric (volume) flow rate of the liquid, P1-P2 is the pressure difference at the beginning and end of the pipe, η is the viscosity of the liquid, L is the length of the tube, and R is the radius.

This is the Hagen-Poiseuille law - the physical law of hydrodynamics for the so-called Poiseuille flow, that is, the steady flow of a viscous, in the particular case of an incompressible, fluid in a thin cylindrical pipe. It relates the flow rate of the liquid through the cross-section of the pipe with the pressure drop at the ends of it for the given parameters of the viscosity of the liquid and the geometric dimensions of the pipe. The law was established empirically in 1839 by G. Hagen, and in 1840-1841 was independently discovered by J. L. Poiseuille. Later, in 1945, J. G. Stokes substantiated this law theoretically.

The Hagen - Poiseuille equation describes a number of characteristics of the fluid flow in a pipe. It has many restrictions, but we are now interested in only one point. It follows from the equation that the volumetric flow is directly proportional to the pipe radius to the fourth power. This is an important point, and it means that even a slight increase or decrease in the radius of the vessel should lead to a significant increase or decrease in blood flow.

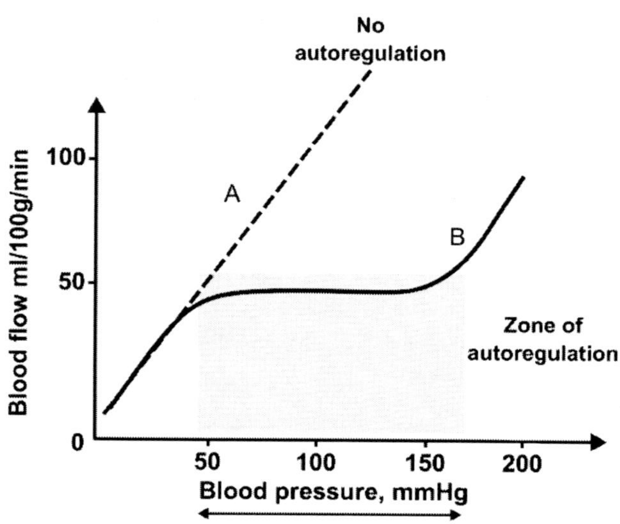

Figure 2. The main principle of blood flow autoregulation – the changes in blood pressure always cause less change in blood flow through vascular bed (B) than it could be in a passive-elastic tube (A). It is clear that the zone of autoregulation has its own limits, determined by the properties of the structural and effector elements of the vascular wall.

Considering that the liquid is practically incompressible, it could be assumed that the regulation of blood flow in a wide range of values is carried out with very insignificant (in quantitative terms) changes in the lumen of the vessels. It is, first, due to changes in the level of isometric tonic tension of the smooth muscles of the vascular wall.

Reactive (vascular response to a temporary occlusion of blood vessels) and exercise (increased blood flow during exercise) hyperemia's are generally accepted models for studying the mechanisms of local blood flow regulation. Exercise hyperemia refers to the increase in skeletal muscle blood flow that occurs during muscular activity. Because this increase in blood flow occurs in response to increased cell metabolism, exercise hyperemia is referred to as active or functional hyperemia, terms which also apply to the increase in flow to any organ that experiences an increase in parenchymal cell metabolism.

The mechanisms of development of working hyperemia are most often described within the framework of the metabolic hypothesis. V. Khayutin was the only onc at that time who dared to abandon the metabolic theory and proposed a new biomechanical mechanism for the formation of exercise hyperemia (Khayutin, 1971).

Briefly, in Khayutin's laboratory, the complete independence of the blood supply of the skeletal muscle from the developed strength and the physical work performed was discovered. Khayutin considered these data fatal for metabolic hypothesis. He believed that the direct cause of the dilation of the terminal arterioles during working hyperemia is a mechanical factor. Such a factor, in his opinion, is a forced change in the shape of the terminal arteries because of the action of contracting skeletal muscle fibers. He supposed that in the resting skeletal muscle, the arterioles are elongated, which is a necessary condition for the generation of impulses that maintain the myogenic tone of the arterioles. Muscle contraction reduces the tension of the arterioles, which leads to a decrease in the degree of deformation of the pacemakers and a weakening of the myogenic tone.

Of course, this hypothesis, like any other, is quite vulnerable to criticism. Especially if we consider the mechanical factor as the only cause of working hyperemia. In any case, supporters of the myocardial and metabolic hypotheses should not consider their views to be the only true and possible ones.

In our own studies, we have more often studied the reactions of local blood flow in response to arterial and venous occlusion. That is, we studied reactive hyperemia. It is important that these vascular reactions were fully reproduced on the isolated and denervated gastrocnemius muscle. We will dwell on this data in more detail.

The results of these studies clearly showed that changes in the vascular tone of the skeletal muscles because of temporary cessation of blood flow are realized due to local regulatory mechanisms and are not associated with external influences on the vessels.

There are several basic theories explaining the mechanisms of formation of these two main local vascular responses: 1) Myogenic hypothesis, in accordance with which vascular tone is a function of intravascular pressure. This explanation is based on the ability of VSMs to dilate in response to decrease in intravascular pressure (the Ostroumov-Beiliss phenomenon). 2) In accordance with the metabolic hypothesis, the vascular tone is a function of the blood flow. This theory explains the tone level by the influence of vasoactive substances released into the bloodstream during the metabolism process. 3) And the last, somewhat exotic, theory, suggesting an effect on the level of vascular tone of extravascular tissue pressure, due to the shifts in the capillary filtration of a liquid when the intraluminal pressure in the vessel changes (Folkow, 1964; Rodbard, 1971; Khayutin, 1964; Konradi, 1973; Soloviev, 1973).

Chapter 6

Evidence of the Existence of Peripheral Mechanisms of Blood Flow Regulation

The peripheral mechanisms of vascular tone were considered only as a kind of reserve, providing a partial restoration of vascular tone sometime after the vasomotor center was switched off or the vasoconstrictor nerves were transected.

In the 19th century, Goltz (1864) wrote that arteries and veins during a person's life are tonically contracted, and this tone is dependent on large nerve centers. What else could say Owvsyjannikov (1873), who found a significant (up to 30-40 mm Hg and below) drop in systemic arterial blood pressure (SBP) after transection of the spinal cord under the medulla oblongata. However, you just had to wait only 30-40 minutes after the transection to see that the vascular tone was completely restored. In 1963, another great expert of the vessels of that time, Bozler (Bozler, 1962) pointed out that smooth muscle activity is triggered in the same way as in skeletal muscles, mainly by impulses from nerves.

However, already in the early works of Bernard (1866) and Konradi (1944) promulgated some interesting facts. In some cases, SBP did not fall below 60-70 mm Hg, despite the transection of the spinal cord. Consequently, vascular tone does not necessarily have to decrease sharply after the vasomotor center is turned off. Even more convincing in this regard were the experiments of Konradi (1944), who showed that a relatively high level of systemic BP (60-80 mm Hg) was preserved in animals after complete dissection of the spinal cord below the sixth cervical segment.

Interestingly, F. Goltz (Goltz, 1874) observed the restoration of the tone of the vessels that expanded after denervation. However, he ascribed this restoration to the action of some small peripheral centers lying in the vascular wall. In addition, he interpreted the expansion itself as the result of concomitant irritation of vasodilating nerve fibers. Yet, he did not deny the fact of restoring tone after denervation.

Deviation 5. *I first saw this amazing phenomenon in 1968 when, as a 2nd year medical student, I was just beginning to study the effects of arterial and venous outflow cessation (arterial and venous occlusion, respectively) in isolated feline gastrocnemius muscle. Muscle denervation did lead to a sharp increase in blood flow, but within 20-40 minutes, the blood flow returned to its initial level.*

Such results did not fit into the ideas that existed at that time about the mechanisms of formation of vascular tone. Record-breaking in this respect the results were obtained by Lebedev in the laboratory of Waldman, and then Lebedev in the laboratory of Konradi (1973). In these experiments, SBP after transection of the spinal cord with an ultrasonic knife for 30 min. recovered to 100-110 mm Hg.

Later it was found that after a complete sympathectomy, transection of the sympathetic fibers of the limb or ear, the blood flow in the denervated vessels after a period of decrease for 10-40 minutes restored to original values. Convincing and complete data of this kind are contained in the last monograph by Konradi (1973) and do not require additional evidence.

In the experiments of Lofstrom et al. (Löfström et al. 1965), an anesthetic was injected into the region of the stellate ganglion. As a result, the blood flow in the forearm increased from 2.6 to 5.5 ml/100 cm^3/min. Then, a strong vasodilator agent, "substance P," was injected into the artery of the forearm. The blood flow increased again from 5.5 to 26.1 ml/100 cm^3/min, i.e. more than 5 times.

Thus, the vascular tone not only remained after denervation, but also did not lose its controllability. Only what is available can be reduced. "Nothing will come out of nothing," said Shakespeare's King Lear, and after him, Professor GP Konradi, so dear to my heart for the rare talent of a scientist and the independence of his judgments.

Moreover, it turned out that even after a complete sympathectomy of a cat, dogs can live, move and even reproduce (Cannon 1939). That is, no vascular catastrophe occurred after switching off the sympathetic nervous system, even in humans (Cobbold, Levis, 1956.).

It is quite clear that local shifts in blood circulation cannot be considered completely isolated from the reactions of the cardiovascular system as a whole, but it must be emphasized that they arise because of the adaptation of each organ to its own needs, determined by the level of functioning and metabolism (Levtov, 1967).

It can be argued that peripheral mechanisms are an independent control circuit of vascular tone, the activity of which, if necessary, is corrected by neurohumoral influences of a central nature. The adaptive-functional capabilities of this control loop are quite large. In the absence of central neurogenic influences, the adaptation of organs and tissues to changes in the external environment is almost not disturbed.

Chapter 7

Reactive Hyperemia in Skeletal Muscles

One of the most important local vascular reactions is reactive hyperemia (RH), i.e., the reaction of increasing blood flow after a period of its temporary cessation (arterial occlusion). Known for over 150 years (Cohnheim, 1872) that if arterial flow stops for some time, then the blood flow through the vessels of the organ in the post-occlusion period increases (Figure 3).

Thus, the term reactive hyperemia (RH) refers to the temporary increase ('hyper') of blood flow ('emia') because of ischemia, or an arterial blockage. This occlusion (blockage) can take the form of any outside force, like a tourniquet wrapped around the arm during a blood draw or a clamp placed on a vessel during surgery, or internal forces, like a buildup of plaque or a blood clot within the vessel that impedes or interrupts blood flow. By the way, a classic example of this is the inflatable arm-cuff for non-invasive measuring blood pressure.

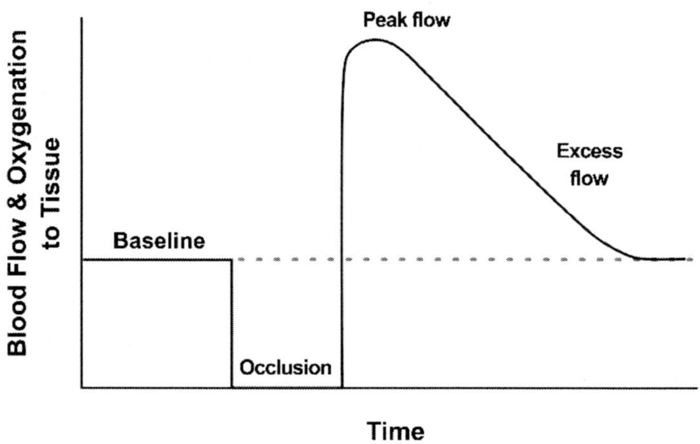

Figure 3. Schematic representation of the course of reactive hyperemia (RH) after arterial occlusion. Restoration of blood flow after arterial occlusion is accompanied by a rapid increase in blood flow to peak values exceeding the initial level, and its subsequent return to baseline. The main parameters of RH are the peak blood flow, the total excess of blood during hyperemia, and the duration of the hyperemia itself.

RH is well expressed both in isolated skeletal muscles and in intact limbs of humans and animals. It reproduces well in the kidney, in the brain, and occurs in the skin, myocardium and intestines.

According to the data obtained in this matter, blood flow through the skeletal muscles of the limbs of humans and/or animals can increase in the post-occlusion period by 2-3 times compared with the initial level. In the next few seconds or minutes (depending on the duration of the cessation of blood flow), hemodynamic parameters return to the pre-occlusive level.

It is important to note that RH develops equally well in both intact and denervated organs. It is well known, for instance, that RH in canine muscle gracilis was identical when using both intact and acutely or chronically denervated muscle. It means that if the nerves are involved in the formation of RH, which is unlikely, then they secrete some yet unknown at the time mediator.

Reactive hyperemia is a good diagnostic method in the clinic of acute and chronic disorders of local blood circulation, and it is a wonderful tool for studying the mechanisms of local blood flow regulation in the experiment.

Thus, a number of local physiological mechanisms may be involved in the origin of RH. Such local causes can be a change in the chemical composition of tissues during ischemia, a drop in intravascular pressure in the ischemic zone, a changing level of oxygen tension in the blood and tissues (pO_2), changes in tissue pressure, etc. The most important of them is the hypothesis of metabolic regulation, the hypothesis of regulation by oxygen deficiency and the hypothesis of myogenic regulation of organ blood flow (Konradi, 1973). We have shown that the participation of one or another mechanism of regulation of vascular tone after arterial occlusion depends on the duration of blood flow arrest. With occlusions lasting up to 30 seconds, the pressure drop in the occlusion zone becomes the determining factor and, accordingly, it is easy to explain by myogenic theory. Occlusions of a longer duration are accompanied by the accumulation of various tissue vasoactive metabolic products, and the theory of metabolic regulation comes first (Soloviev, 1973). The trigger for RG, of course, remains the myogenic mechanism. That is, it is the drop in intravascular pressure distal to the site of occlusion that triggers the process of vascular relaxation and subsequent increase in blood flow.

The metabolic hypothesis will not be the subject of our discussion. The reason is clear; we are discussing hypotheses and possible mechanisms for the formation of basal tone, where there is no place for external humoral influences. Given the fact that, according to Folkow's definition, a smooth muscle cell is a mechanoreceptor with an integrated contractile system, we will restrict ourselves to myogenic regulatory mechanisms, i.e., those that are intrinsic to these cells.

In addition, metabolic theory cannot explain the effect of venous occlusion on peripheral vessels at all. This is the most painful moment for this theory. Since the blood flow stops completely in both arterial and venous occlusion, then, according to the metabolic hypothesis, the same (or close) changes in the balance of vasoactive substances should occur. Therefore, the vascular tone should also change the same way, regardless of the way the blood flow is stopped.

However, it has long been established that venous occlusion either does not give hyperemia at all or leads to an extremely slight increase in blood flow in the post-occlusion period (Gaskell, 1880; Bayliss, 1902). Additionally, Kan, Levtov (1970) discovered that vein occlusion very often leads to a clear decrease in post-occlusive blood flow.

These results are in good agreement with the concept of the so-called veno-arteriolar reaction and are easy to explain from the standpoint of the myogenic regulation hypothesis, according to which intravascular pressure is the main factor in maintaining vascular tone (Hanson & Johnson, 1962). In fact, with venous occlusion, the pressure in the vessels does not decrease (it even slightly increases), but at arterial occlusion – it always falls.

Indeed, in 1962 R. Fales et al. showed that venous occlusion causes a decrease in tissue metabolism, in contrast to arterial occlusion, when such a shift does not occur (Fales et al. 1962). Consequently, changes in blood flow in both cases occur unambiguously with shifts in metabolism. However, Kan, Levtov (1970), after checking the data of Fales et al. (1982) under conditions of complete and partial vascular occlusion, concluded that oxygen consumption increases after both arterial and venous occlusion.

The constancy of the oxygen content in venous blood in the Fales experiments, Levtov explains that they failed to stop the blood flow through the vessels of the muscle during vein occlusion due to the preservation of collateral vessels. However, why does the level of oxygen tension in the isolated gastrocnemius muscle not drop during venous occlusion, even with careful hemodynamic isolation? Below we present our hypothesis of the absence of hyperemia after venous occlusion, based on data on the characteristics of transcapillary fluid exchange and related tissue pressure changes under this condition.

One of the most important aspects of the problem of local regulation of blood flow is the question of the relationship between intravascular pressure and vascular tone. In response to an increase in blood pressure, the vessels always narrow due to the contraction of the smooth muscles of the vascular wall. Ostroumov, which at the end of the 19th century revealed that blood flow through the skin of both normal and denervated limbs did not increase with increasing blood pressure, first pointed out this fact. This could only be explained by the fact that, in response to an increase in intravascular pressure, the vessels reacted by narrowing the lumen.

Later, Bayliss (1902) confirmed these observations, indicating that a decrease in intravascular pressure leads to an increase in vascular wall tension. However, Anrep (1912) categorically rejected all Bayliss' conclusions about the active contraction of the vascular wall in response to an increase in intravascular pressure. He argued that with those methods of increasing blood pressure that Bayliss used asphyxia, vasoconstriction could well be the result of the action on them of adrenaline released during these conditions. Anrep's criticism was very convincing, and Bayliss recognized it (Bayliss, 1923), believing that the issue remains unresolved.

It is interesting that Bayliss proceeded from a comparison of his plethysmographic studies with facts far from the physiology of blood circulation. He brought to the discussion the fact of muscle contractions of a worm in response to disintegration. Anrep did not deal with general biological issues but relied on facts from the physiology of the blood circulation, indicating that the vessels relax when exposed to acidic metabolic products.

In the end, however, Bayliss was right. In addition, it was his data that Folkow (1949) later used to develop his ideas about basal tone and local regulation of tissue blood flow based on the hypothesis of myogenic regulation. Summarizing the results of studies of vascular responses to changes in intravascular pressure, Folkow suggested that the smooth muscle cells of the terminal arteries have the function of pacemakers for myogenic activity (Folkow, 1964).

Thus, theoretically at least two types of control loops can take part in the formation of RH: central (extra organic) and peripheral (intra organic) muscle blood flow regulation loops.

As can be seen from the above, the metabolic and myogenic hypotheses of blood flow regulation, traditionally used to explain the mechanisms of RH, are not able to describe this process in its entirety. This forces us to look for new ways and mechanisms to explain the phenomenon of post-occlusion increase in blood flow. Finally, it is also important for understanding the mechanisms of modulation of basal vascular tone.

We turned our attention to transcapillary fluid exchange, hoping to solve some particular problems of local regulation of blood flow with its involvement. However, data of this kind are still clearly not enough to create a new hypothesis for the regulation of local blood flow. Nevertheless, changes in tissue pressure caused by shifts in transcapillary exchange can fully claim the role of an effective modulator of basal tone.

For a long time in physiological literature, there were no significant articles devoted to RH. At last, Rosenberry and Nelson presented such work (Rosenberry & Nelson, 2020). It should be noted for its special practical significance, since in the clinic the reproduction of reactive hyperemia can serve as a useful diagnostic technique and a marker of the quality and effectiveness of the treatment.

It is important to note that the authors presented a detailed scheme of the mechanisms of the formation of RH, known to date (Figure 4). In accordance with this scheme, a decrease in tissue pO_2 during arterial occlusion stimulates vasodilation through mainly metabolic mechanisms involving prostacyclin (PGI_2), adenosine, nitric oxide (NO), and K^+ channel-mediated hyperpolarization. Adenosine and PGI_2 binding their receptors lead to the activation of adenylyl cyclase (AC), which catalyzes production of cAMP from ATP. This second messenger then activates protein kinase A (PKA), which directly stimulates endothelial NO synthase (eNOS), increasing NO production. Adenosine receptor binding also activates ATP-sensitive K^+ (K_{ATP}) channels, while PKA activates Ca^{2+}-sensitive K^+ (K_{Ca}) channels. K^+ channel activation causes outward K^+ efflux, resulting in hyperpolarization. Endothelial cell hyperpolarization raises the driving force for Ca^{2+} to enter the cell and eNOS activation and NO production. Increased intracellular Ca^{2+} also activates phospholipase A_2 (PLA_2), which catalyzes production of arachidonic acid (AA), which cyclooxygenase (COX) converts to PGI_2. When produced, NO rapidly diffuses into the underlying VSM, where it activates guanylyl cyclase (GC). GC converts GTP to cGMP, which then activates protein kinase G (PKG). PKG mediates vasorelaxation by activating K_{Ca} channels, causing K^+ efflux. The resulting hyperpolarization leads to voltage-sensitive Ca^{2+} channels closure and prevents Ca^{2+}influx. PKG also activates Ca^{2+}-ATPase pumps, increasing the extrusion of Ca^{2+} from the myocyte and sequestration of Ca^{2+} into the sarcoplasmic reticulum (SR). The final result of these actions is decreased intracellular Ca^{2+}concentration, shifting the balance in activity between myosin light chain kinase and myosin light chain phosphatase to favor phosphatase activity (Kitazawa et al. 2009). Some evidence exists that PKG also phosphorylates MLCP and increases its activity (Kitazawa et al. 2009; Rosenberry & Nelson, 2020). This decreases the phosphorylation of myosin and reduces smooth muscle contraction.

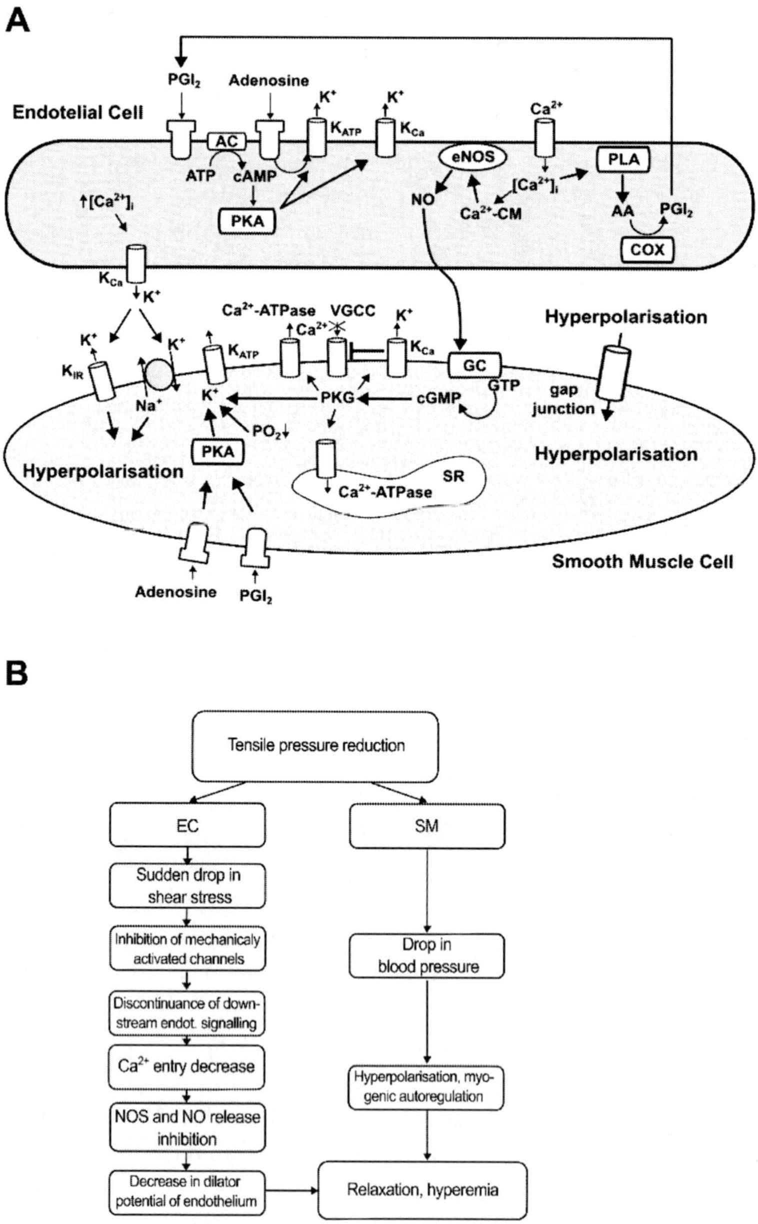

Figure 4. A, cellular mechanisms underlying reactive hyperemia after a relatively long (more than 30 sec) cessation of arterial inflow. B, reactive hyperemia after short arterial occlusion.

Finally, endothelial cell depolarization both directly, via myoendothelial gap junctions, and indirectly, via endothelial cell K^+ efflux, activates Na^+-K^+-ATPase and inwardly rectifying K^+ (K_{IR}) channels.

Rosenberry and Nelson believe that the trigger mechanism for reactive hyperemia is a decrease in oxygen tension in the tissues in the ischemic zone. This is true but for relatively long occlusions only (Rosenberry & Nelson, 2020). With arterial occlusions lasting up to 30 seconds, the main trigger is a decrease in intravascular pressure and, accordingly, the phenomenon of myogenic autoregulation of blood flow.

It is known that the Van't Hoff rule relates the change in the equilibrium constant, Keq, of a chemical reaction to the change in temperature, T, given the standard enthalpy change, Δreaction H⊖, for the process. We studied reactive hyperemia in an isolated calf muscle of a cat under conditions of a decrease in environmental temperature by 10 degrees Celsius. From the Van't Hoff's equation, the temperature coefficient is calculated by the formula:

$$\gamma = (V2\text{-}V1\ )^{10/(T2\text{-}T1)}, \tag{3}$$

where V1 and V2 are reaction parameters at temperatures T1 and T2, respectively.

The temperature Van't Hoff's coefficient, calculated for the main parameters of the range for 15 seconds of occlusion within 1.1 - 1.2. At the same time, the same parameter for 120 sec of occlusion was within 2.2-2.3. Even considering the limitations for the application of Van't Hoff's rule for biological systems, these data convincingly confirm the metabolic nature of hyperemia after prolonged occlusion and the predominance of physical processes in the formation of hyperemia after a short-term stop of blood flow.

Unfortunately, the authors of this helpful work did not take into account that in the clinic, when an artery is clamped, venous outflow almost always stops too. After venous occlusion, as is known, blood flow not only does not increase, but also often decreases. This may affect the interpretation of study results. However, they fulfilled their main task with regard to the practical use of reactive hyperemia properly (Figure 4).

Thus, the authors of the article concluded that the study of the parameters of reactive hyperemia using adequate methods is a well-reproducible and affordable method for use in the clinic. These methods have a good temporal resolution and provide the possibility of obtaining comprehensive data on the state of the peripheral circulation. There must be agreement on some important aspects, including the period during which the occlusion continues and time points when measurements should be made. It is necessary to take into account the role of changes in the metabolic rate of skeletal muscles under the action of an ischemic stimulus and somehow control this variable. Undoubtedly, RH can be a very useful method for assessing the status of microvascular function, VSM and endothelium in both patients and healthy people.

Chapter 8

Transcapillary Water Exchange and Its Role in Local Blood Flow Regulation: Tissue Pressure Hypothesis

Speaking about the mechanisms of regulation of local blood flow, unfortunately, along with the myogenic and metabolic hypothesis, they often forget to mention that blood flow can be a function of tissue pressure. We will not allow such a mistake.

Tissue pressure is formed due to interstitial fluid located in many intercellular spaces. If we remember that this fluid is practically incompressible, it becomes clear that any influx of additional fluid or its outflow can affect the tissue pressure and, accordingly, the vessels.

Fluid exchange between vessels and tissues occurs through the capillary wall. This wall is a complex biological structure through which water, electrolytes and some organic compounds are relatively easy to transport while proteins are much more difficult. As a result, the concentrations of proteins in blood plasma (60-80 g/l) and tissue fluid (10-30 g/l) are not the same. The volume of filtration through the total exchange surface of the capillaries of the body is quite large, about 60 ml / min or about 85,000 l / day.

Capillary blood flow is due to the difference in hydrostatic pressures in the arterial and venous ends of the capillary. The pressure at the arterial end is 30-35 mm Hg which is 8-10 mm Hg higher than the oncotic pressure of the blood plasma, under the influence of this pressure difference, water and many substances dissolved in it (except for high-molecular proteins) pass from the blood plasma into the tissue fluid, bringing to the tissues the substances necessary for vital activity. As the blood moves through the capillary, the hydrostatic pressure drops and at the venous end of the capillary is 12-17 mm Hg, which is about 10 mm Hg below the oncotic pressure of the blood. As a result, water and substances dissolved in it pass from the tissue fluid into the plasma. This ensures the removal of metabolic products from the tissues. The amount of blood flow in the capillaries corresponds to the intensity of metabolism.

Therefore, at rest, there are 30-50 fully perfused capillaries per 1 mm2 of the cross section of the skeletal muscle; with intensive muscle activity, their number increases by 50-100 times.

According to the classical theory of Starling (1896), the processes of water exchange between capillaries and tissues are determined by the following factors: 1) hydrostatic pressure of blood in capillaries and pressure of interstitial fluid; 2) colloid osmotic pressure of blood plasma and tissue fluid; 3) permeability of the capillary wall.

One of the key points of violations of water-salt metabolism is changes in the intensity of fluid metabolism in the circulatory capillary-tissue system. According to Starling's law, due to the predominance of the hydrostatic value over the colloid osmotic pressure at the arterial end of the capillary, fluid is filtered into the tissue, and the filtrate is reabsorbed at the venous end of the microvasculature. Fluid and protein leaving the blood capillaries are also reabsorbed from the intravascular space into the lymphatics. It should be noted here, in fairness, that Levick said that this commonly accepted idea was incorrect, and the fluid is filtered along the entire length of the capillary, just more at the arterial end and much less at the venous end (Levick, 1991).

Acceleration or deceleration of fluid exchange between blood and tissues is mediated by changes in vascular permeability, hydrostatic and colloid osmotic pressure in the bloodstream and tissues. An increase in fluid filtration leads to a decrease in circulating blood volume, which causes irritation of osmoreceptors and includes a hormonal link: an increase in aldosterone production and an increase in antidiuretic hormone (ADH). ADH increases water reabsorption and hydrostatic pressure, which increases filtration. A vicious circle is created this way.

Blood moves in the capillaries at a certain speed and under a certain pressure, because of which hydrostatic forces are created that tend to remove water from the capillaries into the interstitial space. The effect of hydrostatic forces will be greater the higher the blood pressure and the lower the tissue fluid pressure. The hydrostatic blood pressure at the arterial end of a human skin capillary is about 30-35 mm Hg, and in the venous end - 8-10 mm Hg.

Consider now that the pressure of the tissue fluid is a negative value. It is 6 -7 mm Hg below atmospheric pressure and, therefore, having a suction effect of action, promotes the transfer of water from the vessels into the interstitial space.

What does all this have to do with the regulation of local blood flow? Let us think. Thus, an effective hydrostatic pressure (EHD) is created at the arterial end of the capillaries - the difference between the hydrostatic pressure of the blood and the hydrostatic pressure of the interstitial fluid, equal to 36 mm Hg. At the venous end of the capillary, the EHD value corresponds to 14 mm Hg.

Proteins, the concentration of which in the blood plasma is 60-80 g/l, retain water in the vessels and create a colloid osmotic pressure of 25-28 mm Hg. A certain amount of protein is also found in the interstitial fluid. The colloid osmotic pressure of the interstitial fluid for most tissues is 5 mm Hg. Blood plasma proteins retain water in the vessels, and tissue fluid proteins - in the tissues.

Effective oncotic suction force (EOSF) - the difference between the colloid osmotic pressure of blood and interstitial fluid. It is 23 mm Hg (28 - 5). If this force exceeds the effective hydrostatic pressure, then the fluid will move from the interstitial space into the vessels. If EOSF is less than EHD, the process of ultrafiltration of fluid from the vessel into the tissue becomes inevitable. When the values of EOSF and EHD are balanced, an equilibrium point appears. At the arterial end of the capillaries (EHD = 36 mm Hg and EOVS = 23 mm Hg), the filtration force prevails over the effective oncotic suction force by 13 mm Hg (36-23). At equilibrium point A, these forces are equalized and amount to 23 mm Hg. At the venous end of the capillary, EOSF exceeds the effective hydrostatic pressure by 9 mm Hg (14-23 = -9), which determines the transition of fluid from the intercellular space to the vessel.

According to Starling (1896), there is an equilibrium: the amount of fluid leaving the vessel in the arterial part of the capillary must be equal to the amount of fluid returning to the vessel in the venous end of the capillary. Calculations show that such an equilibrium does not occur: the filtration force at the arterial end of the capillary is 13 mm Hg and the suction force at the venous end of the capillary is 9 mm Hg. This should lead to the fact that in each unit of time, more fluid escapes through the arterial part of the capillary into the surrounding tissues than is returned back. This is how it happens - about 20 liters of fluid passes from the bloodstream into the intercellular space per day, and only 17 liters return through the vascular wall. Three liters of fluid go into the general circulation via the lymphatic system. This is a significant mechanism for the return of fluid to the bloodstream, if damaged, so-called lymphatic edema may occur and, it is very likely that this will affect the level of tissue pressure and, accordingly, blood flow.

Thus, a significant decrease in the oncotic pressure of the blood (by at least l/3) is accompanied by the release of fluid from the vessels into the tissues in such quantities that they do not have time to be transported back into the general bloodstream, even despite the compensatory increase in lymphatic circulation. There is fluid retention in the tissues and tissue pressure increases.

This point is also important to understand the formation of edema. For the first time, Starling (1896) obtained experimental evidence of the importance of the oncotic factor in the development of edema. It turned out that the isolated paw of a dog whose vessels were under perfusion with an isotonic saline solution became edematous and gained weight. The weight of the paw and swelling decreased sharply when replacing the isotonic saline solution with a protein-containing blood serum solution.

The factors that determine the exchange of fluid through the walls of the capillaries are the hydrostatic pressure on each side of the vascular wall and the colloid osmotic pressure of the plasma and interstitial fluid. This was shown as early as the 19th and early 20th centuries. Starling (1896) and Landis (1928) confirmed the correctness of the relationship between the hydrostatic pressure gradient and the outflow of water to the outside in a single capillary. Unfortunately, only one of the four filtration-related variables (plasma colloid osmotic pressure) can currently be measured with sufficient accuracy. Even if it is possible to measure the pressure in an individual capillary, then we still cannot assume that it reflects the total pressure in the capillary bed. It is very difficult to make direct measurements of tissue pressure due to the microscopic dimensions of tissue spaces and the errors inherent in measuring instruments (Kitchin, 1963).

Recall that Guyton (1963), measuring tissue pressure inside a perforated capsule implanted in tissue, obtained negative tissue pressure values.

Now back to local vascular reactions. Kitchin found that the capillary filtration rate only increases with increased tissue metabolic activity (Kitchin, 1963). Enhanced capillary filtration, according to Kitchin (1963), occurs also in those areas of the tissue where intravascular pressure is increased. It must be taken into account that the amount of filtrate will be limited by the limited extensibility of the interstitial spaces.

The rate of transition of various substances through the capillary wall in both directions (C), i.e., transcapillary exchange is expressed by the following equation (Renkin, 1959):

$$C = Q\,(1 - e^{-PS/Q}), \qquad (4)$$

where Q - arterial blood flow in ml/min, *e* - base of natural logarithms, P - vascular permeability coefficient for a given substance, S- vessels surface area.

The main variables in this expression are Q and S. Perhaps the only drawback of this formula is that it does not take into account the concentration gradient of the substance between the plasma and the interstitial fluid.

Renkin et al. (1966) showed that the value of PS increases with increasing RG, i.e., the product of the permeability coefficient and the filtration surface. At a constant permeability coefficient, this increase is determined by an increase in the filtration surface due to the opening of precapillary sphincters. According to the author, this effect was due to the action of vasoactive metabolites that reduce vascular resistance. Nevertheless, it is likely that the decrease in vascular resistance is a secondary phenomenon due to changes in transcapillary pressure during arterial occlusion.

Eberhard (1973) demonstrated that filtration of fluid from the vascular bed into tissues can occur when the sum of tissue pressure (TP) and oncotic blood protein pressure (OBPP) is less than the sum of intravascular pressure (IP) and tissue fluid oncotic pressure (TFOP). Reabsorption occurs if TD+OBPP is greater than IP+TFOP. With the same oncotic pressure of blood and tissue fluid, filtration into the lymphatic pathways is possible. Since significant and multidirectional fluctuations in intravascular pressure are noted during arterial and venous occlusion, it can be assumed that this causes a change in the direction and magnitude of the vector of transcapillary filtering forces.

Kovach research demonstrated that with a decrease in intravascular pressure from normal values to 50-60 mm Hg, the capillary filtration coefficient (CCF) decreased by 30%. Further pressure reduction to 30-40 mmHg reduced CCF by 50% of the normal level. Just to such values, the intravascular pressure in the ischemic zone drops when the artery is clamped (Biró et al. 1975).

The first works on the influence of all these processes on peripheral blood flow appeared in the early 1970s. Of particular interest is the Rodbard concept about "capillaron" - a hemodynamic model for studying the role of tissue fluid in the regulation of local blood flow (Rodbard, 1971; Rodbard et al. 1969). The "capillaron" model is one or more capillaries with a soft permeable wall, covered with a capsule along with the extracapillary filtrate. In Kikuchi and Rodbard studies, this model successfully used to study the phenomenon of self-regulatory escape (Kikuchi & Rodbard, 1974). The design was modeled by reducing the diameter of the arteriole, through which blood enters the "vascular system" of the "capillaron" (see Figure 5 below). Narrowing of the arteriole led to a drop in intravascular pressure. As a result, the model's capillary collapsed and the blood flow through it fell. The level of fluid filtration into the extracapillary space also decreased. A decrease in extracapillary pressure led to an increase in transmural pressure, and the capillary reopened. This caused the restoration of blood flow to the previous values, i.e., self-regulatory escape. According to the authors, the phenomenon of self-regulatory escape is due to passive changes in transmural pressure, which depend on the degree of arteriole constriction.

The "capillaron" and its associated vascular compartments were simulated using this model. An 'aortic' reservoir at a height PA delivered water in sequence to a chain of vessels in series, including an 'artery', a 'capillary' in which the pressure declines from the pressure upstream (Pu) to that downstream (PD), a 'venule', and a 'vein' draining into a 'vena cava' reservoir at a height Pv. The zero-reference level was the anatomical level of the capillary. Screw clamps on the arteriole and the venule permitted constriction of the lumen at these sites. In the real Rodbard studies, the capillary was a 9 cm length of soft-walled single-dip latex rubber tubing of 1 cm diameter. For further details of the experiment, see the text.

G. Beer also studied the reactions of "capillaron" and the vascular system of the muscle gracilis of dogs on a sharp change in the rate of perfusion (Beer, 1971). Both in the muscle and in the model, an increase in blood flow resistance was associated with an increase in extravascular pressure and a collapse of capillaries at their distal end. The change in the vascular resistance of the model occurred with a change in pressure in the capsule, due to the transition of fluid between the capillary and extracapillary spaces. These changes in capsular pressure also affected transmural capillary pressure. When the pressure became zero or negative, the segment of the vessel collapsed.

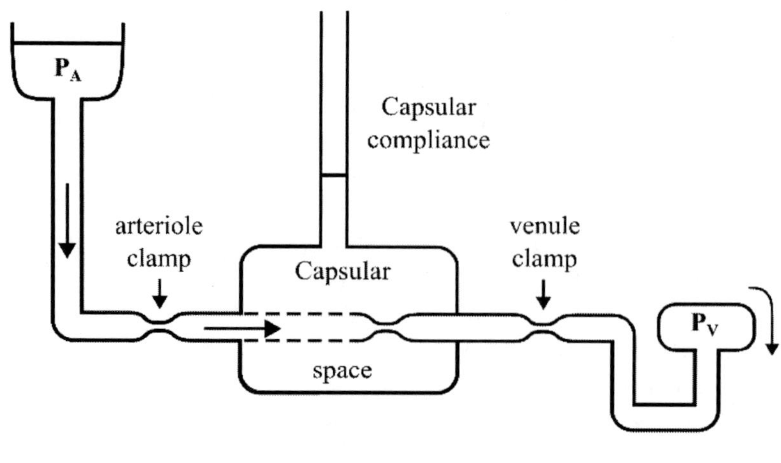

Figure 5. Simplified scheme of Rodbard's "capillaron" model.

G. Beer believes that one should distinguish between an increase in resistance in the proximal and distal parts of the capillary. If the resistance increases in the proximal part of the capillary, then the intravascular pressure distal to this place will fall. At the same time, the rate of fluid filtration from the capillaries decreases and tissue pressure drops. If the resistance of the distal part of the capillary increases, then the capillary pressure increases too and the filtration from the capillaries will increase. This, in turn, increases tissue pressure. Upon careful consideration, it is not difficult to see in these arguments the possible mechanisms for the control of vascular tone during temporary cessations of blood flow - arterial and venous occlusion. However, no one has yet made such an analogy.

Without a doubt, the Rodbard model, which is mechanistic in its essence, very well describes the formation of a real reactive hyperemia. I would call her beautiful and convincing. The only drawback of this model is the passive behavior of smooth muscles.

As a rule, hyperemia usually occurs after arterial occlusion, while venous occlusion does not lead to the development of hyperemia. Although, according to Baylis's concept, hyperemia would be expected after the elimination of venous occlusion, since the pressure in the arterioles falls, the smooth muscles of the vessels should relax, and at least delayed, hyperemia should be expected. However, no one has observed such a delayed hyperemia. Obviously, the accumulation of metabolites should take place both in arterial and venous occlusion. Based on the 'capillaron' model, it can be assumed that when venous outflow is restored, high pressure in the capsule prevents an increase in blood flow. The flow rate then falls below basal values, causing hypoemia rather than hyperemia.

In the course of our own experiments on the study of reactive hyperemia, we noted a very interesting phenomenon. Clamping of the femoral artery of the cat's limb, connected to the body of the animal only through vessels, did not lead to a complete cessation of the outflow from the ischemic organ. We put forward the assumption that the venous outflow (albeit insignificant) that persists during occlusion is a consequence of the inflow of tissue fluid into the vascular bed of the ischemic limb.

It is known that intravascular pressure in the ischemic zone falls exponentially until the arteriovenous pressure gradient is stabilized. Let us assume that the Laplace equation is valid for the vascular wall.

$$(Pi- Po)\ 2r\ \Delta X = T2\ \Delta X, \tag{5}$$

where: Pi – intravascular pressure; Po – tissue pressure; r – vascular radius; ΔX – arbitrarily selected section of the vessel; T – tonic tension of the vascular wall.

Simplifying this expression, we can write:

$$Pi=Po+T \tag{6}$$

In other words, the lumen of the vessel remains constant if the above-mentioned equality is maintained. When changing the values included in this equation, the lumen of the vessel will change until the appropriate ratio between intravascular pressure, tissue pressure, and vascular wall tone is restored. With a decrease in intravascular pressure during arterial occlusion to a critical value, there inevitably comes a moment when tissue pressure relatively increases. In addition, this, in turn, will lead to the inversion of the trans-capillary filtering pressure vector, water filtration into the vessels and a decrease in tissue pressure. In this case, even short-term and insignificant fluctuations in the volume of the limb muscles should be observed. The theoretical expediency of such a mechanism seems obvious; it remains to prove the reality of its existence.

Indeed, occlusion of an artery supplying an isolated cat gastrocnemius muscle for 60 seconds already in the first 5 seconds led to a decrease in the volume of the muscles of the limb by 40 ± 4 mm3. In the next 55 seconds, it remained stable while restoration of arterial inflow led to an increment in muscle volume by 21±1 mm^3 with subsequent recovery (Figure 6). It should be recalled that the experimental conditions were such that collateral blood flow was excluded.

Even if we assume that when the artery is clamped, the venous vessels collapse and a certain amount of blood is displaced from them (Konradi (1973), this does not contradict our reasoning. The fact is that for 3 minutes of arterial occlusion, the blood in the venous outflow catheter sharply brightened. That is, visual data indicated a decrease in hematocrit value.

Then, what force pushes the blood plasma out of the vascular network of the limb, closed at one end? The source of such power may be the influx of an additional volume of fluid from tissue spaces into the vessels of the ischemic zone.

To test this hypothesis properly, we studied the dynamics of the hematocrit value in outflowing blood. If tissue fluid actually enters the vessels during ischemia, then it must certainly lead to a change in the ratio of formed elements and blood plasma. This assumption was confirmed in experiments with the measurement of blood hematocrit. Hematocrit decreased after 60 sec. arterial occlusion from the initial 35 ± 0.5% to 28 ± 1.0% for 45 sec. post-occlusion period, and a significant decrease in hematocrit was observed as early as 30 sec.

Thus, it is likely that the transcapillary exchange during arterial occlusion changes in such a way that tissue water enters the vessels in the ischemic zone. Using the equation 7 (Kaznacheev, Dzizinsky, 1975) it is possible to calculate the loss of tissue water per 100 ml of arterial blood:

$$\pm WL = X - 100;$$

$$X = Ha\ 100/Hv; \qquad WL = (Ha\ 100/Hv) - 100, \qquad (7)$$

where: WL - loss of water per 100 ml of arterial blood; a - arterial hematocrit; Hv - venous hematocrit; ± - mean the direction of the fluid displacement vector, tissue - blood or blood - tissue, respectively.

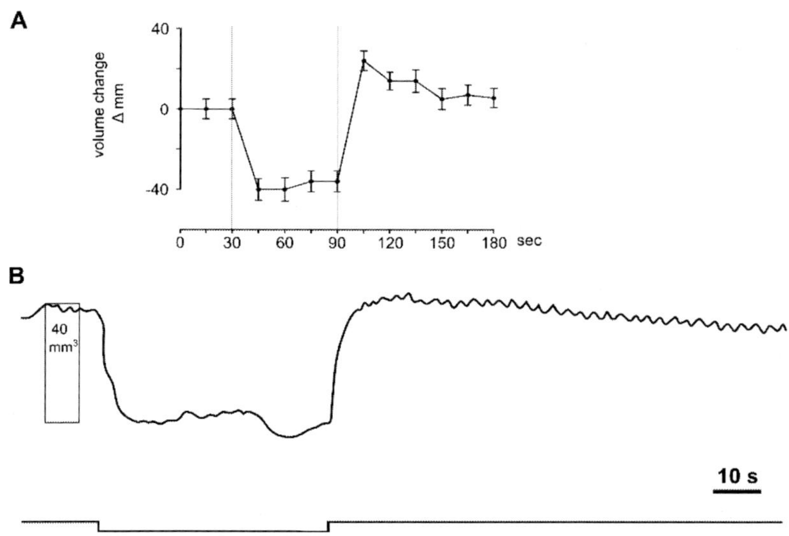

Figure 6. Dynamics of volumetric fluctuations of the cat gastrocnemius muscle during arterial occlusion and in the post-occlusion period. A - averaged data based on the results of 20 observations; B – original experimental recordings dated 04-01-1974. Designations of curves (from top to bottom): plethysmogram, time scale (5 sec.), time interval of occlusion. Please note: this figure first appeared almost half a century ago, back in the pre-computer era, so its quality is not good enough.

The hematocrit of venous blood at 60 seconds of arterial occlusion decreased from 35±1 to 28±1%. Hematocrit of arterial blood - 33±1%. The calculated loss of interstitial water (WL) before occlusion was 6.0 ml, after 60 sec occlusion - 14.0 ml.

If we assume that the blood content in the muscle is 10% of its weight (Konradi, 1973) and the weight of the gastrocnemius muscle in our experiments did not exceed 40 g, then the amount of blood that simultaneously fills the vessels of the muscle should be equal to 4 ml. If we recalculate the loss of fluid by this amount of blood, then the obtained value (+0.56 ml) is in good agreement with the volume of flowing from a hemodynamically isolated muscle during arterial occlusion - 0.65 ml.

Outflow of tissue fluid into the vascular bed should lead to a decrease in tissue pressure. In addition, this way may contribute to vasodilation in the post-occlusion period or even be its direct cause.

This extremely important fact is also interesting in another respect. This filtration mechanism can, to some extent, stabilize the volume of the vascular bed of the ischemic zone and counteract the decrease in intravascular pressure during the cessation of arterial inflow. The possibility of the existence of such a mechanism of auto stabilization confirms not a linear, as one would expect, but an exponential character of a decrease in muscle volume and intravascular pressure during arterial occlusion.

A completely different picture we observed with venous occlusion. The hematocrit value by the 30th second of the post-occlusion period increases to 41 ± 1%. This indicates the transition of fluid from the vascular bed to the tissues during blockade of the outflow of blood. For 90 s of the post-occlusion period, hematocrit values return to normal, i.e., the liquid phase of the blood returns to the vascular bed. Based on the amount of blood contained in the calf muscle, the amount of blood transferred to the tissues is 0.8 ml. Figure 7 shows that the volume of the muscle during venous occlusion increased rapidly and within 30 seconds increased by 40 мм3 and then a second wave of volume increase by 19 ± 3 mm3 is observed. When the outflow was restored, the muscle volume sharply decreased by 20 ± 5 mm3 below the pre-occlusion values and remained at this level for another 20-40 seconds. That is, there is an excellent correlation with blood flow after venous occlusion.

Therefore, the filtration mechanism that affects tissue pressure should be taken into account when analyzing the mechanisms of RH formation, since it can significantly influence vascular tone in arterial occlusion.

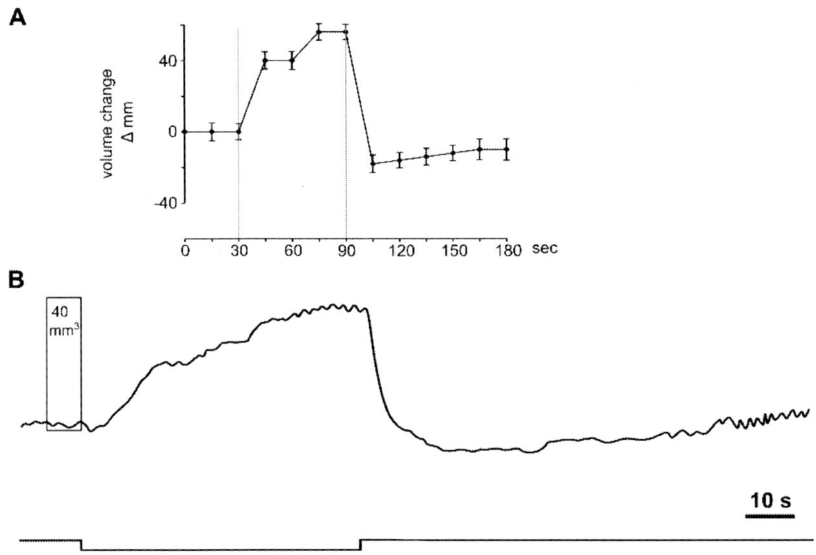

Figure 7. Dynamics of volumetric oscillations of the muscles of a denervated cat limb during venous occlusion and in the post-occlusion period. A - averaged data based on the results of 20 observations; B – experimental traces dated 04-01 -1974. Designations of curves (from top to bottom): plethysmogram, time scale (5 sec.), time interval of vein occlusion.

As for the paradoxical absence of a decrease in the level of oxygen tension in skeletal muscles during venous occlusion, we observed this phenomenon only in experiments on a denervated limb. In the isolated gastrocnemius muscle, the pO_2 level, although insignificant, decreased in some experiments. This made it possible to carry out comparative measurements of the rate constant of oxygen consumption in arterial and venous occlusion. The values of the constants were 0.059±0.002 s-1 and 0.015±0.0006 s-1, respectively. It is likely that the interstitial fluid accumulation caused by venous occlusion would impair oxygen diffusion between plasma and tissue.

Thus, oxygen consumption during venous occlusion significantly decreases compared to the cease of blood flow from the venous side. It is likely that the interstitial fluid accumulation caused by venous occlusion would impair oxygen diffusion between plasma and tissue. The mechanisms of this phenomenon remain unclear to us. A possible reason is the increase in diffusion distances for oxygen molecules.

Summarizing all of the above, we can say the following. According to the tissue pressure hypothesis, local regulation of blood flow occurs mainly in low-pressure vessels due to the pressure of tissue fluid on them. In this case, the regulation of blood flow does not require an active reaction of the smooth muscles of the microvasculature. With increased filtration of fluid in the tissue, the pressure of the interstitial fluid will increase. This increased tissue pressure will act like an outside force on all blood vessels located in this area. Without thinking, these changes in tissue pressure and this external force will affect the resistance of the blood vessels.

As a rule, the regulation of vascular tone under the influence of tissue pressure is considered in connection with the blood flow in the pulp of the kidneys and teeth, since these areas are the vascular networks enclosed in a relatively rigid capsule (A. C. Brown & Yankowitz, 1964; L. B. Hinshaw et al. 1959).

As mentioned above, in 1966 S. Rodbard put forward the hypothesis of tissue pressure, presenting the physical system he developed, called the "capillary." This system was able to simulate critical vascular closure and opening, arterial and venous autoregulation, and various types of congestion. The model was an encapsulated structure that included parenchymal cells, tissue fluid, and a permeable capillary with soft walls (Figure 5).

Studies carried out using this capillary system showed that the local, non-emergency regulation of blood flow could be carried out at the capillary level, without the direct active participation of smooth muscles. We can say that the conductivity of the vessel (the reciprocal of the resistance) is a function of the degree of relative permeability of the segments of the vessel immediately above and below the measurement point. As the permeability changes, so does the extravascular or tissue pressure and, accordingly, the effective transmural pressure, which acts more effectively on the soft-walled vessel.

Beer tried to test the hypothesis about the role of tissue pressure in the regulation of blood flow by comparing the responses to the "capillaron" model and to the dog *m. gracilis* (Beer, 1971). The model was used to measure inlet pressure, capsule volume, and capsule pressure. In the preparation m. gracilis recorded arterial and venous pressure, as well as changes in its volume. Beer subjected both systems to a sudden change in perfusion rate. Both systems showed an equally sharp rise in blood pressure, then a sharp drop in pressure to control values, and finally a slow progressive increase in blood pressure. In the model, the third phase is accompanied by an increase in extravascular volume and pressure. In muscle preparation, the third phase was associated with an increase in muscle volume.

In the case of the capillary model, increased resistance to flow was associated with increased extravascular pressure and possible collapse of the soft-walled "capillary" at the distal end. Therefore, Beer concluded that the increasing resistance to flow in the animal's muscle should also be associated only with increased tissue pressure and capillary collapse.

Hinshaw et al. (L. Hinshaw, 1964; L. B. Hinshaw et al. 1959) analyzed many of the factors involved in the phenomenon of renal autoregulation. They hypothesized that the components of changes in vascular resistance observed with an increase in blood pressure include metabolic response, myogenic response, post glomerular viscosity change, increase in extravascular Bowman's capsule pressure, and increase in tissue pressure. However, despite the variety of counteracting forces, tissue pressure was the main mechanism responsible for the formation of a reaction of reactive hyperemia in response to short (15 s) occlusions.

There is also an opposite point of view by Swann et al. (Swann et al. 1950) who conducted a series of experiments to elucidate the role of interstitial tissue pressure in the regulation of blood flow in the kidneys. Their data showed that tissue pressure did not increase dramatically with increasing blood pressure. They also examined changes in deep vein pressure with increases and decreases in blood pressure. On average, the increase in blood pressure per mm Hg caused an increase in interlobular venous pressure by 0.26 mm Hg.

Additionally, the absence of any disproportionately large changes in venous pressure associated with changes in blood pressure does not support the hypothesis of autoregulation of blood flow by tissue pressure.

The Starling Equation and the Endothelium: Their Roles in Capillary Leak Syndrome Development

Once again about fluid exchange and the special role of the endothelium in this process. Usually, speaking about the endothelium, first, they recall nitric oxide and other vasoactive substances synthesized by the endothelium. Now we will talk about the role of the endothelium in water metabolism and, accordingly, its role in the regulation of tissue pressure in this connection.

According to modern concepts, the endothelium is the inner lining of blood vessels that separates the blood flow from the deeper layers of the vascular wall. This continuous cell monolayer covers the inside of the vessel's lumen. Its total weight in the human body is about 1.5–2.0 kg. It performs not only a barrier-transport function but is also an important secretory organ. The endothelium continuously produces a huge amount of the most important biologically active substances, being at the same time a giant paracrine organ distributed over the entire area of the human body. The endothelium synthesizes substances important for the control of blood coagulation, regulation of vascular tone, and blood pressure. It takes part in the filtration function of the kidneys, the contractile activity of the heart, the metabolic supply of the brain, regulates the diffusion of water, ions, metabolic products, responds to the mechanical effect of the flowing fluid, and changes in blood pressure. The endothelium is sensitive to chemical and anatomical damage, which can lead to increased aggregation and adhesion of circulating cells, development of thrombosis, and sedimentation of lipid conglomerates.

In this case, we are interested in the barrier-transport function of the endothelium. The implementation of this function throughout the microvessels occurs in different ways. The transport of substances through the endothelium of different parts of the vascular bed occurs in different ways. The walls of the venous components of the microvasculature are more permeable to protein than the walls of other microvessels. The permeability of postcapillary venules for water significantly exceeds the permeability of pre capillaries and capillaries. Significant variations in protein transport across the endothelial lining are observed even along a single microvessel.

Transport of intravascular fluid through the endothelium occurs: 1) directly through endothelial cells - through the system of their microvesicles and transendothelial channels (transcytosis, transendothelial transfer), 2) through interendothelial gaps - areas of connection of endothelial cells with each other.

Fluid exchange between the intravascular and interstitial sectors obeys Ernst Henry Starling's law. According to this law, the fluid moves in accordance with the pressure gradient created, on the one hand, by the hydrostatic intravascular pressure and the colloid osmotic pressure of the interstitial fluid, and, on the other hand, by the hydrostatic interstitial pressure and the colloid osmotic pressure of the blood plasma.

According to Starling's classical concept, inside the capillary about 2/3 of the length from its beginning there is a point of equilibrium of all the forces described above, proximal to which fluid extravasation predominates, and distally resorption. At this ideal equilibrium point, fluid exchange does not occur. Real measurements show that a certain zone of the capillary is indeed in a position close to equilibrium, but even in it, the release of liquid still prevails over resorption. That is, there is, as it were, a certain tendency or predisposition to the development of tissue edema. In a healthy body, this excess transudate returns to the blood through the lymphatic vessels.

With an increasc in hydrostatic pressure in microcirculatory exchange vessels, the equilibrium zone shifts towards postcapillary venules, increasing the filtration surface and reducing the resorption area. A drop in hydrostatic pressure leads to a reverse shift of the near-equilibrium zone. The total volumetric filtration rate in an individual region is determined mainly by the total surface area of functioning capillaries and their permeability. A quantitative assessment of the volumetric velocity of the transcapillary movement of a liquid can be made using the formula:

$$Qf + CFC\ [(Pc\text{-}Pi) - \delta\ (\pi c - \pi i)], \tag{8}$$

where: Qf – is the volume of liquid filtered through the capillary wall, per unit area; δ is the osmotic reflection coefficient of the capillary membrane, which characterizes the actual permeability of the membrane for water and substances dissolved in it; primarily protein? Pc is the value of hydrostatic pressure of the intravascular fluid; Pi is the hydrostatic pressure of the interstitium; πi is the value of the colloid osmotic pressure of the intravascular fluid.

CFC is the coefficient of capillary filtration, which characterizes the area of the exchange surface (the number of functioning capillaries) and the permeability of the capillary wall for liquid. The coefficient has the dimension - ml/min/100 g of tissue/mm Hg, i.e., this parameter shows how many milliliters of fluid are filtered or absorbed into 100 g of tissue in 1 minute with a change in capillary hydrostatic pressure of 1 mm Hg.

The value of hydrostatic pressure in the capillaries, squeezing fluid into the tissue, at the arterial end of the capillaries is about 30 mm Hg. In the course of the capillaries, it decreases due to friction up to 10 mm Hg. at their venous end. The average capillary pressure is estimated at 17 mm Hg.

The colloid osmotic pressure of plasma does not coincide with the total osmotic pressure on cell membranes. It is provided only by those particles that do not pass freely through the capillary wall. These are exclusively protein molecules, mainly albumins and a1-globulins. Characteristically, fibrinogen is almost never involved in the creation of oncotic pressure. The total osmotic pressure on the cell membrane is created by both dissolved and suspended particles, and it is 200 times higher than its colloid-osmotic component. However, the protein component of the total pressure is the only significant value that affects the passage of liquid through the vessel wall.

Salt and non-electrolyte components of the total osmotic pressure on both sides of the histohematic barriers are balanced by the diffusion of the corresponding relatively low molecular weight substances, the rate of which is thousands of times higher than the fluid filtration rate. Normally, the plasma concentration of proteins is more than 3 times higher than the interstitial one. In muscles and brain tissues, the concentration of oncotic equivalents is even lower. Therefore, plasma proteins create an oncotic pressure of at least 19 mm Hg, which keeps fluid in the vessel. To this is added about 9 mm Hg. due to the effect of Donnan - electrostatic fixation by anionic protein molecules of excess cations in the intravascular space. Thus, the total holding pressure of 28 mm Hg exists throughout the capillary.

The average oncotic pressure of the tissue fluid is under normal conditions 6 mm Hg and retains water in tissues. If the excess protein that enters the tissue through transcytosis and inflammation were not reabsorbed through the lymphatic system, the oncotic pressure gradient between the blood and tissues would gradually be lost.

The hydrostatic pressure of the interstitial fluid was thought for almost 70 years after Starling to be positive, resisting the release of fluid from the vessel. The experiments of Arthur Guyton showed that under the skin between the vessels, there is a negative (that is, sub-atmospheric) suction pressure. Under normal conditions, free fluid pressure in most tissues is from -2 to -7 mmHg (average value -6 mm Hg).

Suction by tissues of fluid from capillaries and postcapillary venules actually greatly facilitates the work of the heart in tissue perfusion and has a decisive effect on the paths of normal microcirculation. The pressure of the water bound by the tissue gel is also at the sub atmospheric level, but it is 1–2 mm Hg. higher than in the free phase. Positive tissue pressure is only in organs located in a closed volume, for example, in the brain. In other tissues, it becomes higher than atmospheric only with noticeable edema. A partial vacuum under the skin promotes a compact state of cells in healthy tissues, even in the absence of binding connective tissue structures. With its loss in edematous, for example, inflamed tissue, the bonds between cells weaken.

The higher permeability and increased area of the venous ends of the capillaries compared to the arterial ones balances the oncoming flows, despite the almost half the absolute value of the resulting resorption vector compared to the transudation vector. The above mechanism regulates filtration and reabsorption. However, other processes, diffusion and transcytosis, also occur at the histohematic border, which make an important contribution to determining the composition of the tissue fluid.

Diffusion is the main mechanism of transcapillary exchange. The rate of filtration flow is much lower than the rate of capillary blood flow. However, it has been calculated that the rate of histohematic water exchange is very high, therefore, it is not determined by filtration but can only be associated with diffusion. As a result, the exchange of proper water in tissues generally does not correspond to the mechanically variable characteristics of capillary blood flow. The diffusion value depends on the number of functioning capillaries (direct relationship), the concentration gradient of dissolved substances (direct relationship) and the blood flow velocity in the microvasculature (inverse relationship).

Additional protection of the interstitium from excessive accumulation of fluid and the formation of edema is the drainage system of the lymphatic vessels. Edema is a typical pathological process, which consists in the creation of excess fluid in the interstitial sector of the extracellular water space. The term "edema" is not used in relation to intracellular overhydration (the term "swelling of the cell" is more acceptable for its designation). With edema, there is always not only an excess of extracellular tissue water, but also an increase in the sodium content in the tissue fluid. With edema, the suction tissue pressure always decreases, and with severe tissue hyperhydration, it becomes positive. Clinically, the initial edema with negative tissue fluid pressure corresponds to the symptom of fossa formation when pressing on the edematous tissue. If no pressure pit is formed, the pressure in the tissue is positive, which corresponds to "tense," or far advanced, edema. For instance, the same non-pitted edema can also be characteristic of inflammatory exudate.

A. Guyton calculated that the negative pressure in the tissues is equal to 5.3 mmHg, the drainage function of the lymph in relation to the liquid (about 7 mmHg), and the resorption of tissue protein into the blood through the lymph (another 5 mm Hg)) taken together, in total they create a "buffer reserve" of the order of 17 mm Hg. This reserve should protect tissues from the immediate development of edema with an increase in filtering pressure and a decrease in oncotic pressure.

Therefore, edema begins to form when the mean intracapillary pressure increases (or plasma oncotic pressure decreases) by 17–18 mm Hg, i.e., upon reaching at least 35 mm Hg - for capillary hydrostatic or 10 mm Hg - for plasma oncotic pressure. Edema is a manifestation of imperfect adaptation. The adaptive role of edema can be seen in the fact that this phenomenon protects the body from the development of hypervolemia, which can have life-threatening acute consequences, resulting in a violation of systemic hemodynamics. Local edema has a dilutional effect on tissue fluid, which potentially reduces the concentrations of pathogens, toxins, and autacoids when tissue is damaged.

Edema is one of the mechanisms for limiting the zone of inflammation. At the same time, vessels are squeezed in edematous tissues, microcirculation is additionally disturbed, diffusion of nutrients is difficult, and such tissues become infected more easily and heal worse. Like other typical pathological processes, edema is poly etiological.

The interstitium is also by no means a void but consists of a collagen matrix filled with proteoglycan filaments adjacent to each other. Under physiological conditions, the interstitium has little extensibility, and its structure prevents the free movement of fluid. Based on the facts described above, from the standpoint of Starling's theory, it is difficult to imagine the possibility of increasing the amount of fluid in the interstitium by 2-3 times. Meanwhile, a pronounced edematous syndrome is easily modeled in the experiment and is quite common in the clinic in patients with hypovolemic shock, sepsis, and extensive burns.

Thus, even a small increase in interstitial fluid volume during venous occlusion can lead to a significant increase in tissue pressure and prevent vascular relaxation after venous occlusion. It is likely that this mechanism is one of the main reasons for the lack of increase in blood flow after venous occlusion.

Chapter 9

Vascular Basal Tone and Myogenic Automaticity

Every physiologist researching blood circulation knows Folkow's postulate that a smooth muscle cell is a mechanoreceptor with an integrated contractile system. In this definition, the principle of autonomy of the smooth muscle cell is already visible. There is reason to believe that the time will come when the smooth muscle cell will be called a contractile system with a built-in trigger for electrical activity.

Analysis of the results of numerous studies suggests that none of the known factors that can affect the VSMs from the outside, cannot be considered as a unique trigger that ensures the formation and support of vascular tone in its full volume. Attention is drawn to the fact that a common feature for vessels of resistance (characterized as being considered the most pronounced basal tone) is their inherent autorhythmic contractile activity in the form of alternating spontaneous phase contractions or so-called automaticity. "Automaticity refers to the ability of cells to exhibit specific activity (for muscles, the cycle of contraction-relaxation) under the influence of stimuli arising in them, and not under the influence from outside" (Konradi, 1973).

For a long time, VSMCs were classified as multiunit smooth muscles that do not have automatism. The turning point occurred when Bohr and colleagues began to study small, isolated vessels (Uchida et al. 1967).

Deviation 6. *The emergence of new approaches and techniques often leads to breakthroughs in experimental research. Moreover, it does not have to be a device based on new principles of physics and electronics. Often this is simply the emergence of new approaches to the measurement of physiological parameters. In 1967, when I started doing my first physiological research, there were no methods for recording the tone of isolated blood vessels (with the exception of resistography developed by Khayutin). We were forced to develop a new device for measuring the outflow of blood from the gastrocnemius muscle based on a drop photo sensor and a step telephone relay. Eleven years later, in 1978, in the physiology of smooth muscles for* *recording contractile reactions, bulky devices with flasks were still used, where large fragments of animal intestines were placed in Tyrode's solution. We were forced again to develop compact horizontal chambers for working with small isolated vessel fragments. It was on them, working with small branches of the coronary arteries of a pig, that I first saw spontaneous contractions of VSM cells. The portal vein does not count, its ability to autorhythmic activity was already well known to everyone.*

Now the situation is different. Detailed guidelines for working with isolated smooth muscle fragments have appeared. Of the latter, I would like to mention the work of Wenceslau, McCarthy, Early, et al. (2021), which describes in most detail the methods for measuring vascular function in vitro. It is a wonderful guide for students, young researchers and not only them.

Bohr's laboratory worked mainly with perfused vessels with a diameter of 100 to 300 microns (this is a high class!). When the vessels were perfused with a calcium-free solution, the perfusion pressure dropped and stabilized at values that did not change under the influence of papaverine and isoproterenol. Vessels of the mesentery and skeletal muscles were studied. Therefore, when switching to a normal saline solution, the vessels of the mesentery did not narrow, and the vessels of the skeletal muscles quickly returned to the initial level of tone. Brain vessels behaved similarly to skeletal muscle vessels. However, in fairness, the vessels of the mesentery with a diameter of less than 100 μm also reacted to the transition to perfusion with normal saline by contraction.

That is, the autorhythmic activity perfectly reproduced in the complete absence of nervous and humoral influences acting from the outside. The favorite objects of physiologists for the study of automaticity in physiology of circulation in this matter are the heart and portal vein. However, automatic activity is also inherent in the smooth muscles of the digestive tract, the small pelvis, and, most importantly for us, almost all vessels of small diameter, the so-called resistance vessels. The mechanisms of the autorhythmic activity of smooth muscles remain the "hard nut" of modern physiology. Nevertheless, we need to know them in detail. There is no other way to provide the clinic with an effective tool for pharmacological control of vascular tone and blood pressure. For autorhythmic activity, an element of the regulation system called an oscillator is needed. Qualitative analysis can identify the elements essential for generating oscillations and can enhance our understanding of underlying oscillator mechanisms. Two essential elements of a biological oscillator are 1) an inhibitory feedback loop, which includes one or more oscillating variables, and 2) a source of delay in this feedback loop, which allows an oscillating variable to overshoot a steady-state value before the feedback inhibition will be completely effective (Friesen & Block, 1984).

Basal (Intrinsic) Tone Definition and Intrinsic Mechanisms of Its Formation

Above mentioned Bohr's experiments with the removal of extracellular calcium, of course, do not indicate that the basal tone is entirely due to the action of calcium coming from the environment. You cannot say that the functioning of the brain is a consequence of the action of oxygen on the grounds that in the absence of oxygen the brain dies. The necessity of something for this or that activity is not the reason that this something is the cause of this activity. Konradi is often repeated - always after that, does not mean because of that. Calcium, of course, is a necessary link in the contractile component of the basal tone. We also need mechanisms to ensure the energy process, electrogenesis, ensuring the processes of coordinated depolarization. Repolarization, a trigger, and a switching mechanism are needed for each cycle of the process of autorhythmic activity. And, finally, a mechanism is needed to synchronize the contractions of individual cells into a single process of tonic contraction of the vascular wall.

Basal tone is the degree of active tension of the vascular wall, which remains after the elimination of neurogenic and humoral influences. This is the intrinsic myogenic activity of the smooth muscle cells of the vascular wall. Folkov (1964) called smooth muscle cells mechanoreceptors with a built-in contractile system. This means that one of the key reactions of smooth muscle to stretching, the Ostroumov-Bayliss reaction, is realized exclusively through its own intracellular mechanisms.

Basal vascular tone is determined by structural and myogenic components. Its structural part consists of a rigid but elastic vascular "frame" formed by collagen and elastin fibers, which determine the resistance of blood vessels, if the activity of their smooth muscles is completely excluded. This is the skeleton of blood vessels. The myogenic part of the basal tone in a significant part is provided by the tension of the smooth muscles of the vessels in response to the tensile force of arterial pressure.

Thus, even in the absence of nerve influences on the vessels, in the event of their complete denervation, the residual vascular tone, called basal tone, continues to persist. Basal tone is based on intrinsic myogenic mechanisms of smooth muscle cells.

First, it is the ability of VSMCs to spontaneously exhibit bioelectrical activity, i.e., to automation and the spread of excitement from cell to cell through tight contacts. This leads to their contraction and narrowing of the vessel's lumen. The second reason is depolarization and contraction of smooth muscle cells under the influence of the stretching effect of blood pressure on the vessel wall. Basal tone is clearly expressed in the vessels of organs with a high level of metabolism, i.e., in the vessels of the kidneys, heart and brain. It is influenced by humoral factors. Cell metabolites carbon dioxide, organic acids reduce basal tone and dilate blood vessels, and vasopressin, angiotensin, adrenaline circulating in the blood increase basal tone and the vessels narrow. Due to the presence of basal tone and its ability to local self-regulation, the vessels of these areas can maintain the volumetric blood flow rate at a constant level, regardless of fluctuations in systemic arterial pressure.

So, lct us sum up the intermediate results. Even with complete denervation and elimination of humoral influences, a residual vascular tone, called basal, intrinsic or myogenic tone, continues to persist. It is based on the myogenic mechanism, i.e., it is intrinsic to smooth muscle cells. It is due to the ability of the smooth muscle cells of arterioles to exhibit spontaneous bioelectrical activity, i.e., to automation and the spread of excitation from cell to cell. The level of basal tone is influenced/modulated by humoral factors of dilatation and constrictor nature and, of course, nervous regulation. To the greatest extent, basal tone is expressed in the vessels of organs with high metabolic activity (heart, kidneys, brain). It is believed that due to the basal tone, the vessels are able to maintain the volumetric blood flow rate at a constant level, regardless of fluctuations in systemic arterial pressure.

There seems to be a definition of basal tone, but there is nothing in it to indicate how it all works. A classic situation arises with a black box that says, "basal tone." Each of us is free to apply some kind of perturbing influence to the input of this system (each one has his own, depending on the area of physiology / pharmacology / biophysics in which he works), register the output signal and draw the appropriate conclusion. Each one is his own. The classic version with an elephant and blind men studying it (see the last figure in this book).

Is it all the same - basal vascular tone? The physiological reality exists only in our imagination and as a kind of speculative construction. With its structural component, everything is clear - this is the skeleton of a vessel made of collagen, elastin, and muscle. Something like an extensive water supply network in a large house. However, this very smart network has autonomous mechanisms built into it, allowing it to independently regulate and optimize the flow of fluid flowing through it, depending on the demand of consumers. The key word here is self.

Sometimes it seems to me that we are really chasing some chimera created by our imagination. Sometimes it begins to seem to me that the basal tone is an artificially created hypothetical construction made up of functional structures known to us, invented solely to somehow explain the mechanisms of regulation of local blood flow. Something like Maxwell's demons, (we will return to them again later, after all, this is a very useful chimera). There seems to be no well-defined, relatively simple material substrate behind this term, like sodium-potassium ATPase or calcium/potassium channels. I think this is not so and such a construct still exists in reality

Most likely, it exists in the form of an intricate complex of metabolic pathways, and cellular and subcellular structures organized and looped into a single system in such a way as to ensure the maintenance of an optimal level of tonic tension of VSMs in conditions of constantly changing influences from the external environment.

This does not mean that it cannot be identified. Our task is precisely to identify the components and connections/links in this system as reliably as possible in order to subsequently be able to accurately pharmacologically influence them, if necessary, i.e., with the development of a pathological process in this system.

In order to better understand the essence of the basal tone problem, let's try to find analogies in physics. For instance, in telecommunications - a carrier wave, carrier signal, or just carrier, is a waveform (usually sinusoidal form) that is modulated (modified) with an input signal for the purpose of conveying information. It is a fact that most radio systems used frequency modulation (FM) or amplitude modulation (AM) to make the carrier transfer information. This carrier wave usually has a much higher frequency than the input signal does. The frequency of a radio or television station is actually the carrier wave's frequency. The purpose of the carrier is usually to transmit the information through space as an electromagnetic wave (Figure 8).

It is important to understand that the information transmitted by a radio signal is not at the carrier frequency itself but contained in sidebands (one of two frequency bands on either side of the carrier wave, containing the modulated signal) on either side of the carrier, i.e., the energy of the carrier component is not useful in transmitting the information.

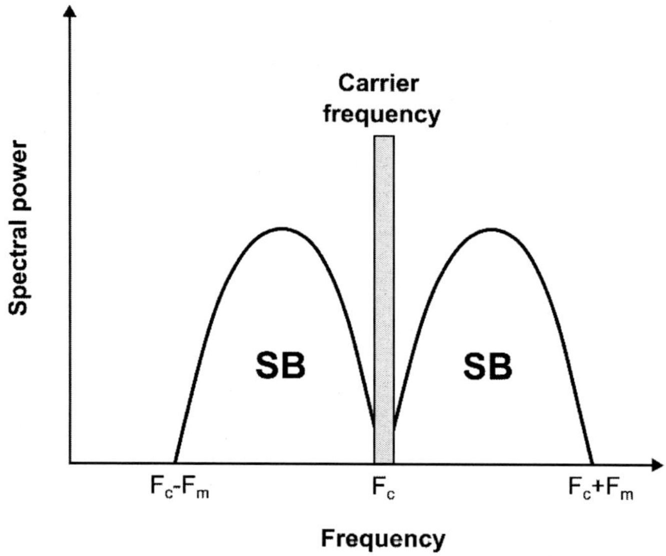

Figure 8 shows the frequency spectrum of a typical radio signal from an AM or FM radio transmitter. It consists of a strong signal (C) at the carrier wave frequency fC, with the modulation contained in narrow frequency bands called sidebands (SB) just above and below the carrier.

We believe that the basal tone with a certain degree of approximation is similar to such a carrier frequency, while external influences (neural and humoral) on it are similar to modulating frequencies. It is they who ensure the adjustment of the blood flow through the vessel to the metabolic needs of the organ or tissue. On the other hand, in the absence of a carrier frequency, the modulating frequencies cannot reach the receiver.

Let me remind you that blood vessels lacking nerve control initially lose the ability to respond adequately to the metabolic demands of tissues but they are able to restore the level of their tonic tension after a shot time and retain the ability to function normally and resist to blood flow (i.e., the Ostroumov-Bayliss mechanism works properly). For instance, the denervation of skeletal muscles increases the blood flow in them about two times, but the subsequent injection of acetylcholine into the bloodstream causes a tenfold increase in blood flow, indicating that the vasodilation capacity of vessels in this case remains (Khayutin, 1964; Konradi, 1973).

Thus, we can say that in order to designate and explain this feature of the behavior of denervated vessels, the concept of "basal tone" of the vessels was introduced. Obviously, the basal vascular tone consists of structural and myogenic components. The structural part is the rigid vascular framework formed by collagen and elastic fibers, which determines the mechanical resistance of the vessels even when the activity of their smooth muscles is completely turned off.

The myogenic part of the basal tone is provided by the tension of the smooth muscles of the vessels, which develops in response to the tension force of the arterial pressure. Consequently, changes in vascular resistance under the influence of nervous or humoral factors overlap (modulate) the basal tone, which is normally more or less constant for a certain part of the vessel and, by analogy with a radio signal, represents a certain basic "carrier frequency." A number of different chemical and mechanical factors can affect basal tone by opening or closing membrane ion channels, activating membrane receptors and their signaling pathways, etc. In conditions where there are no nervous and humoral influences, vascular blood flow resistance is determined only by basal tone.

Bjorn Folkow Hypothesis: Advantages and Weaknesses

In accordance with the hypothesis proposed by Bjorn Folkow (1964), the basal vascular tone is the result of summation of rhythmic phasic contractions of many smooth muscle cells, and its regulation is carried out by changing the frequency, duration and amplitude of these phase contractions. Based on the analysis of phase contractions of single smooth muscle cells, he concluded that the resistance to blood flow is determined by the ratio between the total duration of the periods of its contraction and relaxation. An increase in the frequency of phase contractions, caused by stretching, leads to a decrease in the total duration of cell relaxation periods, and the ratio of the duration of contraction periods to the duration of relaxation periods increases, and the resistance to blood flow increases. At sufficiently high frequencies of phase contractions, their time summation is possible, merging into a tonic contraction. If there are no direct contacts between smooth muscle cells (for example, in metarterioles and precapillary sphincters), the rhythmic phase contractions of such cells are usually not synchronized. In this case, the spatial summation of phase contractions of individual cells is possible. In arterioles, the wall of which in most cases has a continuous smooth muscle layer, the rhythmic contractile activity generated by pacemaker cells is usually synchronized. Since the number and localization of pacemakers can be different, both temporal and spatial summation of phase contractions of a large number of cells is possible with the development as the result of smooth muscle tonic tension.

The logicality and persuasiveness of the hypothesis proposed by B. Folkov for the formation and regulation of the basal vascular tone is such that for more than 60 years it has remained widely recognized without significant changes. Nevertheless, in recent years some facts have accumulated, which are difficult to explain only on the basis of this hypothesis. The data obtained in the Department of Circulatory Physiology at the Bogomoletz Institute of Physiology in Kyiv (Bershtein, Gurevich, Soloviev, 1982) allow us to suggest that the basal vascular tone is formed not only solely due to the summation of the phasic contractions of a large number of smooth muscle cells. After all, if the basal tone is based only on the rhythmic contractile activity of VSM cells, it remains unclear, due to which the initial level of tonic tension continues to be maintained in experimental conditions after pharmacological suppression of phasic contractions in vascular tissues. The same consideration arose in the analysis of data presented by other authors. It was shown that after administration of verapamil to the buffer solution, which blocks the ability to generate action potentials and phase contractions, the tonic reaction of the portal vein smooth muscles to norepinephrine was largely preserved and was at least 40-50% of the response observed in the absence of the calcium antagonist (Golenhofen, 1976).

The existence of varieties of VSM cells that differ sharply in their contractile properties at rest and the ability to respond differently to irritation is beyond doubt. So, Golenhofen (1974, 1976), based on the presence of myogenic automatism, divided the smooth muscles of the vessels into three groups: a) smooth muscles, the cells of which are rhythmically active and not differentiated by the properties of excitation and conduction; b) smooth muscles, the cells of which are rhythmically active, but some of them generate excitation, while others perform a conductive function; c) smooth muscles, the cells of which normally do not have rhythmic activity and are activated predominantly neurogenic. There is reason to believe that such differences are determined not only by the features of the neuroeffector and functional organization of the smooth muscle layer of the walls of different sections of the vascular bed, but also by the features inherent in their constituent cells. Thus, it was shown that VSM cells, characterized by phase contractile activity, contain no more than 2.2% (of the total cytoplasm) of the sarcoplasmic reticulum (Devine et al. 1972), while in smooth muscle cells that have the ability to generate tonic contractions, it is twice as much up to 5.0% (Somlyo, Somlyo, 1976). In this regard, it is obvious that the dependence of contractile reactions on the extracellular concentration of calcium ions in them should be different.

The cells of a rhythmically active VSM, in contrast to the tonically contracting, apparently have a mechanism that ensures the removal of free Ca^{2+} from the cytoplasm at a rate and rhythm corresponding to the frequency of phasic contractions. This refers to a mechanism similar to that, which provides diastolic relaxation in the heart muscle and a clear correlation between contraction and relaxation of the myocardium. Otherwise, it is difficult to explain the mechanism of the formation of phasic contractions with a sufficiently high frequency of their alternation, which is observed in rhythmically active VSM cells.

There is also reason to argue that the transmembrane mechanisms for increasing the concentration of calcium ions in the cytoplasm of smooth muscle cells differ significantly. For instance, K. Golenhofen postulated the concept of phasic (P-system) and tonic (T -system) systems of activation of contractions in smooth muscles, including vascular ones (Golenhofen, 1976). It was based on data about different sensitivity of phase and tonic contractions of smooth muscles to the removal of calcium ions from the perfusate and studying the effect of various calcium current blockers on the tone and membrane potential. Moreover, he believed that smooth muscles are differentiated according to the predominant number of cells in their composition, in which the P - or T - activation system prevails. The idea of a possible differentiation of VSMs according to the mechanism of excitation–contraction coupling in their cells is not new. There is a well-known point of view Somlyo, Somlyo on electromechanical and pharmacomechanical coupling in smooth muscles (Somlyo & Somlyo, 1968). Its essence lies in the existence in VSM the cells membranes of which have not only electrically excitable, but also chemically excitable calcium permeability systems.

According to the terminology adopted later, this corresponds to two types of calcium channels: fast voltage-dependent and slow chemosensitive, that is, channels activated by the influence of agonists on the membrane chemoreceptors associated with these channels. In the early 1980s, M. F. Shuba (1981) suggested the presence in the membranes of smooth muscle cells of the so-called slow voltage-dependent and non-inactivating or slightly inactivating calcium channels. A very interesting idea, which later received confirmation in the form of the existence of the so-called "window currents." These channels differed from fast voltage-gated channels in their sensitivity to calcium current blockers, the absence or weak inactivation, and other activation thresholds. As a result of my frequent conversations with

M. F. Shuba on this subject, I realized that, in accordance with his views, in the smooth muscles of vessels with basal tone, constantly activated slow voltage-dependent calcium channels, and possibly also chemosensitive calcium channels, should be constantly located. Thanks to them, calcium entering the cytoplasm of cells maintains a certain level of basal tone.

Finally, curious data were obtained at the Bogomoletz Institute of Physiology indicating the differences in the cells that form the muscle layer of the same vessel. Using the method of microelectrode measurement of membrane and action potentials, it was shown (Gurevich, Bershtein, Evdokimov, 1976; Gurevich, Bershtein, Soloviev, 1981) that most of the smooth muscle cells of the rat portal vein are characterized by rhythmic electrical activity in the form of slow depolarization waves with amplitudes up to 10 mV and a duration of about 3.0-3.5 s, on top of which action potentials with an amplitude of 15-17 mV ensure. The membrane potential of such cells did not exceed 20–25 mV, and the membrane resistance was of the ordcr of 3–5 MΩ. Along with this, cells that do not possess rhythmic changes in the level of polarization of the membrane were also detected. Unlike rhythmically active cells, they are characterized by a higher membrane potential (30–50 mV) and membrane resistance - up to 50–80 MΩ.

The data obtained serve as the basis for the hypothesis that the VSM contains both the cells capable of generating primarily phase contractions and the cells that are capable of contracting predominantly tonic.

The possibility of differentiation of smooth muscle cells according to their functional characteristics is not so unexpected. So, no one doubts that the structure of skeletal muscles includes the so-called white (fast, phase) and red (slow, tonic) muscle fibers, the predominant content of which allocate red and white skeletal muscles. Fast-phase fibers are capable of developing considerable efforts in relatively short periods of time. The tonic muscles contract approximately twice as slowly as the phase and, although in the end they develop a comparable tension per unit cross-section, the rate of energy expenditure in the skeletal muscle phase fibers is much higher. These features are combined with noticeable differences in the structure and, especially, the metabolism of these two types of skeletal muscle fibers.

If we proceed from the idea of the existence of differentiation of VSMCs according to functional characteristics, then the formation of basal vascular tone cannot be reduced solely to the integration of the phase contractions of many smooth muscle cells, although the participation of this mechanism may even be decisive. At the same time, one cannot fully agree with the ideas that the basal vascular tone is based solely on the tonic contraction associated with the continuous influx of calcium ions into the cytoplasm, provided by the slow voltage-dependent and chemo-sensitive calcium channels being permanently activated (Shuba, 1981).

Obviously, it should be recognized that the basal vascular tone includes two components, the presence of which is due to the presence of two types of smooth muscle cells that are functionally different. By the way, Konradi (1973), holding the opinion that myogenic automatism is the most likely mechanism for the formation of basal vascular tone, wrote: "... this does not exclude the possibility of the possible existence of another, non-tetanic in nature, non-intermittent contractile process."

The idea of basal vascular tone as a state determined by two components - the emerging integration of the rhythmic phase of contractions of smooth muscle cells and the activity of cells that contract predominantly tonic - allows us to explain the results of studies showing the ability of VSMs to maintain a certain level of tonic tension under the condition of sharp inhibition or even the complete absence of phase contractions.

Based on a large amount of our own and literature data on the high sensitivity of rhythmic contractions to external influences, it can be assumed that the basal component of tone, due to their integration, is relatively less stable. It is possible that this component is involved in relatively rapid changes in vascular resistance that occur in the process of adaptation of the blood supply to the current level of functional activity of organs and tissues.

Interstitial Cells of Cajal

One of the first candidates for the role of the generator of rhythmic activity in smooth muscles could be interstitial cells of Cahal, or ICC, named after the famous Spanish neurohistologist, Nobel laureate Santiago Ramon and Kahal (1852 - 1934), who described them in 1893. Ramon-i-Kahal believed that the cells he discovered were special elements of the intramural nerve plexus responsible for the motility of the gastrointestinal tract.

Electrophysiological evidence of the role of these cells in establishing the rhythm of slow waves of the smooth muscles of the stomach and intestines were presented at the end of the 20th century (Takaki, 2003). The interstitial cells of Cajal set the rhythm of contractions (peristalsis) of the hollow organs of the gastrointestinal tract. They are also found in the urinary tract, urinary bladder, ureters, prostate gland, portal tracts of the liver, gallbladder and bile ducts, fallopian tubes, myometrium, mammary gland and, which is especially important for us, in the walls of arteries and lymphatic vessels. The interstitial cells of Cajal have an elongated fusiform shape. The cell length is from 40 to 100 microns, the thickness is 0.2–0.5 microns. ICCs have from 2 to 5 processes of length from several tens to hundreds of microns, some of the processes have secondary and tertiary branching, forming a three-dimensional network. The processes contain specific thin fibril-like segments and extended cistern-like sections.

As pacemakers, they play a key role in the activation and coordination of phases and the propagation of contractions in smooth muscle. Another function of these cells is to control the transmission of excitatory and inhibitory nerve impulses to smooth muscle cells. Interstitial cells of Cajal, located between the circular and longitudinal muscle layers, play an important role in the regulation of motor activity and intestinal sensitivity to mechanical stimuli. In the stomach, the network of Cajal cells begins in the proximal stomach and is regarded as the pacemaker of the upper digestive system. Cajal cells contact with varicose endings of axons of nerve cells and SMC membranes, modulate the transmission of nerve impulses to muscle fibers. At the same time, they are sensitive to mechanical stimuli. Stretching of the walls of the stomach during eating causes depolarization of cell membranes and the appearance of slow-wave activity of the pylorus. Apparently, this underlies the gastrocolic reflex, which is expressed in the appearance of the urge to defecate 20-30 minutes after breakfast. But the role of Cajal interstitial cells in the generation of slow wave potentials in smooth mice of the gastrointestinal tract is best known. It should be noted that the characteristics of these waves in different organs are different, and this fact is central in the diagnosis of motor disorders of the gastrointestinal tract using electrogastroenterography. The interstitial cells of Cajal set the frequencies of slow waves from 2-4 to 10-12 per minute.

The oscillation parameters set by the interstitial cells of Cajal are stable. They do not change under the influence of acetylcholine, histamine, adrenaline, atropine, procaine, morphine, cocaine, but the generating function of Cajal cells depends on the activity of cyclooxygenase-2 - when this enzyme is suppressed, the cells become insensitive to stretching.

The exact location of ICCs as pacemakers is unknown. It is believed that the pacemaker of the stomach is located in the proximal (closest to the esophagus) part of the stomach, and for the small intestine, probably in the confluence of the common bile duct into the duodenum. However, when removing a section of the stomach or intestines, a new pacemaker always appears, being a pacemaker for the underlying parts of the organ.

Some researchers consider the term "interstitial pacemaker cells" (IPC) to be more modern and more correct, leaving the term "interstitial cells of Cajal" to be either narrower or only historical. At the same time, the term "interstitial cells of Cajal" is more common in modern gastroenterology. A new classification (not shared by all) was proposed by Komuro (Komuro, 2006). It was based on ultramicroscopic features of the structure of these cells in comparison with fibroblasts and smooth muscle cells, on the basis of which he subdivided them into 2 groups: the interstitial Cajal cells and fibroblast-like cells. Fibroblast-like cells have a number of pronounced morphological differences: the presence of a well-developed granular endoplasmic reticulum, a small number of mitochondria, the absence of a basal membrane and caveolae. In turn, Cajal cells are divided into 3 types. Type I includes Cajal cells with the least pronounced similarity to smooth muscle cells; type III - Cajal cells with the most pronounced similarity with smooth muscle cells. Type II - intermediate, represented by Cajal cells with signs of cells type I and III.

Depending on the depth of location in the muscle wall, Cajal cells have different morphological characteristics. Thus, the cells of the Cajal of the Auerbach plexus are represented by three (I – III) types, while among the cells of Cajal l of the deep intermuscular neuroplex is dominated by type III cells. Cells located inside the circular and longitudinal muscular layer of the intestinal wall have 2 processes each with orientation along the axis of the intestine, and in cells located near the Auerbach and deep intramuscular nerve plexus, from 3 to 5 processes are observed with a characteristic type of branching: secondary, tertiary and higher order.

All Cajal cells morphologically differ from smooth muscle cells and, most likely, are special specialized pacemakers. Smooth muscle cells, on the other hand, are an independent contractile element with an integrated stretching sensor and a trigger for electrical activity. The fact is that any smooth muscle cell under certain conditions can be forced to contract autonomously. Block the potassium channels of the outward current in the smooth muscles of the aorta (tonic type) and you will observe rhythmic activity that is not typical for it in normal conditions. If in pathological conditions in the smooth muscles of the vascular wall for one reason or another, outward currents are blocked (or inward currents are activated), then the number of cells with an autorhythmic activity can increase dramatically.

Interestingly, following enzymatic dispersion of the guinea-pig mesenteric artery, up to 10% of the cells demonstrated unusual morphology resembling non-contractile cells with thin processes resembling interstitial cells of Cajal (Pucovský et al. 2003). These cells were found in rabbit portal vein, too (Harhun et al. 2004). The pacemaking function of these types of cells in the gut is well known. It is likely that they play an interpolation function between nerves and vascular SM cells, but it is possible that they have some yet unknown functions taking into account their ability to transdifferentiate into SM cells.

Historically, it was generally accepted to divide smooth muscles into tonic and phase types (Golenhofen, 1976; Ozaki & Karaki, 1993). Thus, there are two different, in their electrical and contractile characteristics, types of smooth muscles - one is characterized by a low and unstable membrane potential, the presence of spontaneously generated action potentials and phase contractions (phase type). An example would be the portal vein. For another type of smooth muscle (tonic), spontaneous activity is not peculiar. They react to stimulation by gradual depolarization and often without noticeable changes in the membrane potential (pharmacomechanical coupling). For instance, plasma membranes of pulmonary artery and aorta cells have several times lower conductivity for ions of sodium, potassium and chlorine, as well as more significant resistance than the cell membrane of the portal vein. According to Golenhofen, smooth muscles are composed of both types of cells - capable of generating primarily phase contractions, as well as cells of the tonic type. The predominance of a particular type of cell determines the ability of smooth muscle to contract in phase or tonic inherent manner.

Vasomotions

This type of behavior of smooth muscle cells provides, perhaps, the greatest approximation to understanding the mechanisms of autorhythmic activity. It is assumed that vasomotion (i.e., rhythmic spontaneous oscillation in tone of blood vessel walls, independent of heartbeat, innervation or respiration) play a significant role in supplementing oxygen to tissues in normal and pathological conditions. They are important for controlling blood pressure, and their severity decreases with a number of pathologies, for example, diabetes (Aalkjær & Nilsson, 2005).

Aalkjær and Nilsson, (2005) and Matchkov (2010) presented one of the most detailed studies of vasomotions. He believes that this type of vasomotor reaction is realized through interaction between intracellular calcium, released from the sarcoplasmic reticulum, and changes in membrane potential. In his opinion, rhythmic changes in intracellular calcium, when there is a sufficient concentration of cGMP, cause changes in the membrane potential, activating electrically connected cells in smooth muscle and leading to the development of synchronized phase activity. That is, synchronous depolarization of smooth muscle causes the same synchronous influx of calcium and, thus, leads to rhythmic contractions of blood vessels (Jacobsen et al. 2007, 2008).

Matchkov's merit also lies in the fact that he was the first to clearly identify and describe chloride channels in VSM, which have the properties necessary to synchronize the contractions of the smooth muscle cells of the vascular wall. It is also worth mentioning the high concentration of chloride ions in VSM (around 50 mM) compared to many other cell types.

Prior to this, chloride channels had been studied for many years, but they remained, as they were, in the shadow of cation channels. A special role belongs to the so-called calcium-dependent chloride-activated channels (CaCC). CaCCs were identified in vascular tissue, but mainly at a functional level (Hartzell et al. 2005). Unfortunately, pharmacological agents capable of selectively activating or, conversely, inhibiting these channels are still not known (Bakhramov et al. 1996; Berg et al. 2012).

Thus, based on the study of ionic currents by the patch-clamp method in smooth muscles, chloride currents with unique properties were identified (Machkov, 2010). This chloride current was activated by cGMP, was very sensitive to calcium, and was inhibited by very low concentrations of zinc ions, while traditional CaCC inhibitors only affect this current at very high concentrations. This cGMP-dependent, calcium-activated chlorine current has a linear dependence on potential, which differs from the similar envy for CaCC, usually characteristic of anionic conduction. This type of current is found in intestinal cells, VSM isolated from a number of vascular pools, but not found in the pulmonary artery.

Based on its unique characteristics, it has been proposed that the calcium-activated, cGMP-dependent chloride current can synchronize vascular wall smooth muscle cells and that the protein bestrophin may serve as a molecular substrate for this current. Bestrophin was first identified as a gene whose mutations cause viral macular degeneration (VMD) or Best's disease (Hartzell et al. 2005). There are reasons to believe that bestrophin is the chloride channel (Milenkovic et al. 2008).

It seems that Matchkov was the first to relate the chlorine current to one of the four known isoforms of the protein bestrophin. PCR and Western blot studies of various blood vessels showed the presence of the protein bestrophin-3 in many vessels, with the exception of the pulmonary arteries (where there is also no cGMP-dependent current). This is convincing evidence that bestrophin-3 is necessary for the formation of a cGMP-dependent calcium-activated current of chloride ions.

The presence of an electrical connection between cells of the VSM is important for their successful synchronization and significantly depends on the functioning of the channels between the cells, called gap junctions. Many cardiovascular diseases (e.g., hypertension and atherosclerosis) are associated with defects in intercellular communication and communication. Studies using gap blockers, the so-called gap-junction, heptanol and 18α-glycyrrhetinic acid, 18β-glycyrrhetinic acid and connexin mimetics confirm this in many cases. Matchkov (2010) also suggested that the channels and active ion carriers in the cell membrane do not function independently of each other but interact as functional units. A close functional relationship between the gap junction contacts, Na^+, K^+ -ATPase, Na^+/Ca^{2+} - exchanger and ATP-dependent K^+ channels was demonstrated, and this happens in certain limited spatial compartments of the cell. It was shown that inhibition of the Na^+/K^+ -ATPase with ouabain inhibits calcium release with the help of the Na^+/Ca2+ exchanger and this leads to a local increase in intracellular calcium and inhibition of intercellular communication. It was also found that ATP-dependent K^+ channels are an important player in this functional block. This effect is mutual, since the K^+ channel provides the Na^+/K^+ -ATPase with K^+ ions, while the ATP-dependent K^+ channels, in turn, also affect the activity of the Na^+/K^+ -ATPase.

G. Siegel (1983) proposed a very interesting mechanism for the formation of autorhythmic activity. It is because oscillations of phosphofructokinase-1 activity (i.e., glycolysis) lead to oscillations of ATP concentration and, accordingly, Na^+/K^+-ATPase activity (i.e., ion pump function). The changes in the electrogenic activity of the sodium pump lead to oscillations of the membrane potential, which spreads to neighboring cells. This assumption is supported by the fact that the application of ouabain easily blocks vasomotion.

Thus, in accordance with Matchkov (2010), the following chain of events may be suggested for the initiation of vasomotion. The voltage-independent model where the interaction between phospholipase C (PLC), phospholipase A_2 (PLA_2) and PKC amplifies the IP_3 signal. The elevated IP_3 level can induce oscillation in $[Ca^{2+}]_i$ due to biphasic regulation of the IP_3 channels by $[Ca^{2+}]_i$. Smooth muscle cells can be synchronized by the second messenger links between the cells. The next pathway suggested for voltage-dependent oscillations. CICR can affect two membrane conductances (for example, Ca^{2+}-activated K^+ channels (BK_{Ca}) and Ca^{2+}-activated Cl^- channels (CaCC)) which have opposite effects on the membrane voltage. Neighboring SM cells will be then synchronized by membrane potential changes. The interaction between cytosolic and membrane oscillators occurs as follows: IP_3 induces the local Ca^{2+} release which gives rise to Ca^{2+} waves through CICR. Transiently elevated $[Ca^{2+}]_i$ stimulates a depolarizing membrane current, possibly the Ca^{2+}-activated Cl^- current. The following depolarization opens voltage-dependent calcium channels, induces a global Ca^{2+} influx, which in turn affects the membrane potential and enhances the possibility of oscillations. This model has been experimentally supported when vasomotor activity appeared to be endothelial dependent. This may be due to the dependence of cGMP on Ca^{2+}-activated Cl^- current.

Concerning endothelium-dependence of these processes is however still a matter of debate. This is what Machkov thinks, and he does the right thing. This is unlikely.

I would not unequivocally state that vasomotor activity is the basis of basal tone, but this phenomenon, inherent in smooth muscle cells, is a good model for understanding the essence of basal tone. However, the problem of the high electrical resistance caused by the multiple membranes of smooth muscle cells remains. How can electrical signals be conducted so efficiently through so many cells over such long distances in the arterial wall?

Really, the study of vasomotor activity allowed us to shed light on some of the mechanisms of automatism. Our understanding of vasomotor smooth muscle function has changed dramatically over the past few decades. The classical concept of regulation of the vascular system, regulated solely by circulating hormones and sympathetic innervation, has given way to a vision of local regulation. It turned out that the effector elements of the cardiovascular system have their own regulators of contractile activity built into them. And the researchers faced another task - to understand how they work.

Chapter 10

The Energy Sources of the Cell: The Role of Glycolysis and Oxidative Phosphorylation

First, any system of regulation requires energy for its functioning. The basis of life on Earth is the energy of the sun. In the process of photosynthesis, solar energy is stored in the chemical bonds of carbohydrate molecules, of which the six-carbon sugar glucose plays the most important role. After other living organisms use these molecules for food, the energy stored in them is released and then used for their own metabolism. This occurs during the processes of glycolysis and respiration. The complete chemical process under conditions of normal oxygenation can be briefly described as follows:

GLUCOSE + OXYGEN → CARBON DIOXIDE + WATER + ENERGY

The term "glycolysis" combines the word lysis, meaning "cleavage," with the word glucose. As the name implies, the process begins with the chemical extraction of energy by splitting a glucose molecule into two parts, each containing three carbon atoms. In the process of glycolysis, each molecule of glucose produces two three-carbon molecules of pyruvic acid. In addition, the energy of glucose is stored in molecules that are commonly called the "energy currency" of the cell - two ATP molecules and two NADH molecules. Thus, already at the first stage of glycolysis, energy is released in a form that can be used by the cells of the body.

The further course of events depends on the presence or absence of oxygen in the medium. In the absence of oxygen, pyruvic acid is converted into other organic molecules in the course of the so-called anaerobic processes. For example, in yeast cells, pyruvic acid is converted to ethanol. In animals, which include humans, when oxygen reserves in the muscles are depleted, pyruvic acid turns into lactic acid - this causes the feeling of muscle stiffness so familiar to all of us after heavy exercise stress.

In the presence of oxygen, energy is released during aerobic respiration, when pyruvic acid is split into carbon dioxide and water molecules with the simultaneous release of the remaining energy stored in the carbohydrate molecule. Respiration occurs in a specialized cell organelle, the mitochondria. First, one carbon atom of pyruvic acid is cleaved off. This produces carbon dioxide, energy (it is stored in one NADH molecule), and a two-carbon molecule - an acetyl group. Then the reaction chain enters the metabolic coordination center of the cell - the Krebs cycle.

The Krebs cycle (also called the citric acid cycle or tricarboxylic acid cycle) is an example of a well-known phenomenon in biology - a chemical reaction that begins when a certain incoming molecule combines with another molecule that acts as a "helper." This combination initiates a series of other chemical reactions in which product molecules are formed and at the end a helper molecule is recreated, which can start the whole process again. In the Krebs cycle, the acetyl group formed during the breakdown of pyruvic acid plays the role of the incoming molecule, and the four-carbon oxaloacetic acid molecule plays the role of the helper molecule. During the first chemical reaction of the cycle, these two molecules combine to form six-carbon molecules of citric acid (the cycle owes one of its names to this acid). Then eight chemical reactions take place, in which first energy-carrier molecules and carbon dioxide are formed, and then a new oxaloacetic acid molecule. To process the energy stored in one glucose molecule, the Krebs cycle must be completed twice. The net profit is equal to two ATP molecules, four carbon dioxide molecules, and ten other energy-carrying molecules. Carbon dioxide eventually diffuses out of the mitochondria and is released during exhalation.

The Krebs cycle is fundamentally important for life, not only because it generates energy. In addition to glucose, many other molecules that also form pyruvic acid can enter into it. For example, when you are on a diet, the body does not have enough of the glucose you consume to maintain metabolism, so lipids (fats) enter the Krebs cycle, after preliminary splitting. That is why you are losing weight. In addition, molecules can leave the Krebs cycle to take part in the construction of new proteins, carbohydrates, and lipids. Thus, the Krebs cycle can take energy stored in various forms in many molecules and produce a variety of molecules as output.

From an energetic point of view, the net result of the Krebs cycle is to complete the extraction of energy stored in the chemical bonds of glucose, transfer a small part of this energy to ATP molecules, and store the rest of the energy in other energy-carrying molecules. Speaking about the energy of chemical bonds, we must not forget that in order to separate the connected atoms, it is necessary to do work. During the final stage of respiration, this remaining energy is released from the carrier molecules and is stored in ATP.

Molecules that store energy move within the mitochondria until they collide with specialized proteins embedded in the inner membranes of the mitochondria. These proteins take electrons from energy carriers and begin to pass them along a chain of molecules - like a chain of people passing buckets of water on a fire - extracting the energy stored in chemical bonds. The energy extracted at each stage is stored in the form of ATP. In the final step, electrons combine with oxygen atoms, which then combine with hydrogen ions (protons) to form water. At least 32 ATP molecules are formed in the electron transport chain - 90% of the energy stored in the original glucose molecule.

The transformation of energy in the Krebs cycle involves a rather complex process of chemiosmotic conjugation. This term indicates that along with chemical reactions, osmosis is involved in the release of energy - the slow seepage of solutions through organic partitions. In fact, the electrons from the energy carriers that are the product of the Krebs cycle are transferred along the transport chain and enter the proteins immersed in the membrane that separates the inner and outer compartments (compartments) of the mitochondria. The energy of the electrons is used to move hydrogen ions (protons) into the outer compartment, which serves as an "energy store" - like a reservoir formed in front of a dam. When protons flow across the membrane, energy is used to form ATP, similar to how water in front of a dam is used to produce electricity when it falls on a generator. Finally, in the inner compartment of the mitochondria, hydrogen ions combine with oxygen molecules to form water, one of the end products of metabolism.

Deviation 7. *The surprising common property of all cancer cells seems to be only one thing - the replacement of the three-step process of cellular respiration with the more ancient and primitive glycolysis. Back in 1926, Otto Warburg, investigating the formation of lactic acid in healthy and malignant (tumor) cells found that cancer cells break down glucose into lactic acid much more easily and quickly than normal cells do. According to Warburg, tumor tissue produces lactic acid at a rate eight (!) times faster than a working muscle. The production of lactate at this rate fully provides the tumor tissue with energy (although there are only two ATP molecules for two lactate molecules). Based on these data, Warburg suggested the existence of the so-called "cancer exchange." He believed that a defect in mitochondria is formed in cancer cells, which leads to irreversible disturbances in the aerobic stage of energy metabolism and subsequent dependence on glycolytic metabolism. In this case, glycolysis compensates for the energy deficiency of the damaged respiration. He showed that cancer cells continue to use glycolysis for energy* *even when there is sufficient oxygen in the tissues. This phenomenon is called the Warburg effect. What is the reason for this choice of tumor cells?*

What are the possible benefits of glycolysis as an energy source? Consider this question on the example of unicellular organisms. Unicellular structures consist of only one cell, but this cell is essentially a whole organism leading an independent existence. Single-celled organisms are well adapted to the environment in which they grow and reproduce. The main evolutionary pressure on single-celled organisms to reproduce is the availability of nutrients.

Therefore, the metabolism of unicellular organisms developed in such a way that the reserves of nutrients and free energy were directed, first, to building the structures necessary for the emergence of a new cell. Most single-celled organisms reproduce using the energy of glycolysis, even in the presence of sufficient oxygen. Therefore, despite the low efficiency (two ATP molecules versus 36), glycolysis can provide enough energy for cell proliferation.

With a deficiency of oxygen, the final electron acceptor in the redox chain of mitochondria, there is a pronounced hyperreduction of all components of the terminal oxidation link. The transport of electrons along the respiratory chain and the process of formation of macroenergy phosphates associated with it are stopped. We know that under conditions of normoxia, the NAD link of the mitochondrial respiratory chain accepts reducing equivalents from various sources:

1. From substrates of the Krebs cycle with the participation of specific dehydrogenases;
2. Hydroxy acyl-CoA dehydrogenases supply hydrogen ions to the NAD-link during the oxidation of fatty acids;
3. A complex system of pyruvate dehydrogenase, splitting off hydrogen ions in oxidative decarboxylation reactions, transfers them to the NAD link of the redox chain;
4. Extramitochondrial NAD-H, formed in the central reaction of glycolytic oxidoreduction, also donates its protons to the mitochondrial respiratory chain.

A powerful flow of reducing equivalents under conditions of oxygen deficiency is not realized due to hyper reduction of the NAD-dependent region of the respiratory chain. At the same time, the main energy system of the cell is switched off from functioning, and ATP production is sharply reduced.

Under anaerobic conditions, the cell seeks to make up for the energy deficit by activating glycolysis. Despite the fact that almost 20 times less ATP is produced during anaerobic glycolysis than during the complete combustion of glucose in the Krebs cycle, the potential rate of the process can mainly provide the energy consumption of the body. However, for the implementation of glycolytic reactions, a constant influx of the oxidized form of NAD (NAD +) is required, which, under normoxia, is provided by the operation of specific shuttle mechanisms. Glycolytic NADH penetrates mitochondrial membranes through the functioning of α-glycerophosphate, β-hydroxybutyrate, and other mechanisms of transfer of reducing equivalents. Oxybutyrate and glycerophosphate shunts are the main competitors of the lactate dehydrogenase mechanism for the oxidation of glycolytic NADH, whose activity at normal oxygen concentration in the cell is suppressed by the more active mechanisms mentioned above.

Thus, if the electron transport function of the redox chain is impaired and its NAD link is hyper-reduced, the cell is forced to find other ways of reoxidizing cytoplasmic NAD-H. Under conditions of acute hypoxia, the end product of glycolysis, pyruvate, does not undergo decarboxylation and is not involved in the Krebs cycle, but, taking reductive equivalents from cytoplasmic NAD-H, turns into lactate with the release of new portions of the oxidized form of NAD. Glycolysis includes chemical rearrangements of the following type:

- splitting of the six-carbon skeleton of glucose into two three-carbon pyruvates;
- phosphorylation of ADP to ATP, carried out by abstraction of phosphate from compounds with a high phosphate transfer potential formed during glycolysis (thus, ATP during glycolysis is formed due to substrate phosphorylation, in contrast to the oxidative phosphorylation of the respiratory chain, where ATP is formed due to the transfer of electrons and protons along the carrier chain);
- transfer of the H^+ ion to NAD^+ with the formation of reduced NADH.

The overall equation for glycolysis is:

$$\text{Glucose} + NAD^+ + 2ADP + 2Pi \rightarrow$$
$$2\ \text{pyruvates} + NADH + 2H^+ + 2ATP + 2H_2O$$

With prolonged and severe hypoxia, activation of the lactate dehydrogenase mechanism of NAD supply for glycolysis ultimately leads to the depletion of glycogen stores and tissue acidosis due to the accumulation of acidic metabolic products (lactate, pyruvate, oxybutyrate, glycerophosphate, etc.). Excessive concentrations of the final substrate of anaerobic glycolysis lactate inhibit the last reaction of the glycolytic cycle.

The regeneration of NAD stops, namely, the deficiency of the pyridine nucleotide stops glycolysis and anaerobic ATP production. Cellular acidosis contributes to the disruption of membrane permeability, up to the destruction of lysosomes. Autolytic enzymes enter the cytoplasm. The process of autolysis of cells develops, accompanied by damage to tissues and organs. Irreversible changes are formed in the body.

One of the recognized hypotheses for the regulation of local blood flow is, at least partially, the regulation of oxygen deficiency. Why do vessels begin to react even to a slight decrease in the level of oxygenation in the environment? Why is oxygen so important for the functioning of living systems?

Many hypotheses have been put forward to explain the mechanism of oxidative phosphorylation. The chemiosmotic theory proposed by Mitchell in 1961 is currently generally accepted (Figure 9).

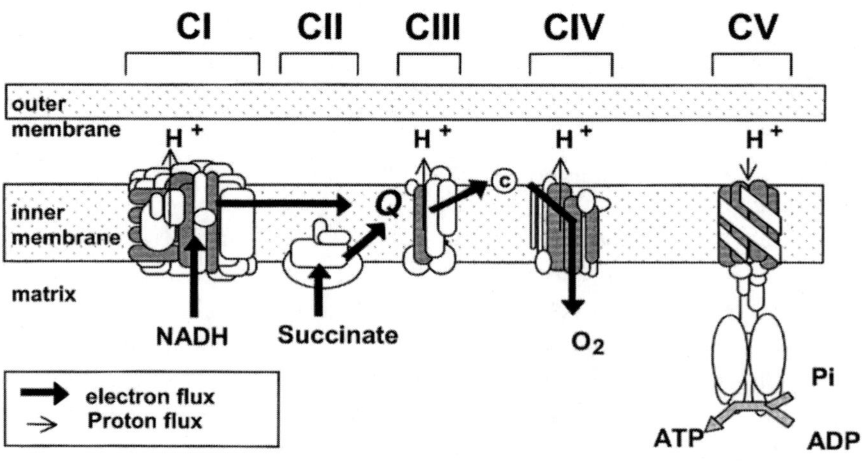

Figure 9. Scheme of coupling of respiration and phosphorylation according to Mitchell 's chemiosmotic theory. See explanations in the text.

1. This process takes place on the inner membrane of mitochondria, where the respiratory chain of enzymes is located.
2. The inner membrane is impermeable to protons (and most cations). This property makes it possible for charged particles to be distributed unevenly on both sides of the membrane. The motion of protons and electrons has a strictly defined direction.
3. Carrier enzymes of the respiratory chain are arranged in a zigzag pattern in the membrane. They are able not only to accept atomic hydrogen from oxidized substrates, but also to transport it in the transverse direction through the membrane.

Reaching the opposite (outer) layer of the membrane, the carrier releases protons into the water space outside it, and electrons, with the participation of additional carriers, are sent back to the inner layer of the membrane. Then they transferred to the next enzyme of the respiratory chain. To restore enzymes, in addition to electrons, protons are needed, which come from the internal space due to the forced dissociation of water. In total, during the transfer of a pair of electrons along the respiratory chain, three pairs of protons are pushed into the intermembrane space.

Thus, protons are transported from the inner layer of the membrane from the side of the matrix to the outer layer from the side of the intermembrane space, and electrons are transferred along the enzyme chain, reaching the final electron acceptor, oxygen:

$$2e^- + \frac{1}{2} O_2 + H_2O = 2OH^- \quad (9)$$

Because of this redistribution of electrical charges, the inner membrane on the side of the matrix becomes negatively charged and alkaline (an excess of OH- ions accumulates in it). From the side of the intermembrane space, it is acidified and becomes positively charged (due to the transport of protons). An electrochemical proton gradient appears, in the form of energy concentrated on a closed membrane. The electrochemical potential is denoted ΔμH+ and consists of electric potential (ΔΨ is the difference in electric potentials) and osmotic potential (ΔpH is the difference in proton concentrations):

$$\Delta\mu H+ = \Delta\Psi + \Delta pH \quad (10)$$

The main component of this value (4/5) is the electric potential. Due to the difference in concentration and electric potential, a force acts on the protons located in the outer space, tending to transfer them through the membrane into the inner space.

The return of protons to the matrix is carried out using the enzyme adenosine triphosphatase (ATPase or ATP synthase). This enzyme is embedded in the inner membrane. The resulting changes in the membrane (electrochemical potential) are transferred to ATP synthase, which activates and catalyzes the synthesis of ATP.

ATPase is an integral protein consisting of two types of subunits: F0 - consists of four polypeptide chains that pass through the entire inner membrane and form a channel for protons; F1 - mushroom-shaped catalytic subunit located on the inner membrane from the side of the matrix, which, in fact, carries out the reaction:

$$ATP + H_2O = ADP + H_3PO_4 \quad (11)$$

The current of protons creates an electric field in the catalytic subunit, which shifts the reaction towards ATP synthesis. In the matrix, protons combine with hydroxide ions. Water is formed - the end product of oxidative phosphorylation. The membrane is discharged, and the energy of the electrochemical potential is converted into the energy of macroergic bonds of ATP. Under the conditions of the organism, about 60% of the energy of the electrochemical potential is accumulated in the macroergic bonds of ATP, the rest of it is dissipated in the form of heat, due to which the body temperature is maintained. It should be noted that the proton gradient on biomembranes can be used not only for the synthesis of ATP, but also for other purposes: for transport of nucleoside di- and triphosphates through membranes, for maintaining osmotic pressure, for transport of substances through membranes against a concentration gradient, and, as indicated above, for heat production.

Thus, oxidative phosphorylation is the synthesis of ATP from ADP and inorganic phosphate due to the energy of the electrochemical potential.

The role of oxygen in life on Earth is decisive, and it is difficult to overestimate its importance. However, it was not always so. The exact composition of the Earth's primary atmosphere is currently unknown, however, as a rule, scientists believe that it was formed because of degassing of the mantle and was of a restorative nature. It was obviously based on carbon dioxide, hydrogen sulfide, ammonia, and methane. This is evidenced by:

- Existence of non-oxidized deposits on the earth's surface (for example, river pebbles from oxygen-labile pyrite);
- No known significant sources of oxygen and other oxidizing agents;
- Study of potential sources of the primary atmosphere (volcanic gases, composition of other celestial bodies).

Oxygen catastrophe (or oxygen revolution) - a global change in the composition of the Earth's atmosphere, occurred at the very beginning of the Proterozoic during the Siderian period about 2.45 billion years ago. The result of the oxygen catastrophe was the appearance of free oxygen in the composition of the atmosphere and a change in the general character of the atmosphere from reducing to oxidizing. In general, the biological properties of molecular oxygen are at least twofold. This happens in nature, for example, the famous nitric oxide. The molecule is a two-faced Janus. So oxygen, on the one hand, is a powerful oxidizing agent, with which you can get a lot of useful energy, and at the same time a strong poison that freely passes through cell membranes and activates the reoxidation process (Sessions et al. 2009).

All living systems of organisms that deal with oxygen must have special enzyme systems in their arsenal that can minimize its toxic effects. Those who do not have such enzyme systems are doomed to be strict anaerobes, surviving only in an oxygen-free environment. On modern Earth, these are some bacteria and archaea.

Almost all oxygen on Earth is of biogenic origin, that is, it is released by living beings (we are talking about free oxygen and not about oxygen atoms that make up other molecules). The main source of O_2 is oxygen photosynthesis; there are simply no other known reactions capable of producing it in comparable amounts. From the school biology course, we know that photosynthesis is the synthesis of glucose $C_6H_{12}O_6$ from carbon dioxide and water, which occurs with the help of light energy. The main "actor" here is carbon dioxide, which is restored by water; oxygen in this reaction is nothing but a by-product, a waste. Not everyone knows that photosynthesis may not lead to the release of oxygen if some other substance is used as a reducing agent instead of water - for example, hydrogen sulfide H_2S, free hydrogen H_2, or some iron compounds; such photosynthesis is called anoxic.

No one knows for sure, but, almost certainly, oxygen-free photosynthesis appeared much earlier than oxygen. Therefore, in the first billion(s) years of the existence of life on Earth (although photosynthesis was going on, there was no saturation of the Earth's atmosphere with oxygen. The oxygen content in the atmosphere at that time was a maximum of 0.001% of the modern one. In fact, for a temporary organism, this is a hard anoxia.

Everything changed when blue-green algae, or cyanobacteria (a typical representative is oscillatoria), entered the scene. Subsequently, they became the ancestors of plastids, photosynthetic organelles of eukaryotic cells. Cyanobacteria are a very ancient evolutionary branch. By the standards of earthly history, they are surprisingly unchanged. For example, the blue-green Alga Oscillatoria (Oscillatoria), which is widespread in modern reservoirs, has fossil relatives that lived 800 million years ago.

At first, cyanobacteria were few in number, since the oxygen photosynthesis they mastered did not provide serious advantages over the oxygen-free photosynthesis that other groups of microbes possessed. But the chemical environment of these microbes gradually changed. The moment has come when the "raw materials" for oxygen-free photosynthesis simply ceased to be enough. Then the hour of cyanobacteria struck.

Oxygen photosynthesis has one undoubted advantage - a completely unlimited supply of the initial reducing agent (water) and one big drawback - the high toxicity of the by-product (oxygen). Not surprisingly, this type of exchange was not "popular" at first. But with the slightest shortage of other substrates, except for water, the owners of oxygen photosynthesis should immediately receive a competitive advantage, which happened. This was followed by an epoch about a billion years long, during which the appearance of the Earth was determined primarily by cyanobacteria. Recently, it has even been proposed to informally name it "cyanozoic" after them (Lyons et al. 2014).

It was cyanobacteria that started the oxygen revolution 2.4 billion years ago or, if you like, the oxygen catastrophe, or the Great Oxidation Event (GOE). Strictly speaking, this event was neither instantaneous nor absolutely unique (Lyons et al. 2014) .

Therefore, 2.4 billion years ago something new happened. For a short time by the standards of earth's history (a few tens of millions of years), the concentration of oxygen in the atmosphere increased by about a thousand times and remained at this level; it never sank back to its former insignificant values. The biosphere irreversibly became oxygenated.

For the vast majority of ancient prokaryotes, this level of oxygen was deadly. Therefore, the first result of the oxygen revolution was mass extinction. Mostly those who managed to create oxygen-protecting enzymes survived, and sometimes thick cell walls to boot (including cyanobacteria themselves had to do this). There is reason to believe that in the first 100-200 million years of the "new oxygen world," oxygen was only poison for living organisms and nothing more. Then the situation changed. The biota's response to the oxygen challenge was the appearance of bacteria, which included oxygen in the chain of reactions decomposing glucose and thus began to use it for energy.

It immediately turned out that the oxygen oxidation of glucose (respiration) in terms of energy is much more efficient than anoxic (fermentation). It provides several times more free energy per molecule of glucose than any arbitrarily complicated version of oxygen-free metabolism. At the same time, the initial stages of glucose breakdown among users of respiration and fermentation remained common: oxygen oxidation served as a superstructure over the already existing ancient biochemical mechanism, which in itself did not need oxygen.

A group of microbes that have mastered the risky but efficient way of obtaining energy with the help of oxygen is called proteobacteria. According to the now generally accepted theory, it was from them that the respiratory organelles of eukaryotic cells - mitochondria - originated.

According to genetic data, the closest modern relative of mitochondria is the purple helical alpha-proteobacterium *Rhodospirillum rubrum* (Esser et al. 2004). *Rhodospirillum* has both respiration, fermentation, and anoxic photosynthesis, in which hydrogen sulfide is used instead of water, and can switch between these three types of exchange depending on external conditions. Undoubtedly, such a symbiont - that is, in this case, an internal cohabitant - was very useful to the ancestor of eukaryotes.

Glycolysis and oxidative phosphorylation, despite the seeming difference in terms of oxygen dependence, represent a dual mechanism for supplying the body with energy. Glycolysis supplies pyruvate for the Krebs cycle. At the same time, to maintain the cycle of glycolysis, a constant influx of the oxidized form of NAD (NAD^+) is required, which, under normoxia, is provided by the operation of specific shuttle mechanisms.

Let us sum up the intermediate results of this section. The structure of mitochondrial membranes is very complex, and this complexity is justified by their high degree of importance for the respiration process. The outer membrane of mitochondria is smooth, while the inner membrane is repeatedly folded. These folds (or cristae) make it possible to increase the working area of the membrane necessary to accommodate the entire complex of respiratory proteins there. First, the carbon atoms of carbohydrates, fatty acids and amino acids are oxidized to CO_2 (glycolysis, Krebs cycle, β-oxidation of fatty acids), and the electrons thus obtained are used to form NADP. Next, NADP is oxidized by molecular oxygen to form water. The NADP-oxidase reaction is accompanied by the release of a very large amount of free energy (about 1.1 eV during the transfer of one electron from NADH to oxygen), which can be stored by the respiratory chain in the form of a transmembrane difference in the electrochemical potentials of H^+ ions, i.e. protons.

The work of respiratory proteins-enzymes is similar to the work of pumps: passing electrons to each other, they pump protons into the intermembrane space. As a result, the inner membrane of the mitochondria is charged like a capacitor. Potentials are created: electric (positive charges are outside the mitochondrial membrane, negative charges are inside the organelle) and chemical (there is a difference in proton concentrations: there are fewer of them inside the mitochondria, more outside). It is known that the electric potential on the mitochondrial membrane, which serves as a good dielectric, reaches 200 mV at a membrane thickness of only 10 nm. For comparison: the action potential on the membranes of nerve cells during signal transmission reaches only 30 mV, and the membrane potential of smooth muscle cells reaches 40-50 mV.

Having accumulated in the intermembrane space, protons, like an electric current, rush back to the mitochondria - there their concentration is lower. However, they can only pass through special ATP synthase channels built into the inner membrane: the proton channel (rotor) of this enzyme is fixed in the membrane, and the catalytic complex protrudes into the mitochondria, into the matrix. The flow of protons spins the rotor, like a river spins a water mill. As a result, the molecular rotor rotates at an incredible speed - 300 revolutions per second! This rotation leads to the formation of a high-energy molecule - ATP. It is estimated that about 40 kg of ATP is synthesized and consumed per day in an adult human body, while the life of each molecule is very short.

The electrical polarization of the inner mitochondrial membrane largely determines the electrochemical potential of hydrogen ions, thus being a significant factor in the conversion of the oxidation energy of respiratory substrates and its storage in the form of newly synthesized ATP. However, the electrical potential gradient across the mitochondrial inner membrane ($\Delta\Psi m$) performs a number of functions unrelated to energy production. Even under conditions of severe hypoxia, which excludes the formation of ATP in mitochondria due to oxidative phosphorylation, mitochondria retain their $\Delta\Psi m$ due to the hydrolysis of cellular ATP, which indicates the exceptional value of $\Delta\Psi m$ for non-energetic functions of mitochondria. Among these functions, it is very important to ensure the transport of metal cations and proteins carrying positively charged amino acid sequences into mitochondria, which are necessary for maintaining the mitochondrial structure and metabolism. $\Delta\Psi m$ is a powerful regulator of the generation of reactive oxygen species by mitochondria, which perform important physiological and pathophysiological functions. In addition, finally, $\Delta\Psi m$ is a critical element in the mechanism for recycling faulty mitochondria, the so-called mitochondrial quality control machine. Violation of this mechanism leads to an increase in the heterogeneity of the mitochondrial population in the cell, and the degree of such heterogeneity can be considered as an indicator of the cellular pathological phenotype.

What happens to the cell when glycolysis is blocked? Let's start with nerve cells, which are considered the most sensitive to any energy metabolism disorder.

There is evidence that, for example, in young granular neurons of the cerebellum, inhibition of glycolysis by replacing glucose with 2-deoxy-D-glucose causes a slowly developing mitochondrial depolarization (MD) that is resistant to removal of external Ca^{2+} and blockade of glutamate-activated channels. Based on these data, it was concluded that the observed MD is not a consequence of the release of endogenous glutamate from neurons or glial cells.

MD caused by blockade of glycolysis, in turn, is inhibited by oligomycin and was prevented by the addition of pyruvate to a glucose-free medium. Therefore, MD is caused by an ADP-dependent increase in the flow of protons through mitochondrial ATP synthase against the background of weakened respiration.

Thus, the functioning of the glycolytic cycle and respiration are coupled and coordinated.

Oxygen Sensors in Smooth Muscle Cells

How do VSMCs "know" that the oxygen content in the environment has changed, and they need to contract or relax to maintain normal blood supply to organs and tissues? Why do some vessels contract in response to a decrease in oxygenation, while others relax?

The answer to the first question most often sounds like this - there is a certain structure called an oxygen sensor, which can detect changes in pO_2 and further transmit information to the contractile apparatus of cells. The identification of all elements of such a system of control and regulation is an important task for physiologists.

The answer to the second question is that everything depends on the localization. It is generally accepted that the vessels of the systemic circulation respond to hypoxia by relaxing and increasing blood flow to compensate for the lack of oxygen. In contrast, pulmonary vessels contract in response to a decrease in oxygenation is necessary to maintain a normal ventilation-perfusion relationship and redistribute blood flow from poorly ventilated to well-ventilated areas of the lungs. Everything is in the interest of the body. These are our reasonable bodies!

Thus far, everything seems to be logical and understandable. However, why, then, in the event of a breakdown of the body (disease), can we not correctly identify a poorly functioning element in the system of regulation and effectively influence it with one or another pharmacological agent? It turns out that we have a well-drawn, logically justified scheme, but it is purely phenomenological. Pharmacological interventions such as "shooting on the squares" are ineffective. It is necessary to identify the pharmacological target as accurately as possible. In this case, this is the structure responsible for receiving and processing the corresponding signal, i.e., oxygen sensor.

Another problem is that the same vessel may respond differently to hypoxia under different conditions. For instance, the portal vein of the rat, if previously incubated in a hypoxic environment, will contract in response to hypoxic exposure, although before that it always relaxed. If the hypoxic effect continues for a sufficiently long time (up to 20 minutes), then the level of tonic tension of the same portal vein begins to slowly but significantly increase.

In general, hypoxic contraction is quite easily explained based on the concepts of Mitchell's chemo-osmotic hypothesis. Any delay in the transport of electrons along the respiratory chain must be accompanied by the loss of Ca^{2+} ions by mitochondria and the appearance of their excess in the cell myoplasm.

The situation with the coronary arteries is especially indicative. Oxygen tension is a major regulator of blood flow in coronary circulation. Everyone knows what angina pectoris is and how unpleasant and deadly it is when the coronary arteries contract excessively.

More than 40 years ago, evidence has been found that SM cells in large epicardial coronary arteries react to hypoxia or anoxia by contraction. The data obtained clearly indicate that hypoxia augments the contractile responses to different agonists in a number of blood vessels (Borda et al. 1980; Rubanyi & Paul, 1985). Similar results were also obtained in experiments on isolated rat hearts (Karmazyn et al. 1984).

The contraction of coronary SM under hypoxia is, indeed, a surprising discovery, since the physiology of blood circulation firmly confirms the view that vascular SM are relaxed under hypoxia (lung vessels are the only exception). The suggestion that the contraction of coronary arteries as a result of O_2 deficit is an artifact that only occurs in isolated vascular preparations was quashed when, in our laboratory it was shown (Soloviev, Braquet, 1992) that inhalation of hypoxic gas mixture (8% O_2 - 92% N_2 mixture) by anesthetized dogs leads to a biphasic dilation-constriction response in the coronary vessels. Blood flow increased from 60.2 ± 7.9 to 72.0 ± 10.0 ml/ min ($P > 0.05$) followed by a significant reduction, over 10 min, to 37.6 ± 10.0 ml/min ($P < 0.01$).

Rubanyi and Paul studied the relationship between pO_2 and vascular tone in isolated annulus of the porcine left descending coronary artery (Rubanyi & Paul, 1985). The porcine left descending coronary artery, isometrically mounted and equilibrated in Krebs bicarbonate solution (37°C, pH 7.4, gassed with 95% oxygen + 5% carbon dioxide), demonstrated spontaneous basal tone. Decreasing pO_2 in the bath by 40%, 20%, and 12% caused a sustained increase in basal smooth muscle tension activated by 40 mM potassium chloride. A further decrease in pO_2 almost to zero (anoxia) led to relaxation to the initial level. Cyclooxygenase inhibitors indomethacin, aspirin and meclofenamate reduced vascular tone and completely prevented coronary vasoconstriction caused by a decrease in pO_2 in the bath to 12% or 40 %, but did not affect anoxic vasorelaxation.

According to these authors, the data indicate the existence of two different mechanisms of the regulation of vascular tone, sensitive to oxygen, in the coronary arteries of pigs. One of them is activated at relatively high pO_2 values (10-40%), and the vasoconstriction caused by this mechanism is mediated by the action of vasoactive prostaglandins. The other works at low values of pO_2 (close to zero), and the inhibition of mechanical activity by this mechanism may be due to the limitation of the oxidative energy exchange.

Now it is well documented that the mechanical tension of VSM is very sensitive to environmental oxygen tension (pO_2), and muscle cells in the vascular wall depend on oxygen supply for maintenance of their isometric force. The effect of low pO_2 (hypoxia) on VSM is quite well investigated, but, nevertheless, there is little data about the cellular mechanisms of oxygen lack on membrane and cytosolic structures in VSM.

The most urgent problem now is the identification of the so-called 'oxygen sensors' in VSM, i.e., cellular structures directly involved in the reception of pO_2 changes and realization of corresponding contractile response. It has been shown that low pO_2 can alter myofilament responsiveness to Ca^{2+} and this effect may be related to cAMP-dependent phosphorylation of myosin light chain kinase, its inactivation and subsequent uncoupling between Ca^{2+} and contractile machinery in VSM (Soloviev & Basilyuk, 1993). However, alternative sensor mechanisms by which low pO_2 may affect VSM tonic tension cannot be excluded. It should be remembered that it is the plasma membrane with ion channels built into it that first encounters the effect of the hypoxic factor.

There are some experimental data that the effects of hypoxia on contractile activity in VSM are mediated via plasma membrane mechanisms, particularly its permeability to some cations. Results obtained in many studies Soloviev, Bazilyuk (1981); Greenidge and Keatinge (1983) allow to suggest that the VSM plasma membranes may be involved in the response to hypoxia primarily, and that the mechanisms of contractile machinery energy supply take not so great part in this process (Hellstrand et al. 1977; Sigurdsson et al. 1981; Soloviev et al. 1996).

Another point of view is that the inhibition or activation of cellular function by an acute decrease in pO_2 may be the consequence of two different processes: 1) a sensor (which one?) that monitors the decrease in pO_2, and 2) systems that mediate the contractile response to hypoxia. Using the model of aortic smooth muscle contracted by norepinephrine during relaxations induced by a decrease in pO_2 it was shown that the phosphorylation potential, i.e. the kinetic energy required for ATP hydrolysis, was reduced to 30% of control at the onset of relaxation and gradually fell as the muscle relaxed. The intracellular concentration of free inorganic phosphate ([Pi]) increased by about 0.6 mM during the transients that followed the rapid decrease in pO_2. Relaxations to 80% of maximal force were faster under conditions of increased [Pi] than in control rings, and they occurred at a higher phosphocreatine concentration and phosphocreatine to free creatine ratio, but at the same phosphorylation potential. The authors suggest that this supports the role of the cytochrome aa3 O_2 sensor in the mechanism of relaxations induced by decreased pO_2, and suggests an increase in [Pi] and a decrease in kinetic energy in the transduction mechanism directed at the rate-limiting reactions that control force (Katayama et al 1994).

Among the other potential 'candidates' for an oxygen sensor in VSM plasma membrane, a special role is attributed to the Ca^{2+} channels. This conclusion is based on several lines of evidence. Firstly, for a long time, Ca^{2+} was found to play a decisive role in excitation-contraction coupling in VSM. Secondly, it is a fact that activation of slow (L-type) Ca^{2+} channels in VSM cells requires ATP, and phosphorylation and/or energy-requiring steps (Ohya & Sperelakis, 1989) may exert this effect. Finally, approximately 15% of suprabasal oxygen consumption in VSM is not dependent on tension and has been loosely ascribed to such 'activation processes' such as Ca^{2+} translocation (Paul, Hellstrand and Krisanda, 1984).

Thus, one may envisage a close interrelationship between Ca^{2+} passive transport in vascular SM cells and pO_2 in the ambient medium. It is likely that hypoxia may affect K^+ permeability in SM cells as well. Intracellular recordings of membrane potential demonstrated that vasodilation in arteries under oxygen deficiency can be attributed to a membrane hyperpolarization which, in turn, due to an increase in passive K^+ permeability of plasma membranes (Siegel & Grote, 1988).

For a long period, the inhibition of vascular SM contractility by low pO_2 (hypoxia) was considered primarily the result of decrease of oxidative phosphorylation rate and related restriction of contractile machinery energy supply. The critical level of pO_2 in the cell, when the lack of oxygen begins to limit the transport of electrons along the respiratory chain, is about 1-2 mm Hg. Simple calculations show that an intracellular pO_2 value close to the critical mitochondrial level is achieved at pO_2 in the organ bath perfusate of the order of 10–15 mm Hg. Thus, at pO_2 over 15–20 mm Hg in the myoplasm of cells, oxygen should be sufficient for the functioning of mitochondria and ensuring oxidative metabolism. The decrease in the tonic tension and contractile activity of SMCs observed by us with a decrease in pO_2 only to 100 mm Hg can hardly be associated with the limitation of oxidative phosphorylation processes under this condition.

The critical oxygen pressure is defined as the partial oxygen pressure, pO_2, below which aerobic catabolism (respiration or oxygen consumption) declines significantly. Oxygen pressure for half-maximum respiration, p50, in isolated mitochondria at state 4 was 0.025 kPa (0.2 Torr; 0.3 μM O_2), whereas p50 in endothelial cells was 0.06-0.08 kPa (0.5 Torr).

Our microelectrode polarographic studies using the portal vein of a cat (wall thickness of about 250–300 μm) under *in vitro* conditions showed that with a decrease in the degree of oxygenation of the buffer solution, pO_2 drops especially sharply in the so-called non-stirred layer directly at the surface of the vascular preparation. Its thickness is about 100 μm and the pO_2 level in it falls by 70 mm Hg lower than in the buffer solution at a distance of 5 mm from the surface of the vascular tissue. The experimental data in this case agreed quite well with the calculated ones. Thus, the measured experimental gradient between the surface of the vascular wall and the middle of the media turned out to be 15 mm Hg, and the calculated one was from 27 to 33 mm Hg.

Theoretical calculation of pO_2 levels in the vascular wall during hypoxia turned out to be impossible. Even at pO_2 in the buffer solution equal to 55 mm Hg, the pO_2 value in the tissue at a depth of 50 μm acquired negative values. In the experiment, with a decrease in pO_2 from 145 to 22 mmHg pO_2 in the middle of the media does not fall below 14 mm Hg, which is much higher than the critical level for mitochondria (Soloviev, 1987).

Thus, either the decrease in smooth muscle contractility during hypoxia is not directly related to the restriction of aerobic metabolism, or the critical level of mitochondria is much higher than expected.

Then, estimation of content and dynamics of consumption of ATP and creatine phosphate by smooth muscles of portal vein enabled to conclude that even at complete cessation of oxidative phosphorylation, the stock of high-energy phosphagenes in the VSM is great enough to maintain its contractility for at least 40 s (Hellstrand et al. 1977). At the same time, we have shown that both myogenic activity and developed force were significantly inhibited within the first seconds of hypoxic impact and these responses were started at bath pO_2, values greater than 75-105 mm Hg (Soloviev,1987).

An experiment provided by Namm and Zucker demonstrated that the ATP content in aortal SM cells begins to decrease at bath pO_2 equals to 13.65 mm Hg. At the same time the level of isometric tension developed by SM falls only up to pO2 97.5 mm Hg (Hellstrand et al. 1977; Namm & Zucker, 1973). According to Hellstrand et al. the ATP content in the portal vein falls by 30% only, even after 20 min anoxia in contrast to sharp decrease (by 75%) of intracellular PCr content. Later these data were completed by the experiments showing that with reduced pO_2 the tissue content of PCr decreased whereas ATP remained constant for mean of contractile activity $<$ 10% of control (Lövgren & Hellstrand, 1985).

The fact that the intracellular ATP content in VSM at hypoxia is high enough to provide the contractile process in smooth muscle cells we have confirmed in our experiments where initial (pre hypoxic) amplitude of isometric force developed by VSM at transmural electrical stimulation was almost completely restored at higher frequency and amplitude of electrical stimulation (Soloviev et al. 1996). The most likely is that hypoxia preferentially affects the membrane mechanism of excitation-contraction coupling in VSM cells but not force generation. Incidentally, this is consistent with the well-known idea that smooth muscle uses a lot of ATP during the tension phase, but very little during sustained contraction – the so-called "latch state," which may also be related to sensitization of smooth muscle contraction to Ca^{2+}. Strictly speaking and considering the fact that these data were obtained on the portal vein, this statement can be fully attributed only to smooth muscles with autorhythmic activity. But it is precisely they that are mainly responsible for the formation of basal tone!

Phosphocreatine (PCr) plays an important role in intracellular transfer of energy from mitochondria to myofibrils and other cellular energy-dependent components (McClellan et al. 1983). Energy of phosphagenes phosphate link is transferred from mitochondrial ATP on PCr, which diffuses into the myoplasm where local creatine phospho kinases transfer phosphate link from PCr to ADP with ATP formation.

It is obvious that ATP content is important in the regulation of the slow (L-type) Ca^{2+} channels in VSM and phosphorylation of the channel's protein might be involved in this regulation. In this case, metabolic intervention that lowers ATP or PCr content, such as metabolic poison or hypoxia may lead to rapid inactivation of Ca^{2+} channels and electromechanical uncoupling. If ATP, used for Ca^{2+} channel phosphorylation, is the product of PCr reactions, then the intracellular PCr content reflects the number of active (open) Ca^{2+} channels in VSM cell plasma membrane.

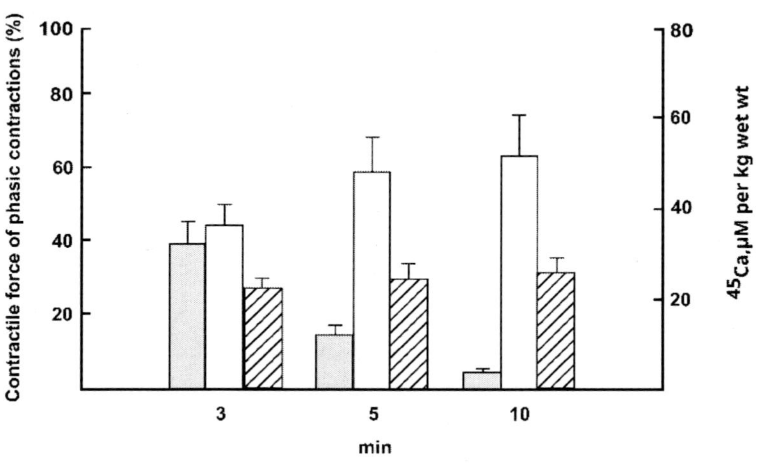

Figure 10. Uptake of ^{45}Ca in the isolated rat portal vein over a 3-, 5- and 10-min incubation period in normoxic (white columns) and hypoxic (black columns) solution containing ^{45}Ca. Related changes in contractile force (dashed columns) during hypoxia were expressed in the percentage of average amplitude of phasic contractions under normoxia.

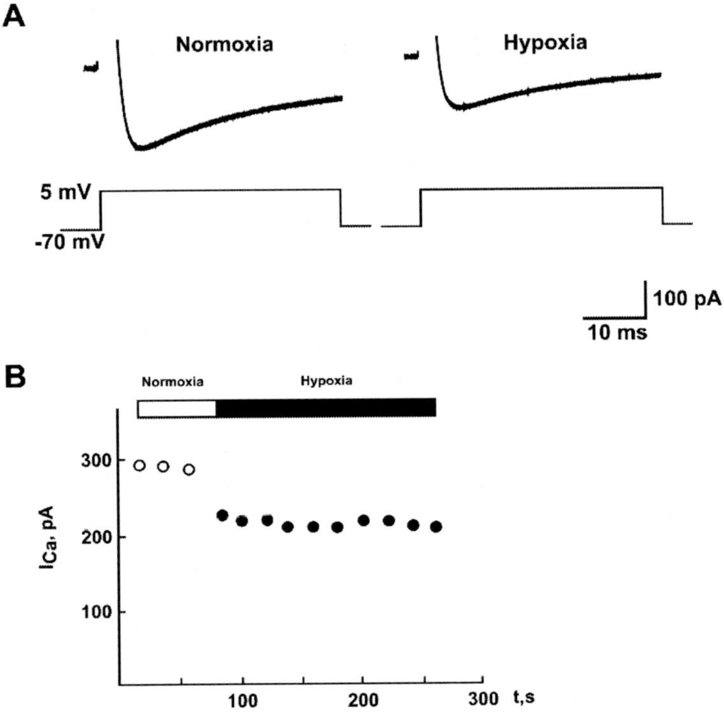

Figure 11. Effect of hypoxia (68 mm Hg) on whole cell calcium current (lCa) in a single cell from rat portal vein. (A) Current traces before and after 1 min hypoxic impact are shown. Holding potential was - 70 mV and test potential was +5 mV. (B) Time courses of the hypoxia effect on I_{Ca} are demonstrated.

The results of our experiments with simultaneous measurement of ^{45}Ca uptake and contractile activity in portal vein at normoxia and hypoxia are shown in Figure 10.

Decrease of bath pO_2, from 141 to 29 mm Hg caused gradual reduction in amplitude of phasic spontaneous contractions. Over 3, 5 and 10-min hypoxic impacts, the amplitude of phasic contractions fell to about 41 ± 3, 15 ± 3 and 5 ± 1% of control (pre hypoxic) value, respectively. At the same time, uptake of ^{45}Ca by smooth muscle cells falls by half. Namely, ^{45}Ca uptake by smooth muscle cells significantly decreased also from 3.6.0 ± 0.4 to 2.2 ± 0.2 µmol per kg wet weight ($P < 0.05$, $n = 6$) at the end of the third minute of hypoxic treatment.

Thus, the suppression of Ca^{2+} current and ^{45}Ca uptake by VSM cells at low pO_2 in our experiments may be a consequence of the inactivation of Ca^{2+} channels, which occurs for various reasons. First, it may be a disturbance in

Ca^{2+} channel phosphorylation. There is direct evidence of a decrease in Ca^{2+} transients in rat portal vein smooth muscle upon inhibition of oxidative metabolism (Swärd et al. 1993). The data obtained shows that hypoxic inhibition of spontaneous contractions in the rat portal vein may also be associated with the involvement of ATP-dependent K^{+}-channels (Lydrup et al. 1994).

Similar data on ^{45}Ca uptake under hypoxic conditions were obtained by Ebeigbe (1982) on the smooth muscles of the rabbit aorta. It is interesting that ^{45}Ca uptake during hypoxia decreased only if the smooth muscles were pre-activated by norepinephrine. If there was no such activation, ^{45}Ca uptake by the muscles increased. In our experiments, the smooth muscles of the rat aorta relaxed during hypoxia only after their preactivation by potassium chloride or electrical stimulation. If they were not preactivated, they either did not respond to hypoxia at all or the hypoxic relaxation was preceded by a transient contraction.

Then, we decided to provide our own experiments to investigate the effect of low pO_2 on transmembrane calcium currents in single enzymatically isolated vascular SM cells.

Figure 11 shows representative records of whole cell total Ca^{2+} current in enzymatically dispersed rat portal vein smooth muscle cells obtained using the patch clamp technique in the whole cell modification. Currents were registered when pO_2 in the bath was 141- and 68-mm Hg, respectively. Command pulses up to +5 mV with a duration of 40 ms were applied every 25 s to the cell clamped at a holding potential of -70 mV. The average peak value of Ca^{2+} current decreased during hypoxia from 284 ± 20 to 202 ± 14 pA ($P < 0.05$, $n = 7$). Similar results were obtained using isolated rat aortic cells (Figure 12) (holding potential -70 mV, command pulses +5 mV): the peak value of the current decreased from 202 ± 21 to 110 ± 11 pA ($P < 0\ .05$, $n = 6$). The influence of low pO_2 on calcium currents completely disappeared within 3-4 minutes after reoxygenation (Soloviev et al. 1996).

Thus, a decrease in the Ca^{2+} permeability of the SM plasma membrane is accompanied by a decrease in the of ^{45}Ca uptake and inward Ca^{2+} current, a disturbance of the generation of action potentials and phase contractions and, finally, to decrease in the isometric force of the SM developed under hypoxic conditions (Soloviev, et al, 1996).

Then, the effects of oxygen deficiency on Ca^{2+}-activated outward potassium currents (IKCa) in single cells from the portal vein were studied (Figure 13).

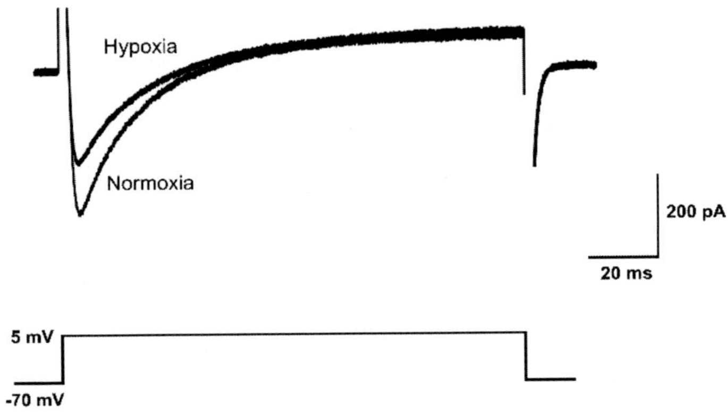

Figure 12. Two traces of I_{Ca} superimposed before and after 1 min application of hypoxic (70 mm Hg) bath solution to single smooth muscle cell from rat aorta. Holding potential was -70 mV and test potential was +5 mV.

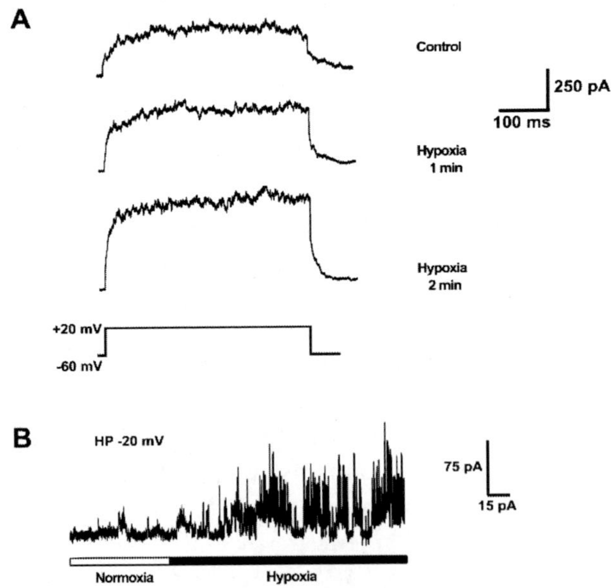

Figure 13. Effects of hypoxia (70 mm Hg) on (A) outward Ca^{2+}-activated potassium current (IK_{Ca}) and (B) spontaneous transient outward currents (STOCs) in single cells from rat portal vein. (A) Holding potential was - 60 mV and test potential was 20 mV. (B) Holding potential was - 20 mV. All recordings of membrane currents were carried out at room temperature (20-22°C).

The membrane depolarization to +20 mV from holding potential -60 mV evoked total IK_{Ca} with transient IKCat, sustained IKCas and oscillatory IKCao components. Lowering of bath pO2 from 141 to 70 mm Hg led to an increase of two components of IK_{Ca} preferentially, i.e., IKCat and IKCao. In the cells held at -20 mV, the discharges of spontaneous transient outward currents (STOCs) were usually seen. Hypoxia significantly enhanced the amplitude and frequency of STOCs, thus indirectly indicating the possible involvement of maxi K channels.

Thus, our results indicate that one of the most vulnerable links in the chain of coupling of excitation and contraction SM cells during hypoxia is the system of passive transmembrane Ca^{2+} transport. Inhibition of oxidative phosphorylation caused by a lack of oxygen is not a limiting factor for the energy supply of the contractile apparatus (at least in the initial stages of hypoxia), but even a slight decrease in the intracellular PCr content can lead to a decrease in the number of open Ca^{2+} channels as a result of impaired phosphorylation.

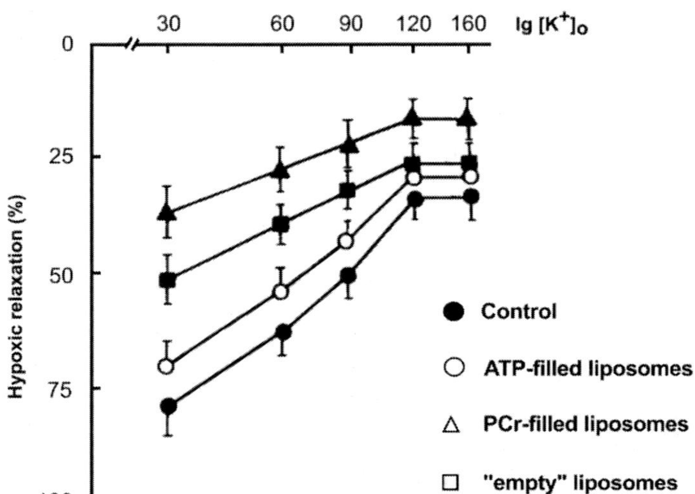

Figure 14. Effects of ATP - (open circles) and PCr-filled (triangles) liposomes on hypoxia-induced (29 mm Hg) relaxation of rat portal vein preactivated with different K^+ concentrations. Abscissa, $\log[K^+]_o$ in bath solution; ordinate, amplitude of hypoxic relaxation in percent to maximal amplitude of K^+-activated tonic component at normoxic condition (142 mm Hg).

Figure 14 illustrates the part of experiments in which ATP - and PCr-filled liposomes were used to make clear the role of high-energy phosphate depletion in hypoxic relaxation of VSM. Out of two substances, only PCr had a distinct antihypoxic effect. For instance, within the 5th minute of hypoxia the amplitude of portal vein phasic contractions decreased in the presence of PCr-filled liposomes by 40% as compared to 80% in liposome-free bath solution (not shown in Figure 14).

Another reason for the decrease in the permeability of SM cells for Ca^{2+} may be a transient increase in intracellular Ca^{2+}, which may be due to impaired ATP-dependent transport of Ca^{2+} outward and sequestration of intracellular Ca^{2+} during hypoxia. This can lead to activation of Ca^{2+}-dependent potassium channels of high conductivity and hyperpolarization of the membrane.

In parallel with us, our Spanish colleagues obtained similar data on the inhibitory effect of hypoxia on calcium currents in vascular SMCs (Franco-Obregon, Lopez-Barneo, 1996). They showed that oxygen tension acts as a major regulator of blood flow in coronary circulation. It turned out that hypoxia can cause vasodilation due to the activation of ATP-regulated K_{ATP} channels in the myocyte membrane, which leads to hyperpolarization and closure of voltage-dependent Ca^{2+} channels. However, there are other oxygen-sensitive mechanisms inherent in VSM, since hypoxia can relax vessels that have been previously contracted by high levels of extracellular K^+, which prevents the development of hyperpolarization after the opening of K^+ channels.

Later, the data were obtained that hypoxic exposure to about 20 mm Hg leads to relaxation of the endothelial-free rings of the coronary arteries of the pig, previously reduced by a high content of K^+ in the presence of glibenclamide (5 μM), a blocker of K_{ATP} channels. In enzymatically isolated human and porcine myocytes, low pO_2 tension reduced basal cytosolic $[Ca^{2+}]_i$ and transmembrane Ca^{2+} influx regardless of activation of K^+ channels. (Smani et al. 2002).

The high sensitivity of smooth muscles of resistance vessels to stretching underlies the phenomenon of myogenic autoregulation. In this regard, it was interesting to find out whether the level of oxygenation affects the implementation of this mechanism. Our studies have shown that rapid stretching of the portal vein SM leads to an increase in the amplitude of phase contractions without visible changes in their frequency. With a decrease in pO_2 to 30 mm Hg, the amplitude of phase contractions during stretching slightly increased only in 7 out of 29 experiments. In other cases, it did not change or even decreased. Similar data we obtained on extra-abdominal segments of the human umbilical vein, which are known to be devoid of sympathetic innervation (Bershtein, Gurevich, Soloviev, 1984).

Therefore, the level of environmental oxygenation can be an effective modulator of vascular tone, and the restriction of oxidative metabolism is not a necessary component of this regulatory mechanism.

In conclusion of this section, a few words about the portal vein as a model of resistance vessels. This very unique vein has a pronounced autorhythmic activity and even plays the role of the heart in the cyclostome fish - hagfish. Both morphologically and functionally, its smooth muscle cells resemble those of small resistance vessels. And, of course, it is much more convenient to work with it. In short, it has long been generally accepted that the experimental analogue of resistance vessels is the VSM of the rat portal vein, which has been thoroughly studied in this regard (Mellander and Johansson, 1968; Pegram, 1980; Gestrelius, Borgstrom, 1986).

The Special Role of Glycolysis in Smooth Muscle Cell Activity: How Do Cellular Oscillators Work?

Undoubtedly, the oscillatory nature of processes is an evolutionary invention of nature, and its functional role has several different aspects. First, fluctuations make it possible to separate processes in time, when several different reactions occur simultaneously in one cell compartment, organizing periods of high and low activity of individual metabolites. Secondly, the characteristics of oscillations, their amplitude and phase carry certain information and can play a regulatory role in the cascades of processes occurring at the level of a cell and a living organism. Finally, oscillatory (potentially or actually) systems serve as local elements of distributed active media capable of spatio-temporal self-organization, including the processes of morphogenesis.

All oscillations associated with stable limit cycles are called self-oscillations. In appearance, they are divided into quasi-harmonic (i.e., sinusoidal or close to them; for example, this is how the vessels of the human umbilical cord contract) and relaxation oscillations of an arbitrary structure (contractions of the rat portal vein). To start self-oscillations, an energy source and the presence of a feedback mechanism that regulates the flow of energy into the system depending on the phase of the oscillations are required.

The emergence of stable undamped oscillations is a fundamental property of nonlinear systems and the basis of the vital activity of living systems. Membrane potential fluctuations underlying autorhythmic activity may be the result of metabolic fluctuations, fluctuations in membrane permeability or fluctuations in the activity of the Na^+/ K^+ - pumps (Barajas-López, Chow, Den Hertog, Huizinga,1989).

Glycolysis, which is a typically oscillatory process, is a sequence of enzymatic reactions leading to the conversion of glucose into pyruvate with simultaneous formation of ATP. Under aerobic conditions, pyruvate penetrates into the mitochondria, where it is fully oxidized to CO_2 and H_2O. If oxygen delivery is limited, as may be the case in an actively contracting muscle, pyruvate is converted into lactate. Anaerobic glycolysis is a complex enzymatic process of the breakdown of glucose that occurs in the tissues of humans and animals without oxygen consumption. The end product of glycolysis is lactic acid. In the process of glycolysis, ATP is also formed, which is necessary to ensure the normal processes of electrogenesis and contractile activity.

Glycolysis is not only the main pathway for glucose utilization in cells, its uniqueness lies in the fact that it can occur not only in the absence of oxygen (anaerobic conditions - anaerobic glycolysis), but continues to function under conditions of normal oxygenation (aerobic conditions - aerobic glycolysis). Under anaerobic conditions, glycolysis is the only real energy supplying process in the animal body. It is thanks to glycolysis that human and animal bodies can perform a certain period of a number of physiological functions in conditions of oxygen deficiency. In cases where glycolysis occurs in the presence of oxygen, they speak of aerobic glycolysis.

It is well known that in resting skeletal muscle with normal oxygenation, the level of lactate formation is very low, on average 20-25 nmol / (min x gram of tissue) (Kushmerick & Crow, 1982). At the same time, they are distinguished by a high rate of oxygen consumption, on average 175 nmol /(min x gram of tissue). The contribution of glycolysis to the total amount of ATP formed at rest is no more than 5%. With intensive work, the formation of lactate increases by 2-4 times, while oxygen consumption can increase by 100 times.

Another thing, VSMs. Even under conditions of normal oxygenation, the level of lactate formation in them seems to be excessively excessive (Kirk et al. 1954). It was a surprising discovery. In addition, this is typical for smooth muscles of many types, such as the uterus, intestines, trachea, etc.

Thus, for VSMs, a high level of glycolytic reactions is a typical characteristic even under conditions of sufficient oxygenation. There is an interesting point of view, that ATP, synthesized during glycolysis, goes directly to ensuring the functioning of Na^{+}/ K^{+} - ATPases (Campbell & Paul, 1992; Paul et al. 1979), i.e., on electrogenesis. While the energy of ATP, which is formed during oxidative metabolism, goes to ensure the contractile function of smooth muscles. At the same time, the compartments of the smooth muscle cells, in which the processes of glycolysis and gluconeogenesis take place, are clearly demarcated (Vallejo & Hardin, 2004). The redox potentials of these compartments are maintained at equilibrium, and thus the cytoplasmic potential of NADH/NAD is kept stable despite query changes in the cytosolic Na^{+}/K^{+}-ATPase compartment (Barron et al. 2000).

Glycolysis is a classic example of an oscillatory biochemical reaction. In the process of glycolysis, the decomposition of glucose and other sugars is carried out, while compounds containing six carbon molecules are converted into tricarboxylic acids, including three carbon molecules. Due to an excess of free energy in the process of glycolysis per molecule of six-carbon sugar, two molecules of ATP are formed. The main elements in the generation of the observed fluctuations in the concentrations of the components of these reactions are: fructose-6-phosphate, fructose-1,6-biphosphate and reduced NAD (nicotinamide dinucleotide); a key enzyme of the glycolytic pathway - phosphofructokinase.

Instability and fluctuations in the membrane potential may be associated with the activity of cytoplasmic oscillators, i.e., due to the instability of metabolic processes in the cell. Or are these events the result of the activity of membrane oscillators, i.e., generated directly in the membrane itself? I think that such a division is undoubtedly very arbitrary, since fluctuations in metabolic processes will certainly affect the operation of ion channels and pumps. This is how, for example, the glycolytic oscillator, first identified in yeast cells (Chance et al. 1964). An important feature of such an oscillator is its dependence (sensitivity) on the rate of substrate supply. Thus, an increase in the concentration of glucose in a cell-free yeast medium (extract) leads to an increase in the oscillation frequency (Boiteux, Hess, 1974).

Madsen, Danø, Sørensen (Madsen et al. 2005) also studied the phenomenon of glycolysis fluctuations in intact yeasts and extracts. Glycolysis oscillations have been found to be controlled by turning on/off the enzyme phosphofructokinase, a key enzyme in the glycolytic pathway! In the case of intact yeast, it was found that the instability leading to oscillations is due to the stoichiometry of the ATP-ADP-AMP system and the allosteric regulation of phosphofructokinase, with the oscillation frequency distributed throughout the system. It is important to note that the $NAD^+/NADH$ ratio affects the modulation frequency without affecting system instability. These data are very important for understanding the synchronization of oscillations in a single yeast cell.

A growing amount of research suggests that important links of molecular controls of the lactate pathway may serve as novel therapeutic targets (Liu et al. 2021). These authors provided an overview of lactate metabolism in cancer and discuss three important contributors to lactate metabolism (lactate dehydrogenase, monocarboxylate transporters, and mitochondrial pyruvate carrier), and present data that inhibition of these three pathways can lead to radiosensitization. The last conclusion in itself, although indirectly, indicates that the blockade of glycolysis leads to an increase in respiration in the tumor tissues and, obviously, the appearance of an excess of reactive oxygen species associated with this. It is clear that glycolysis and lactate production are the main players in cancer metabolism and development.

Isolated mitochondria also exhibit oscillatory activity (Boiteux and Hess, 1974). These fluctuations are most likely generated by internal mitochondrial causes, and not by external causes, as occurs, for example, under the influence of pyruvate during glycolysis. In any case, the release of calcium from mitochondria under the influence of phosphoenolpyruvate suggests a connection between mitochondrial fluctuations and the glycolytic oscillator.

According to Mitchell's chemiosmotic hypothesis, oxidative phosphorylation is controlled by a stationary proton gradient resulting from the release of hydrogen ions from the mitochondrial matrix during the passage of electrons through the respiratory chain (Crompton, Capano, Crafoli, 1976). This proton gradient is then used to either generate ATP or control calcium homeostasis. If the intracellular level of Ca^{2+} rises above the normal "working" level, mitochondria may even partially switch from ATP production to Ca^{2+} transport. Naturally, in this case, the level of mitochondrial oscillatory activity will decrease, since it strongly depends on the value of the ADP/ATP ratio.

When the mitochondria are involved in the regulation of calcium homeostasis, oscillatory changes in the intracellular pH are a side effect of this. It was found that the introduction of calcium into the cytoplasm of Helix cochlea neurons leads to a transient decrease in the intracellular pH with the subsequent restoration of the initial pH level due to the removal of H^+ from the cell (Meech, 1974).

As for the oscillations of the membrane potential, they are most likely associated with fluctuations in the activity of the electrogenic Na^+/ K^+ plasma membrane pumps (Connor et al. 1974). This question is almost resolved. The problem is the identification of the energy source and the trigger of oscillations. The energy source is obviously glycolysis. Trigger - not yet known.

Oscillations of membrane conductivity are closely related to oscillations of the membrane potential. In general, any increase in the outward (potassium) current leads to a hyperpolarization of the plasma membrane, a decrease in excitability and, accordingly, inhibition of the autorhythmic activity. In addition, on the contrary, the result of increasing the inward (sodium, calcium) current will be the activation of myogenic automaticity. That is why, if you want to get an autorhythmic activity in a vessel that does not usually manifest it, simply add to the buffer solution the outward potassium current blocker, i.e. shift the balance of the transmembrane current to the predominance of the outward current.

How does a membrane oscillator work? Baseline - the membrane potential must be maintained within certain limits. An increase in the inward current leads to depolarization and a compensatory increase in the outward current, leading to repolarization, etc. It is clear that such a scheme works only if it involves the electrogenic Na^+/K^+ - pumps that ensure the restoration of ionic concentrations on both sides of the plasma membrane. Another question is how do changes in potassium, calcium and sodium permeability occur? Calcium can play the role of a peculiar potassium permeability switch. Entering from the extracellular space or releasing from the intracellular depots (sarcoplasmic reticulum, mitochondria), it has the ability to activate calcium-dependent potassium conductivity. It follows that all compounds, for example, cyclic nucleotides that affect calcium homeostasis, can also affect the processes of change in potassium conductivity.

Autorhythmic activity is registered in the smooth muscles of the stomach, small intestine, urinary tract, and in the vascular system. The spectrum of this activity differs very significantly - from high-frequency (about 1 contraction per second) to waves with a frequency of about 3-20 contractions per 1 minute.

Slow waves in smooth muscles are almost certainly associated with cyclical fluctuations in the activity of the Na^+/K^+ pump (Barajas-López, Chow, Den Hertog, Huizinga, 1989). This is simply proved by trivial experiments with ouabain. The problem may lie in finding out the reasons for such cycling. The fact that NADPH fluorescence oscillates in phase with slow potential waves in intact smooth muscle certainly fits into this concept. And, nevertheless, following them does not necessarily mean, consequently. It is likely that Na^+/K^+ pumps are sensitive to changes in the intracellular Ca^{2+} concentration, and that an increase in $[Ca^{2+}]_i$ may contribute to the temporary inactivation of the pump, followed by depolarization of the cell membranes. Activation of the plasma membrane Ca^{2+}-ATPases and the calcium uptake into the intracellular depots leads to a decrease in $[Ca^{2+}]_i$, reactivation of Na^+/K^+ pumps and the restoration of membrane potential.

The main oscillator can be the sarcoplasmic reticulum, which periodically releases calcium, leading to the appearance of regenerative calcium waves. In the presence of cyclic GMP (cGMP), this calcium is also capable of activating chloride channels in the plasma membrane. If these currents are activated in a sufficient number of cells, then they, i.e., the cells, will be depolarized. In addition, cells that are not active at this moment will also be depolarized, because all cells are electrically interconnected. Depolarization will cause an influx of calcium through L-type calcium channels, which not only initiates the contraction, but also the release of calcium from intracellular deport, thus activating their intracellular oscillators. As a result, the probability that a sufficient number of cells will become active at the same time becomes very high, i.e., cellular activity is synchronized.

Therefore, there is a reason to believe that the basal vascular tone is formed, at least partially, due to activity of smooth muscle cells of a "phase" type, with a high level of aerobic glycolysis and an autorhythmic activity. The development of hypercontractility of vessels is a consequence of the "awakening" of "silent" cells of a "tonic" type due to a decrease in the outward current and their transition to an autorhythmic mode of activity. Because of the summation of these contractions, the level of basal tone increases, which leads to an increase in blood pressure.

This means that any decrease in the outflow of potassium, caused by certain pathological factors of the external and internal environment, must inevitably lead to an increase in the basal vascular tone and the development of unwanted hypercontractility. There are so many such factors, some of which we will consider below.

The Special Role of Glycolysis in VSMs Responses to Hypoxia

We know that hypoxia triggers vasodilation in systemic vessels to increase oxygen delivery to the hypoxic tissues. The pulmonary vasculature is also sensitive to hypoxia, but, in contrast to the systemic vascular bed, pulmonary SM responds to the lack of oxygen by vasoconstriction.

Hypoxic pulmonary vasoconstriction (HPV) is a unique property of pulmonary artery smooth muscle cells, which constrict in response to reduced airway/alveolar pO_2 level (Evans et al. 2011a; Sommer et al. 2008; Sylvester et al. 2012). HPV develops at pO2 levels below about 60 mm Hg, reducing the blood supply to poorly ventilated regions of the lungs (and vice versa), and thus ensuring the achievement of an optimal ventilation/perfusion ratio in a highly dynamic manner. This mechanism contrasts sharply with the systemic circulation where hypoxia-induced vasodilation occurs to provide an adequate blood supply to tissues lacking oxygen.

This principal difference in responses of the systemic and pulmonary circulation to hypoxia may be explained by different functional demands put on these vascular beds. Namely, the systemic circulation evolved to increase the supply of hypoxic regions with oxygenated blood, while constrictor vascular responses in the lungs help improve arterial oxygenation by means of selective redistribution of blood to maximize perfusion via better-ventilated alveoli. However, this conclusion provides no clues as to the underlying cellular mechanisms.

Thus, we know that reversible hypoxic pulmonary vasoconstriction (HPV) is the mechanism that matches local lung perfusion to ventilation, i.e., serves as an adaptive mechanism for diverting blood flow from poorly ventilated to better ventilated regions of the lung.

Unfortunately, precise cellular machinery underlying this phenomenon is so far poorly understood until this time (Sylvester et al. 2012).

In addition, surprising for us was the fact of complete reversal of the hypoxic contraction of the pulmonary vessels (and not only the pulmonary ones!) against the background of a selective blockade of glycolysis (Figure 15).

Hypoxic contraction of the pulmonary artery disappears after removal of the endothelium. Interestingly, after damage to the myoendothelial gap junctions, blockade of glycolysis no longer affected the hypoxic reactions of the pulmonary artery (that is, blockade of glycolysis did not eliminate hypoxic vasoconstriction in denuded blood vessels) (Figure 16). It is likely that glycolysis in endothelial cells and myoendothelial gap junctions interact in some way to contribute to the development of hypoxic pulmonary vasoconstriction. It is possible that this occurs due to the formation and conduction of depolarizing electrical signals from endothelial cells to smooth muscles and causes their contraction under hypoxic conditions.

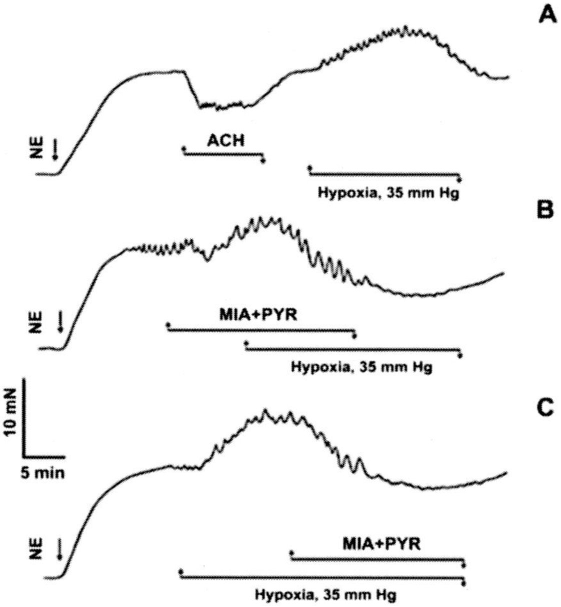

Figure 15. Effect of selective glycolysis blockade on hypoxia-induced contractile responses in guinea-pig pulmonary artery preactivated with norepinephrine (1 μM). A – Control, B- monoiodacetic acid (MIA, 0.1 mM) and pyruvate (PYR, 10 mM) were added to the bath solution before hypoxia influence, C – both above mentioned compounds were added at the plateau of hypoxic contraction. The myoendothelial gap junctions (GJ) inhibitors 18b-glycyrrhetinic acid (18b-GA, 20-30 μM), heptanol (3.5 mM), or 2-aminoethoxydiphenyl borate (2-APB) (75 μM) had little effect on the transient phase 1 of HPV, but abolished the sustained phase 2 which is associated with Ca^{2+} sensitization of myofilaments (Kizub et al. 2013).

It is clear that depolarization of smooth muscle cells takes place, and the ion channels responsible for this process have been identified (Gurney, Joshi and Manoury, 2010). Gurney and co-workers studied smooth muscle cells that regulate the diameter of pulmonary arteries and the resistance to blood flow in the pulmonary circulation in health and disease. The authors postulate that normally these smooth muscle cells are in a relaxed state to maintain low intrinsic vascular tone, but they contract during the development of hypoxic pulmonary vasoconstriction (HPV). It is likely that potassium channels help to maintain low tone in pulmonary VSM cells by polarizing the membrane and preventing Ca^{2+} influx through voltage-operated Ca^{2+} channels. There is a loss of K^+ channel activity in HPV, so drugs that open K^+ channels are predicted to have a beneficial effect, provided their action can be restricted to the pulmonary circulation.

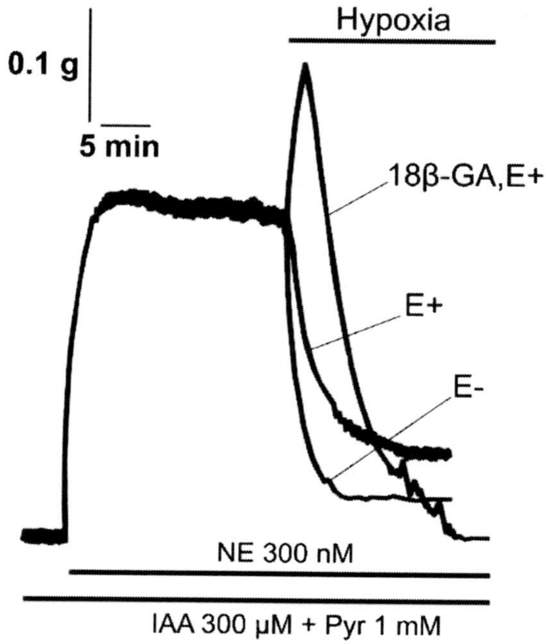

Figure 16. Effect of selective glycolysis blockade with iodoacetic acid (IAA, 10 μM) combined with sodium pyruvate (Pyr, 1 mM) on the hypoxic pulmonary vasoconstriction in intact (E+), denuded (E-) and treated with with 18β-glycyrrhetinic acid (18β-GA, 20 μM) isolated rat thoracic aorta rings precontracted with norepinephrine (NE, 300 nM).

Finally, they concluded that members of the KCNQ family of K^+ channels, the most recent K^+ channels to be discovered in pulmonary arteries, may be a useful therapeutic target for the treatment of HPV. KCNQ channels appear to be preferentially expressed in pulmonary arteries and drugs that modulate their activity have potent effects on pulmonary artery tone.

It is only unclear why in the smooth muscle cells of the vessels of a large circle the reaction to the lack of oxygen has the opposite direction. The trigger for this process in the vessels of the lungs has not yet been fully identified. Of particular interest are the recent news presented by Yan et al. (Yan et al. 2023). They concluded that mitochondrial ROS participate in the development of chronic hypoxia-induced pulmonary hypertension. Furthermore, in their opinion mitochondrial ROS signaling in pulmonary artery smooth muscle cells is centrally involved in enhanced pulmonary arterial constriction following chronic hypoxia, a response potentiated by endogenous endothelin-1.

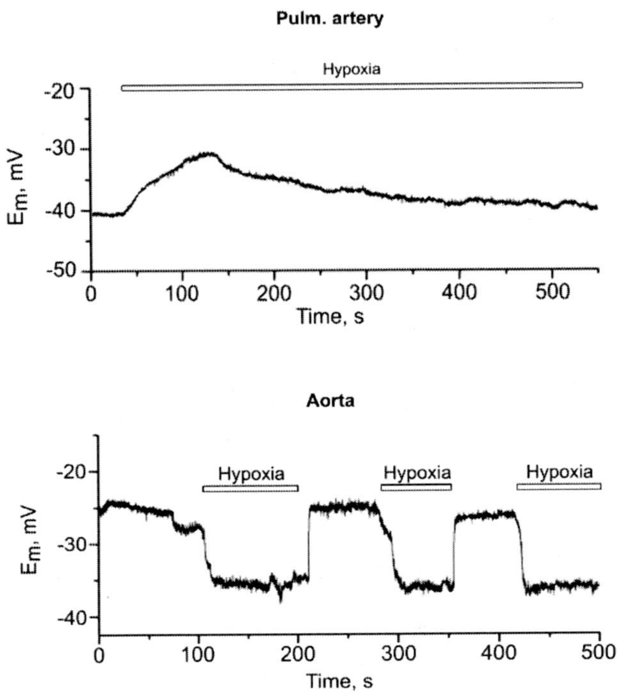

Figure 17. Hypoxia-induced electrical responses in intact endothelium of the guinea thoracic pig aorta A) and pulmonary artery (B). Abscissa - time, sec; ordinate – the membrane potential, mV. Bars above the traces indicate hypoxic (30 mm Hg) solution application.

Surprisingly, under conditions of selective blockade of glycolysis (monoiodoacetate in combination with sodium pyruvate), the smooth muscles of the rat portal vein (this vessel always responds to hypoxia under normal conditions by inhibition of autorhythmic activity and relaxation) respond with a distinct tonic contraction (Gurevich, Bershtein, Soloviev, 1981, 1984). Moreover, this reaction of smooth muscles was fully reproduced in a calcium-free solution with the addition of EGTA. Synchronous registration of contractile and electrical active (sucrose bridge technique) showed that if monoiodoacetate alone caused depolarization of smooth muscles of the portal vein by a maximum of 3 mV, then under conditions of oxygen deficiency, depolarization increased to an average of 19 ± 3 mV.

It turns out that smooth muscles in which glycolysis is compromised are not able, for some reason, to realize the process of hyperpolarization and relaxation under conditions of oxygen deficiency. Later, we confirmed these data and demonstrated that acute hypoxia causes depolarization of pulmonary artery endothelial cells in contrast to hyperpolarization observed in aortic endothelial cells (Soloviev et al. 2012). Selective glycolysis blockade reverses contractile responses to acute hypoxia (10-15 mm Hg) in pulmonary arteries to relaxation and leads to a reversal of depolarization in endothelial cells to hyperpolarization (Figures 17, 18).

It is clear that glycolysis is the key player in this process and may be responsible for the opposite responses of pulmonary and systemic vascular beds to oxygen deprivation.

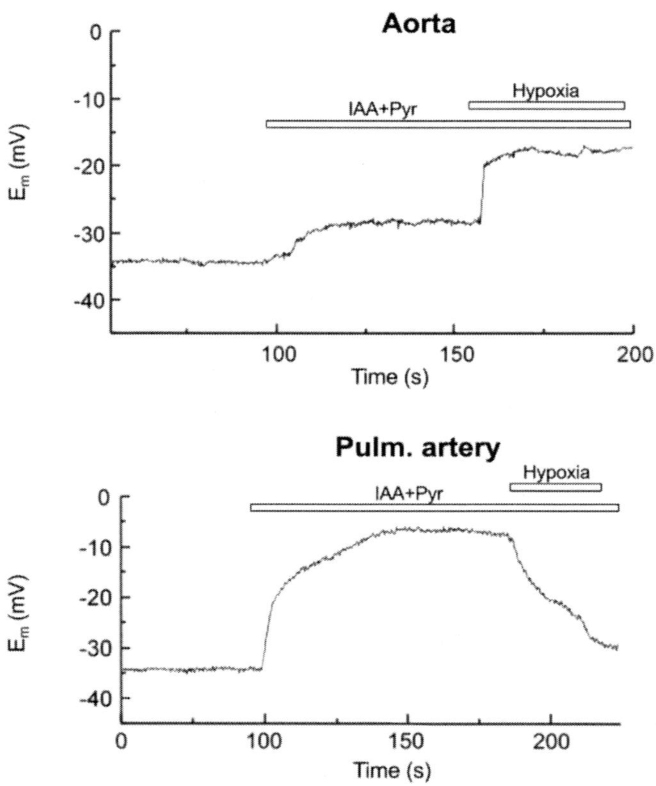

Figure 18. Hypoxia-induced electrical responses in intact endothelium of the guinea pig aorta A) and pulmonary artery (B) under selective glycolysis blockade (IAA, 10 μM plus Pyr, 10 mM). Bars above the traces indicate time intervals of hypoxic solution application and selective glycolysis blockade action.

Thus, the presence of glycolysis is a necessary and indispensable condition for the realization of a normal vascular reaction to hypoxia. Interestingly, in rats with experimental diabetes in which, as is known, glycolysis is compromised, the severity of HPV is sharply reduced (Soloviev, Ivanova, Melnyk et al. 2019).

The mechanisms of HPV have now been fairly well studied, and the main components of this physiologically important phenomenon have been identified. It became clear that functional elements of not only smooth muscle, but also endothelial cells are involved in the formation of HPV. They control calcium dynamics in vascular myocytes and calcium entry through voltage-dependent L-type Ca^{2+} channels, calcium release from calcium stores in the ryanodine-sensitive sarcoplasmic reticulum, and release of vasoconstrictive agents by endothelium (Grimmer & Kuebler, 2017).

In this scenario, several different types of K^+ channels, including ATP-dependent potassium channels (KATP), various voltage-dependent potassium channels (KV) and Ca^{2+}-activated potassium channels (especially BK_{Ca}) play important roles in controlling both the resting and hypoxia-induced changes in membrane potential, and thus Ca^{2+} entry via L-type Ca^{2+} channels during hypoxia. In addition, accumulating evidence shows the importance of cation channels, such as TRPC6 (Fuchs et al. 2011; Weissmann et al. 2006).

We have recently identified a major dysfunction of the pulmonary circulation in type 1 diabetes mellitus (DM), which manifested itself not only by the lack of HPV, but also by a significant vasorelaxation of rat intrapulmonary arteries (iPAs) in response to both physical and chemical hypoxia with pO_2 of 7–10 mm Hg (Soloviev, Ivanova, Melnyk, et al. 2019).

To this end, we found that the lumen area of non-diabetic iPAs as measured in situ using lung slices was strongly reduced under hypoxic conditions, but was increased following STZ-induced (65 mg mg/kg of body weight, i.p.) experimental diabetes. Notably, this abnormality became evident 15 weeks after STZ injection (blood glucose at this time was 27 mM on average), but not at earlier stages of diabetes induction. Regarding possible ion channel mechanisms that could explain this phenomenon, we found that current density of net outward potassium currents in isolated diabetic iPAs myocytes was about two-fold greater compared to non-diabetic cells, and, most interestingly, the current in diabetic myocytes was unaffected by hypoxia. This was in contrast to healthy cells, in which the net outward current was reduced to about 65% of its control amplitude under hypoxia (Soloviev, Ivanova, Melnyk et al. 2019).

It became clear why the smooth muscles of the pulmonary artery of rats with experimental diabetes are not capable of forming normal HPV. Electrophysiological studies have shown abnormally high values of the output current in the isolated smooth muscle cells of the pulmonary artery under normal oxygenation. It is a potassium shunt. Under conditions of hypoxia, this shunt prevents the development of depolarization and contraction.

While it is evident that such dysfunction of the pulmonary circulation could be an important risk factor for patients with diabetes suffering from acute or chronic pulmonary diseases, more studies are required to understand the underlying mechanisms. In this connection, recent reviews of the literature highlight gap in our knowledge of the impact of DM on the vast network of the pulmonary vasculature, contrasting this with the better studied systemic macro- and microvascular dysfunctions in DM (Abernethy et al. 2015).

Nevertheless, people with DM are more likely to develop pulmonary hypertension, while their survival is markedly worse (Abernethy et al. 2015; Movahed et al. 2005; Poms et al. 2013). Chronic hypoxic pulmonary vasoconstriction is one of the major causes of pulmonary hypertension, which, if left untreated, leads to right ventricular hypertrophy and right-sided heart failure – the major life-threatening factor of such pathology. As an adaptive mechanism, cardiac output is reduced under these conditions (Lumb, 2017).

Another relevant avenue of research relates to the possible role of sensory and autonomic innervation in pulmonary dysfunction in DM. Although neuronal input in HPV is normally minimal, DM-induced neuropathies are considered one of the most prevalent chronic complications of diabetes (Evans et al. 2011b). This group of pathologies is very heterogeneous, and they involve virtually every part of the nervous system. There is substantial experimental evidence for the role of neuroinflammation in the pathogenesis of pulmonary hypertension (Hilzendeger et al. 2014) and thus it is entirely possible that nervous system dysfunction will begin to affect pulmonary vascular tone in DM such that vasodilation begins to prevail.

The importance of developing our knowledge of the mechanisms underlying abnormal hypoxic pulmonary vasodilation in DM is highlighted by the pivotal role of HPV in acute respiratory pathologies, such as acute asthma, pneumonia, pulmonary edema etc., where HPV plays a protective role via redirection of blood supply to the better-ventilated regions of the lungs. Furthermore, such research is relevant to other clinical settings such as general anesthesia, that negatively affect HPV (Lennon & Murray, 1996). The situation can be especially dangerous for diabetic patients with already impaired HPV (Soloviev, Ivanova, Melnyk et al. 2019). Within the context of the current COVID-19 pandemic, cases of severe pneumonia requiring artificial (mechanical) lung ventilation are becoming more common than ever, further highlighting the need to understand HPV impairment in DM. Indeed, it is now established that the risk of dying from COVID-19 is much higher for patients having DM. Namely, 2- to 3-fold in patients with type 2 or type 1 DM) (E. Barron et al. 2020).

Based on the already presented evidence (Soloviev, Ivanova, Melnyk, et al, 2019) it is plausible that diabetic patients may greatly benefit from pharmacological interventions aimed at reducing or reversing their abnormal PA vasodilation, especially during general anesthesia, in pneumonia and under mechanical lung ventilation.

Preliminary in vitro tensiometry experiments on vascular rings dissected from main PA have confirmed the abnormal vasodilation of diabetic! tissues in response to hypoxia (5-7 mm Hg), as originally found in small-diameter intrapulmonary arteries (Soloviev, Ivanova, Melnyk et al, 2019). Thus, a significant decrease in constriction and an increase in relaxation in response to hypoxia compared to PA from healthy rats were observed. Incubation with the potent BK_{Ca} channel blocker paxilline restored the response of diabetic PA to hypoxia to control values, except for a transient contraction during the first phase (Figure 19).

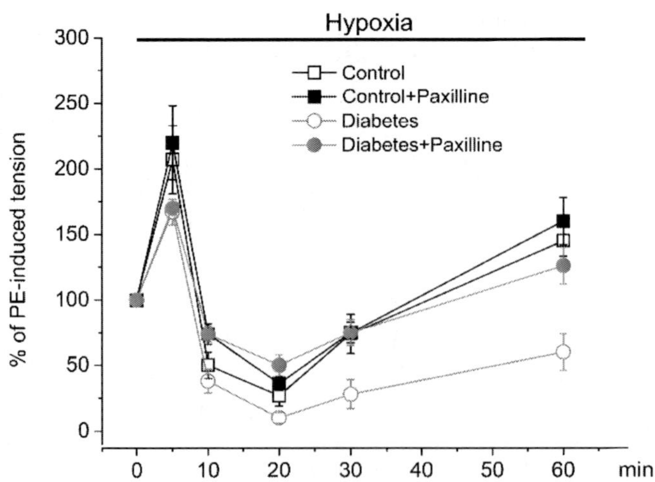

Figure 19. The effect of the paxilline (0.5 μM) on HPV in rat main PA rings, obtained from healthy and diabetic (15 weeks after STZ injection) animals. PA rings were pre constricted with phenylephrine (1 μM). Symbols represent the mean ± SE. *P < 0.05.

Thus, the data obtained clearly indicate that glycolysis plays a critical role in the formation of HPV. It also cannot be ruled out that glycolysis and oxidative phosphorylation are jointly involved in the formation of HPV. Leach et al. (2001) concluded that complex III of the mitochondrial electron transport chain acts as the hypoxic sensor in HPV, and initiates the rise in smooth muscle $[Ca^{2+}]_i$ by a mechanism unrelated to changes in cytosolic redox state per se, but more probably by increased production of superoxide. Additionally, it has been established that glucose and glycolysis are essential for the sustained phase 2 of HPV development. The data obtained support the idea that an endothelium-dependent Ca^{2+} - sensitisation pathway rather than the rise in $[Ca^{2+}]_i$ is involved in this process (Leach, Hill, Snetkov et al, 2001).

Chapter 11

Other Built-in Modulators of Basal Tone: The Role of Perivascular Tissues and the Endothelium

The arterial wall is a heterogeneous three-layered structure composed of an intima, media and adventitia. The second half of the last century was a prelude to the EDRF-nitric oxide age that has occupied vascular scientists for nearly 30 years. Endothelial cells are revealed to have the ability to generate numerous mediators besides prostacyclin and nitric oxide (NO). The need to classify these substances led to the coining of the terms: endothelium-derived relaxing, hyperpolarizing and contracting factors, which included various prostaglandins, thromboxane A2, endothelin, as well numerous candidates for the hyperpolarizing factor. The opposite layer of the vascular wall, the adventitia, eventually and for a quite short period enjoyed the attention of some vascular physiologists. Adventitial fibroblasts were recognized as paracrine cells to the smooth muscle because of their ability to produce some substances such as superoxide. Remarkably, this took place before our awareness of the functional potential of another adventitial cell, the adipocyte. Most small blood vessels in the body are surrounded to some degree by adipose tissue. Possibly, because the perivascular adipose tissue (PVAT) was systematically removed during the experiments as considered a non-vascular artifact tissue, it took quite a long time to be considered a major source of paracrine substances. They are now integrated into a vast pool of mediators synthesized by adipocytes known as adipokines. These include hormones involved in the regulation of metabolism, such as leptin or adiponectin; classical vascular mediators such as NO, angiotensin II or catecholamines; and inflammatory mediators or adipocytokines. The first substance to be studied was an anti-constrictor factor called the fat-relaxing factor of uncertain chemical nature, but it is possible that some of the relaxation mediators mentioned above are behind this factor. The time has come to consider vascular regulation in a complex manner, in terms of paracrine control exercised by all cells present in the vascular wall, namely endothelial, muscle, adventitial, adipocyte and vascular stromal cell (Nava, Llorens, 2019).

Adventicia

Each layer exhibits specific histologic, biochemical and functional characteristics, and, as such, each contributes in unique ways to maintaining vascular homeostasis and to regulating the vascular response to stress or injury. The adventitia, the outer layer of the blood vessel wall, may be the most complex layer of the vascular wall and may be the master regulator of wall physiology and pathobiology. Unlike the normal intima and media, which are composed of endothelial and smooth muscle cells respectively, the normal adventitia is comprised of a wide variety of cell types, including fibroblasts, resident progenitor cells, immunomodulatory cells (dendritic cells, macrophages, T-lymphocytes), vasa vasorum endothelial cells and adrenergic nerves.

The data obtained by (Stenmark, Yeager, Kasmi, Nozik-Grayck, Gerasimovskaya, Li, Riddle and Frid, 2013) clearly indicate that the vascular adventitia acts as a biological processing center for the retrieval, integration, storage, and release of key regulators of vessel wall function. It is likely that it is the most complex compartment of the vessel wall and is comprised of a variety of cells including fibroblasts, immunomodulatory cells (dendritic and macrophages), progenitor cells, vasa vasorum endothelial cells and pericytes, and adrenergic nerves. In response to vascular stress or injury, resident adventitial cells are often the first to be activated and re-programmed to then influence the function (tone) and structure of the vessel wall. Adventitia is able also to initiate and perpetuate chronic vascular inflammation, and to stimulate expansion of the vasa vasorum, which can act as a conduit for continued inflammatory and progenitor cell delivery to the vessel wall.

The adventitial fibroblasts (AF), being the most abundant cellular constituent of the adventitia, has been shown to be a critical regulator of vascular wall function. In response to vascular stresses including hypoxia, the AF undergoes epigenetically fixed functional changes, which include proliferation, differentiation, production of extracellular matrix proteins, adhesion molecules, release of reactive oxygen species, growth factors and metalloproteinases (MMPs), which affect medial smooth muscle cell tone and growth directly. This activated AF phenotype is also characterized by generation of chemokines and cytokines that are capable of recruiting, retaining, and activating circulating and resident inflammatory and progenitor cells. Bidirectional interactions between activated fibroblasts and resident and recruited macrophages, dendritic cells, and progenitor cells can thus create a microenvironment that is conducive to promoting a persistent and nonresolving inflammatory response that includes expansion of the vasa vasorum. The last one acts as a conduit for further delivery of inflammatory/ progenitor cells, with the end result of irreversible functional and structural remodeling of the vessel wall.

The review of Tinajero and Gotlib (2020) proposes a look at adventitia from a functional point of view, and not just as a structural unit. Human and experimental in vivo and in vitro studies show that the adventitia is a dynamic microenvironment in which adventitial and perivascular adipose tissue cells initiate and regulate important vascular functions in disease, especially intimal hyperplasia and atherosclerosis.

Although well away from the bloodwall interface, where much pathology has been identified, the adventitia has a profound influence on the population of intimal and medial endothelial, macrophage, and smooth muscle cell function. Vascular injury and dysfunction of the perivascular adipose tissue promote expansion of the vasa vasorum, activation of fibroblasts, and differentiation of myofibroblasts. This regulates further biologic processes, including fibroblast and myofibroblast migration and proliferation, inflammation, immunity, stem cell activation and regulation, extracellular matrix remodeling, and angiogenesis. A debate exists as to whether the adventitia initiates disease or is just an important participant. (Tinajero and Gotlieb, 2020).

Perivascular Adipose Tissue, A New Era in Vascular Research

The role for perivascular adipose as a source of neurohumoral regulators was first proposed more than 20 years ago (Soltis, Cassis, 1991). A potential role for perivascular adipose tissue as a neurohumoral regulator of vascular responsiveness was studied. Thoracic aortae obtained from male Sprague-Dawley rats are cut into rings for use in a standard in vitro smooth muscle bath set-up. The vessels were either carefully cleaned of surrounding adipose tissue or left intact as a control group. It is important that contractile responses to KCl and phenylephrine as well as relaxation responses to acetylcholine, isoproterenol and sodium nitroprusside are not different between cleaned and intact tissues. However, a significant decrease in the sensitivity to norepinephrine was observed in intact vessels. This altered response was corrected by prior treatment with desipramine plus deoxycorticosterone. Contractile responses of aortic ring preparations to tyramine and a potassium-free physiological solution were significantly greater in intact tissues.

Electrical stimulation resulted in no response in cleaned tissues; however, a frequency-dependent contraction was elicited in intact vessels. Phentolamine blocked the contractile responses generated by these manipulations, which activate the sympathetic neuroeffector system. Responses evoked by electrical stimulation in intact vascular preparations were significantly attenuated by prior exposure to the selective angiotensin II antagonist SarI-Ile8-AII.

Thus, these observations demonstrate that perivascular adipose tissue significantly influences vascular responsiveness in the in vitro setting.

Later, Meyer, Fredette, Barton, Prossnit (2013) unexpectedly found that in the aortic preparations obtained from obese mice, perivascular adipose tissue potentiates vascular contractile responses to serotonin and phenylephrine, indicating activity of a factor generated by perivascular adipose. They designated it as "adipose-derived contracting factor" (ADCF). Inhibition of cyclooxygenase (COX) fully prevented ADCF-mediated contractions, whereas COX-1 or COX-2-selective inhibition was only partially effective. By contrast, inhibition of superoxide anions, NO synthase, or endothelin receptors had no effect on ADCF activity. Perivascular adipose as a source of COX-derived ADCF was identified by detecting increased thromboxane A2 formation from perivascular adipose-replete aortae from obese mice. Taken together, this study clearly identifies perivascular adipose as a novel source of vasoconstriction influences due to the release of COX-derived ADCF. Excessive ADCF activity in perivascular fat under obese conditions likely contributes to increased vascular tone by antagonizing vasodilation. ADCF may thus propagate obesity-dependent hypertension and the associated increased risk in coronary artery disease, potentially representing a novel therapeutic target.

Obesity and AH are known as important risk factors for atherosclerosis and coronary artery disease. They are characterized by an increase in vascular tone. While obesity leads to increased vasoconstrictor prostanoid activity in endothelial cells, fewer known factors are released from fat tissue surrounding arteries (perivascular adipose). Using lean controls and mice with either monogenic or diet-induced obesity, Meyer et al. (2013) determined whether and through which pathways perivascular adipose affects vascular tone. They unexpectedly found that in the aorta of obese mice, perivascular adipose potentiates vascular contractility to serotonin and phenylephrine, indicating activity of a factor generated by perivascular adipose, which we designated ''adipose-derived contracting factor'' (ADCF). Inhibition of cyclooxygenase (COX) fully prevented ADCF-mediated contractions, whereas COX-1 or COX-2-selective inhibition was only partially effective. By contrast, inhibition of superoxide anions, NO synthase, or endothelin receptors had no effect on ADCF activity. Perivascular adipose as a source of COX-derived ADCF was further confirmed by detecting increased thromboxane A2 formation from perivascular adipose-replete aortae from obese mice.

Taken together, this study identifies perivascular adipose as a novel regulator of arterial vasoconstriction through the release of COX-derived ADCF. Excessive ADCF activity in perivascular fat under obese conditions likely contributes to increased vascular tone by antagonizing vasodilation. ADCF may thus propagate obesity-dependent hypertension and the associated increased risk in coronary artery disease, potentially representing a novel therapeutic target (Szasz, Webb, 2012; Meyer et al. 2013).

The Possible Role of the Endothelium in the Basal Tone Formation

Writing about the role of nitric oxide in the regulation of vascular tone is a thankless task. Molecule of the century! So much has already been written that any review will be fragmentary. Let me pass this task on to one of the Nobel Prize winners in this field – Louis Ignarro. Somehow, I happened to attend his lectures at the Jagiellonian University in Krakow, Poland. By the way, it was a conference dedicated to the anniversary of Professor Richard Gryglevsky. He was one of those people who, on their own merit, could also qualify for this award. It is a pity, but there is only one prize, and there are always more contenders.

In his lecture, L. Ignarro said: "Looking back, basic research in the field of NO and cyclic GMP over the past two decades seems to have followed a logical course, starting with the conclusion that NO and cyclic GMP are VSM relaxants that nitroglycerin relaxes smooth muscles by metabolism to NO, progressing to the discovery that mammalian cells synthesize NO, and finally the discovery that NO is a neurotransmitter mediating vasodilation in specialized vascular beds. Since the discovery that EDRF is NO, there has been a large body of basic and clinical research on the physiological and pathophysiological role of NO in cardiovascular function. New knowledge about NO should allow researchers in this field to develop new and more effective therapeutic strategies for the prevention, diagnosis and treatment of numerous cardiovascular diseases. Since NO has a protective and beneficial effect in many disease states, new NO donors for clinical use should prove to be very effective drugs for the treatment of essential hypertension, stroke, coronary heart disease, vascular complications of diabetes, impotence, and other diseases associated with the vascular system" (Ignarro, 2002).

The endothelium is important in maintaining vascular homeostasis and preventing the development of atherosclerosis. However, perturbation of its activity may lead to endothelial dysfunction that, if left untreated, could progress to atherosclerotic lesion formation and subsequent cardiac events. Therefore, assessing endothelial function in patients at risk of cardiovascular disease is important to identify vascular abnormalities and may help monitor strategies and interventions that can improve endothelial function and lower cardiovascular disease risk.

A few years ago, I observed an interesting phenomenon - the appearance of autorhythmic activity in deendothelyzed smooth muscles of the rat aorta in response to the administration of norepinephrine. Spontaneous activity in the vessels of the tonic type is a precursor to the development of spasm. Obviously, the role of the endothelium is to prevent an exccssive increase in the inward current and to prevent an unwanted decrease in the outward one.

Endothelium undoubtedly plays an important role in the regulation of vascular tone. This is a widely known fact that does not require special comments. On the other hand, both the endothelial cells themselves and the products of their activity are too vulnerable and not stable so that they can make a real contribution to the formation of basal tone (Sandoo, Jet, van Zanten, Metsios, Carroll and Kitas, 2010).

Endothelial Dysfunction and Hypercontractility of Smooth Muscle

In the past, endothelium was thought to be only a mechanical barrier. Today, endothelium is known to be a tissue regulating vascular tone due to its electrical and humoral coupling to overlying (or underlying?) smooth muscle cells, cell growth and the interaction between the leukocytes, thrombocytes and the vessel wall. It also synthesizes different growth factors and regulatory molecules and responds to physical and chemical signals. Even though the term "endothelial dysfunction" is generally used for deterioration of endothelium-dependent vasodilatation, the term also includes the abnormalities between endothelium and leukocytes, thrombocytes and regulatory molecules and conditions resulting in aberrant endothelium activation. Healthy endothelium is essential for cardiovascular control. Thus, it plays an important role in the pathogenesis of many diseases and cardiovascular problems such as atherosclerosis, systemic and pulmonary hypertension, cardiomyopathies and other vascular diseases. The aim of this chapter is to explain endothelial dysfunction and the circulating molecules of endothelial cells, as they become potential targets of therapeutic approaches for hypertension.

The role of the endothelium in the triggering of smooth muscle cells automatic activity is significant, apparently, in those vessels where there are clearly pronounced gap junctions, i.e. where they serve to synchronize the oscillations of intracellular calcium and conduct excitation from the endothelium to the underlying muscle layer. Recently, we mentioned (unpublished data) that the removal of the endothelium leads to the disappearance of the phase activity that appears in the smooth muscles of the rat aorta when activated by their norepinephrine. This phenomenon requires special study but the role of endothelial cells in the formation of myogenic activity appears to be not decisive. It is likely that endothelium plays the role of a kind of modulator of the activity of smooth muscle cells, i.e. providing the so-called tuning of vascular tone.

Konukoglu, Uzun (2017) presented a detailed review of the role of endothelial dysfunction in hypertension, considering the nature of its relationship with diseases, as well as different options for antihypertensive therapy on endothelial function. In addition to these, the role of endothelial dysfunction in white coat hypertension has been discussed. They indicate that a key connection between hypertension and endothelial dysfunction is vitally important for future studies to permit new interventions to be designed and released.

Thus, vascular endothelium plays an important role in cardiovascular physiology, forming an interface between blood and adjacent tissues and it is involved in nutrients and metabolites transport as well as in the interaction with circulating cells, hormones, and cytokines. Endothelial cells regulate the vascular tone through the synthesis of nitric oxide (NO), prostaglandins and other relaxing factors. Moreover, healthy endothelium provides antioxidant, anti-inflammatory, and antithrombotic functions and contributes to the maintenance of vascular tone, serving as a gatekeeper for organ/tissue homeostasis and blood pressure control.

Endothelial dysfunction is characterized by a shift of the actions of the endothelium toward reduced vasodilation, cell proliferation, platelet adhesion and activation and proinflammatory and prothrombotic state. Endothelial dysfunction occurs in association with several cardiovascular risk factors, including hypertension, hypercholesterolemia, and insulin resistance. Endothelial dysfunction, also contributing to inflammation in the vascular wall, increased lipoprotein oxidation, smooth muscle cell proliferation, extracellular matrix deposition, cell adhesion, and thrombus formation in conducting arteries It should be noted that the manifestations of endothelial dysfunction may precede the development of hypertension. Essential hypertension is characterized by functional and structural alterations in resistance arteries that lead to increased peripheral vascular resistance.

Endothelial dysfunction may contribute to the increased peripheral resistance by several mechanisms that leads to the enhanced constriction and vascular remodeling (i.e., structural, mechanical, and functional alterations) of resistance arteries, which is associated with the development and complications of hypertension. In particular, endothelial dysfunction may participate to the increased myogenic tone of resistance arteries through the activation of the renin-angiotensin system, endothelin-1, catecholamines, and growth factors production, leading to vasoconstriction, vascular remodeling and then to increased resistance to blood flow and ultimately to increased peripheral blood pressure. The induction of inflammatory processes in the vascular wall may be associated with endothelial dysfunction and may contribute further to the remodeling of resistance arteries, and conduit arteries, which is associated with the increased risk of cardiovascular diseases (Gallo. Volpe, Savoia, 2022).

The PKC enzyme plays a special, possibly trigger role, in the development of hypercontractility of VSMs and the role of the endothelium in this process is undoubted. It is known that aortae from spontaneously hypertensive rats (SHR) demonstrate a decreased relaxant response to acetylcholine (ACh) as compared to aortae from normotensive Wistar-Kyoto (WKY) rats, while papaverine lowered the force of aorta to a similar degree in both strains of rats. PKC inhibitors, H-7 (5×10^{-6} M) and chelerythrine chloride (10^{-6} M), produced a greater decrease in the force developed by the aortae from SHR vs. WKY rats both in intact and chemically permeabilized tissues. In SHR, aortae PKC inhibitors enhanced relaxation to ACh to a greater extent as compared to WKY aortae. Furthermore, in the presence of PKC inhibitors, the constrictor responses of SHR aortae to ACh were transformed into relaxant responses, and the concentration-response curve to Ach was shifted to the left. The sensitivity of aortae from SHR to authentic nitric oxide (NO) was lower compared to WKY rats. EC_{50}s for authentic NO in SHR and WKY rat aortae were different: $-2.9 \pm 0.15 \times 10^{-6}$ M and $4.58 \pm 0.1 \times 10^{-7}$ M (n = 15,

$p < 0.001$), respectively. Bioassay experiments using SHR aortae showed that the addition of chelerythrine (10^{-6} M) to the detector superfusate caused relaxation during treatment of the donor segment with Ach, indicating that the sensitivity of the aortae to NO had been restored. When SHR detector ring was substituted for denuded aortae from WKY rats and PKC inhibitors were not added to the detector superfusate, the relaxation of the detector aortae was also close to the normal ACh-induced relaxation. WKY aortae demonstrated a positive relationship between Ach-stimulated NO release and relaxant response amplitudes (correlation coefficient $r = 0.905$, $p < 0.001$, $n = 10$). In contrast, there was a significant negative correlation in SHR aortae ($r = -0.712$, $p < 0.05$, $n = 10$). Detection of NO release by chemiluminescence showed no significant difference in NO release in SHR and WKY aortae. Taken together, these data suggest that the blunted endothelium-dependent relaxation observed in the aortic SHR is mainly associated with a decrease in the sensitivity of VSM to EDRF/NO under the influence of increased PKC activity (Soloviev, Parshikov, Stefanov, 1998). It is likely that NO activity is inhibited by production of reactive oxygen species and PKC may be involved in their production.

It is likely that the endothelium in the vascular wall plays the role of a kind of fuse, a mechanism that protects smooth muscles from excessive contraction. In our experiments, an interesting phenomenon was often observed - the smooth muscles of the rat aorta began to spontaneously contract after removal of the endothelium (unpublished data). This is very similar to the effect of tetraethylammonium, which blocks the outward potassium currents and provokes the development of spontaneous activity. The role of endothelium in the formation of basal tone is obviously insignificant, but the modulating role is obvious. At least, the role of basal nitric oxide release in the formation of muscle tone is quite logical and probable.

Chapter 12

Calcium Sensitivity as a Basal Tone Supporter

It is well known that intracellular free calcium $[Ca^{2+}]_i$ in smooth muscle cells is one of the main factors determining the contractile force development - contractile activity in VSMCs is initiated by a Ca^{2+}-calmodulin interaction to stimulate phosphorylation of the light chain of myosin (MLC). This classical and well-known scheme of SM contraction and relaxation is presented in Figure 20.

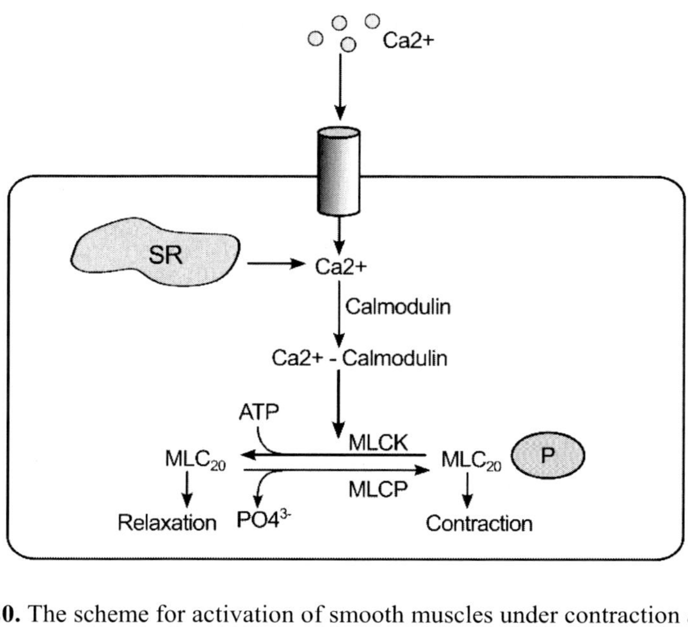

Figure 20. The scheme for activation of smooth muscles under contraction and relaxation SR- sarcoplasmic reticulum, MLC – myosin light chain kinase, MLCP – myosin light chain phosphatase, ATP – adenosine triphosphate. Adapted from Klabunde (2004).

Alternatively, it has been suggested that a Ca^{2+}-independent mechanism or Ca^{2+}-sensitization of contractile elements may participate in smooth muscle contraction. Experiments carried out on smooth muscle from bladder detrusor demonstrated that SM incubated in Ca^{2+}-free solution containing ethylene glycol bis (-aminothylether)-N, N, -tetraacetic acid (EGTA), carbachol and phorbol ester produced sustained contractions. Additionally, depletion of Ca^{2+} stores by caffeine did not affect Ca^{2+}-free contraction induced by carbachol. Finally, W-7 (calmodulin inhibitor) and ML-9 (MLC kinase inhibitor) did not show inhibitory effects on Ca^{2+}-free contraction. Please note that H-7, PKC inhibitor, abolished this contraction.

These data presented by Yoshimura, Yamaguchi (1997) clearly indicate that stored Ca^{2+} and Ca^{2+} -calmodulin-MLCK systems are not required elements of the carbachol-induced Ca^{2+}-free contraction of SM. They decided that this Ca^{2+}-independent contraction was mediated by the activation of PKC coupled with agonist stimulation of the muscarinic receptor.

The main conclusion from this work is that the contractile activity of SMCs and, hence, vascular tone may also vary over a wide range without significant changes in $[Ca^{2+}]_i$. Thus, alterations in the myofilament Ca^{2+}-sensitivity may be very important in the regulation of muscle activity in both health and disease (Figure 21).

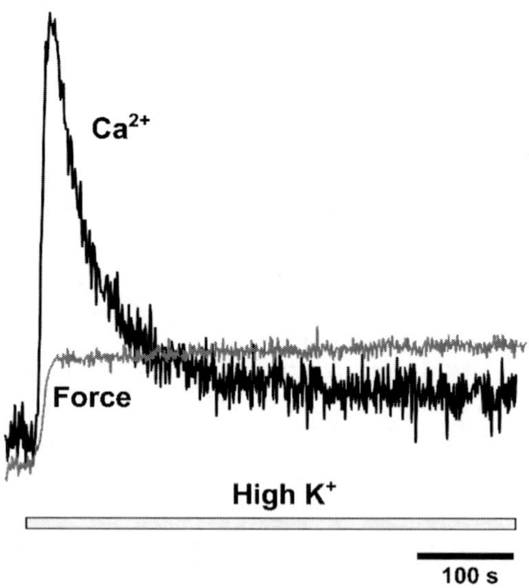

Figure 21. Intracellular Ca^{2+} and force in intact rat aorta upon depolarization from 4.7 mM K^+ to 120 mM K^+. Please note, substitution of potassium chloride for norepinephrine or vice versa does not affect the overall behavior of smooth muscles.

It is generally accepted that Ca^{2+}-sensitization usually requires a receptor-linked vasoconstrictor, but it is interesting to know that KCl can also cause

Ca^{2+} sensitization involving translocation and activation of RhoA kinase. Rather than complicating the Ca^{2+} sensitivity story, this surprising finding is already providing novel insights into mechanisms regulating Ca^{2+} sensitivity of smooth muscle contraction. KCl as a "simple" stimulus promises to remain a standard tool for smooth muscle cell physiologists, whose focus is to understand mechanisms regulating Ca^{2+} sensitivity (Ratz et al. 2005).

Thus, from the classical point of view VSM is known to contract in response to an increase in $[Ca^{2+}]_i$. The increase in $[Ca^{2+}]_i$ activates the calmodulin dependent myosin light chain (MLC) kinase which catalyzes the phosphorylation of the 20,000 dalton MLC. MLC phosphorylation in turn activates the myosin molecule, which can then interact with actin and contract (Kamm and Stull, 1985). In addition to this primary regulatory pathway, several modulatory pathways exist in smooth muscle that can alter the magnitude of force that is developed for any given level of cellular Ca^{2+}. Alterations in myofilament Ca^{2+} sensitivity can be either positive or negative depending on the pathways stimulated.

For increases in myofilament Ca^{2+} sensitivity, two primary hypotheses have been proposed: G-protein dependent activation of Rho kinase and PKC-dependent phosphorylation of a cellular protein called CPI-17 (Somlyo and Somlyo, 2003). Both proposals have a common endpoint, that inhibition of the MLC phosphatase results in a greater level of MLC phosphorylation for any given level of Ca^{2+} and activity of the MLC kinase.

Thus, it is likely that Ca^{2+} sensitization of the contractile proteins in VSMs is signaled by the protein kinase C/Rho kinase's pathways to inhibit the dephosphorylation of the light chain by myosin phosphatase, thereby maintaining force generation. Removal of Ca^{2+} from the cytosol and stimulation of myosin phosphatase or decrease the sensitivity of myofilaments to Ca^{2+} initiate the process of VSMC relaxation.

A number of experimental evidence confirms the existence of such a mechanism of vascular regulation. At first, hypoxia shifts the" pCa-tension'' curves in chemically permeabilized SMCs to the right and decreases the maximal developed SMC force, indicating that myofilament Ca^{2+}-sensitivity and responsiveness have been decreased (Soloviev, Bazilyuk, 1998). Secondly, leftward shift of the "pCa-tension" relationship and dissociation between contractile force and $[Ca^{2+}]_i$ was demonstrated in SM cells obtained from both spontaneously hypertensive (Soloviev, Bershtein, 1992; Soloviev, Parshikov, Stefanov, 1998) and irradiated rats (Soloviev, Tishkin, Zelensky et al. 2005) as compared to non-irradiated normotensive rats (Figure 22).

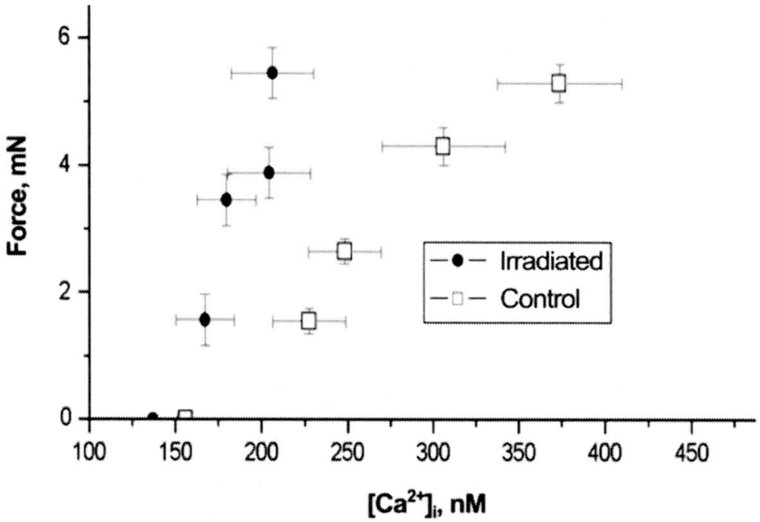

Figure 22. Effect of irradiation (6 Gy) on the KCl-mediated $[Ca^{2+}]_i$-tension relationship in the thoracic aorta. Rings loaded with Fura-2 were subjected to the cumulative addition of KCl and levels of force and the simultaneous measurement of $[Ca^{2+}]_i$ recorded. The results are shown as (open square - control) and (closed circles - irradiated). The slope (mN tension/nM $[Ca^{2+}]_i$) was significantly increased in irradiated tissues as compared to control, indicating that Ca^{2+} - sensitivity of the myofilaments had increased.

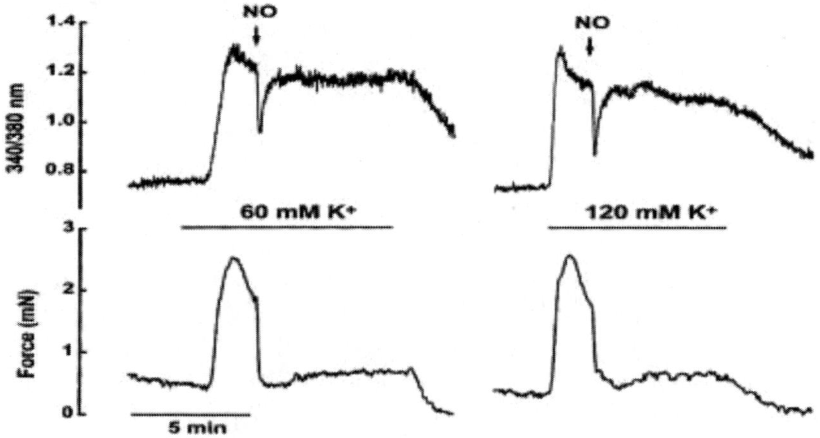

Figure 23. Effect of authentic nitric oxide (NO, 10^{-6} M) on 60 - and 120 mM potassium chloride-induced tension (force, mN) and intracellular Ca^{2+} (ratio) in rat tail artery.

These data clearly confirm the role of changes in calcium sensitivity of myofilaments in vascular tone regulation under hypoxia and AH.

And finally, the nitric oxide (NO) – induced reduction in $[Ca^{2+}]_i$ was transient while related vascular relaxant response was sustained (Soloviev, Lehen'kyi, Zelensky, Hellstrand, 2004) indicating decreasing NO-induced calcium sensitivity (Figure 23).

Please note that MLCK is inhibited by the calcium /calmodulin-dependent protein kinase II, whereas the activity of MLCP is increased by cGMP and perhaps also cAMP-dependent protein kinases. In either case, this results in a decrease in the calcium sensitivity of rMLC phosphorylation and force production. The activity of MLCP is inhibited by Rho-associated kinase, one of the effectors of the monomeric GTPase Rho, and protein kinase C, leading to an increase in calcium sensitivity. Thus, smooth muscle tone appears to be regulated by a network of activating and inactivating different intracellular signaling pathways (Pfitzer, 2001).

Chapter 13

Ion Channel and Vascular Tone

Increased pressure in the lumen of a blood vessel causes vasoconstriction, which is especially prominent in resistance arteries. The ensuring myogenetic tone, which is a critically important common contributor to basal vascular tone, is further adjusted by the action of various vasoconstrictors and vasodilators (neurotransmitters, hormones, nitric oxide etc.) to match current physiological requirements for the intensity of blood flow. It is commonly associated with membrane depolarization to about -40 mV. This necessarily leads to the opening of voltage-dependent Ca^{2+} channels, while the resulting Ca^{2+} influx causes the myogenic response. Indeed, myogenic vasoconstriction largely depends on the activity of these channels as it is significantly reduced in Ca^{2+} external solution and in the presence of selective L-type VGCC blockers, as well as by membrane hyperpolarization of any origin (Abd El-Rahman et al. 2013; Bolton, 1979; El-Lakany et al. 2023; Hill & Meininger, 1994; Jackson, 2020, 2021; Kotecha & Hill, 2005; Nelson et al. 1990, 1991; Potocnik et al. 2000; J. Zhang et al. 2007).

Thus, the two main questions to be answered regarding the ionic nature of vascular tone, including its important myogenic component, are (i) What causes membrane depolarization of vascular myocytes? and (ii) What are the pathways of Ca^{2+} entry into the cell triggering and/or maintaining its state of contraction?

Voltage-Gated Ca^{2+} Channels Are the Major Determinants of Smooth Muscle Contractility

Based on diverse and numerous observations made during the "classical" era of smooth muscle physiology, biophysics and pharmacology, M.F. Shuba proposed his original concept of smooth muscle contraction (Shuba, 1981). It was framed in the context of the prevailing at that time framework of the so-called electromechanical and pharmacomechanical coupling in smooth muscles (Somlyo & Somlyo, 1968), as well as "Theory of P and T systems for calcium activation in smooth muscle" (Golenhofen, 1976) (P meaning phasic and T – tonic contractions).

The main pathways and mechanisms of transmembrane Ca^{2+} influx into smooth muscle cells postulated to exist by M.F. Shuba are shown in Figure 24. Accordingly, M.F. Shuba proposed the existence of fast inactivating VGCCs and slow non- or weakly inactivated VGCCs, as well as a separate class of chemosensitive Ca^{2+} channels, which are activated by receptor agonists (neurotransmitters or various physiologically active substances). These three types of Ca^{2+} entry pathways have been considered to be the ionic channel mechanisms underlying electromechanical and pharmacomechanical coupling, respectively, the latter not necessarily accompanied by membrane depolarization. Notably, an additional mechanism that encompasses both types of coupling has also been proposed, namely dual control of VGCCs by voltage and by the activated receptors, which can either potentiate or inhibit Ca^{2+} entry via VGCCs.

At that time, direct evidence was largely lacking (patch-clamp techniques became available only in 1981). However, with the introduction of the patch-clamp-techniques to recordings of ion currents in isolated voltage-clamped smooth muscle myocytes it was soon confirmed that, indeed, inactivation of VGCCs had a complex nature. The current did not inactivate completely even during long-lasting depolarizations, in some studies of to 5 s duration (Ganitkevich et al. 1986; Smirnov et al. 1992; Zholos et al. 1991).

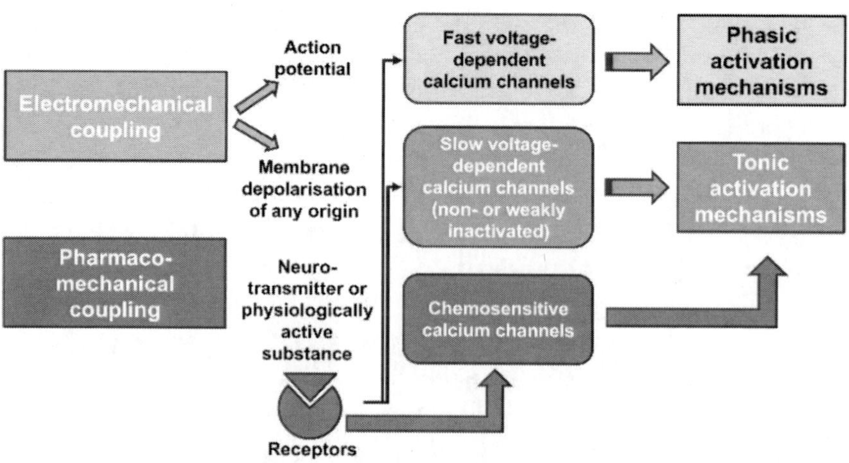

Figure 24. Classical concepts of Ca^{2+} entry mechanisms activating smooth muscle contraction.

In the late 1980s, it became evident that different types of VGCCs were present in smooth muscle myocytes, which differed in their voltage dependence, inactivation kinetics and pharmacological properties. These were suggested to be similar to L- and T-type Ca channels that have been previously identified in neuronal and heart cells (Yoshino et al. 1989). Although these were initially identified in intestinal myocytes, soon enough V.Ya. Ganitkevich and G. Isenberg made similar observations in single myocytes from guinea-pig coronary artery (Ganitkevich & Isenberg, 1990). In particular, they found that at negative potentials, close to the normal resting potential, T-type Ca^{2+} channels were completely inactivated, while L-type calcium channels could be active. The authors thus concluded that "openings of L-type calcium channels can occur at the resting membrane potential of these cells and most probably serve as a pathway for calcium influx into the resting cell." The next question was – how was it possible that the same Ca^{2+} channel type, specifically L-type VGCC, could be both fast and slow voltage-dependent Ca^{2+} channel (Figure 25)?

This apparent paradox was resolved in studies looking at the so-called Ca^{2+} "window current" (Figure 25). "Window current" is a well-known phenomenon, which is present even in the case of fast voltage-gated neuronal Na^+ channels that show very rapid, yet incomplete inactivation (e.g., some neurones can generate persistent Na^+ current). Its amplitude and voltage dependence are determined by channel's steady-state activation and inactivation properties, denoted in the formalism of Hodgkin and Huxley as m_∞ and h_∞, respectively.

To work out steady-state activation and inactivation properties of Ca^{2+} conductance, a standard two-pulse protocol is employed. The first step (the sol-called preconditioning pulse) is applied to a wide range of potentials. The activation curve is then constructed by plotting Ca^{2+} current amplitude divided by the electrochemical driving force for Ca^{2+} as a function of membrane potential at this step. The duration of the preconditioning step should be sufficiently long to evoke steady-state inactivation of Ca^{2+} channels. The second pulse (test pulse) is applied with a short delay (several ms) to allow Ca^{2+} channels to regain their activation gating mechanism, but not long enough to induce any significant recovery of Ca^{2+} channels from inactivation. Finally, plotting the ratio of peak Ca^{2+} currents at these two steps allows the steady-state inactivation curve to construct.

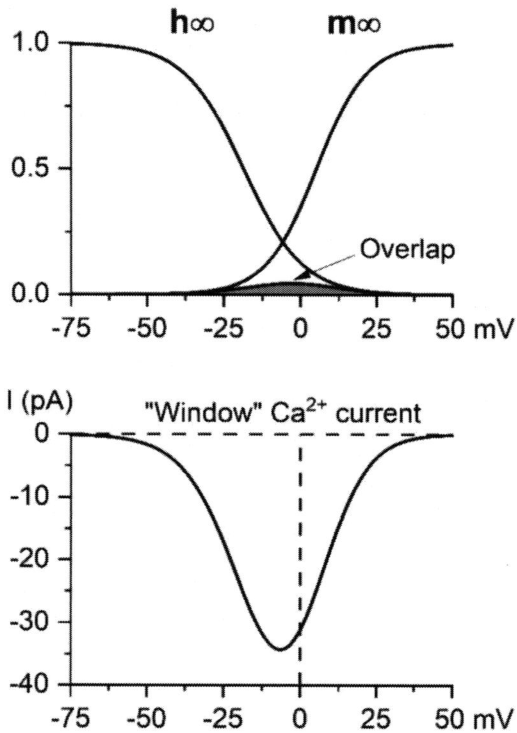

Figure 25. Calcium "window current." Top – the overlap (shaded area) between steady-activation and inactivation curves, both approximated by the Boltzmann equation, is calculated as the product of m_∞ and h_∞ parameters, this way defining a region on the voltage axis where Ca^{2+} channel is already activated, but not yet completely inactivated. Bottom - this predicts a nonzero steady-state current at membrane potentials where the curves overlap (gray region), giving what is called the ''window current.''

Experimentally, non-inactivating inward currents via VGCCs have been described in different SM types (Imaizumi et al. 1989). The authors used prolonged depolarizations for up to 1 min duration and noted that the peak amplitude of the steady-state Ca^{2+} current was in the range from 5 to 25 pA, depending on the type of smooth muscles as they used cells isolated from guinea pig urinary bladder, ureter, *vas deferens*, taenia caecum, and rabbit portal vein.

Ca^{2+} currents via L-type VGCCs are typically much smaller in vascular compared to visceral smooth muscles, as VSMCs are typically non-excitable, while most visceral smooth muscle cells can generate action potentials.

Intrestingly, albeit much smaller, but persistent Ca^{2+} current is present in vascular myocytes at potentials about 17 mV more negative compared to visceral myocytes, i.e., in the membrane potential range typically achieved during the myogenic contraction (A. V. Zholos, personal communications). Thus, in contrast to intestinal smooth muscles, in which tonic contraction may be even physiologically detrimental, in vascular myocytes at their normal resting potentials there is a possibility of either increasing or decreasing this current by even small changes in membrane potential if this happens to occur around the mid-point of the steeply ascending limb of the I-V curve (Figure 25, bottom panel).

It this context, it should be noted that the "chemosensitive calcium channels" postulated by M. F. Shuba may, in fact and at least partially, be the Ca^{2+} "window current" via the same L-type channels providing that vasoconstrictors favorably affect their voltage-dependent properties to induce a larger persistent Ca^{2+} entry, e.g., via phosphorylation of channel-forming proteins. Such scenarios are well known in heart physiology, e.g., an increased area and negative shift of the Ca^{2+} "window current" during β-adrenergic stimulation of cardiac myocytes (Antoons et al. 2007). An elegant computational model based on canard theory was developed allowing to interpret the role of the Ca^{2+} "window current" size and its voltage region in heart arrythmia (Kimrey et al. 2020), but similar insights with regard to its role in vascular tone are lacking. It is also possible that there may also be structural differences that can result in changes of the Ca^{2+} "window current" in vascular myocytes (Figure 25). For example, a $Ca_V1.2$ splice variant that activates at more hyperpolarized potentials was identified in thoracic aorta, cerebral basilar arteries, and mesentery arteries (Liao et al. 2007).

Deviation 8. *Voltage-gated Na^+ channels can also be expressed in arteriolar smooth muscles. Ulyanova and Shirokov investigated the ionic nature of the depolarizing phase of action potentials in the 4th order arterioles of mouse skeletal muscle (Ulyanova & Shirokov, 2018). They found that action potentials could occur in nominally Ca^{2+}-free external solution or after addition of nifedipine, which blocks L-type Ca^{2+} channels. Hower, these actions potentials were sensitive to tetrodotoxin, a specific blocker of voltage gated Na^+ channels, albeit at very high concentration.*

The authors concluded that not only T- and L-type Ca^{2+} channels are expressed in skeletal muscle arterioles, but also tetrodotoxin-sensitive Na^+ channels contribute to the upstroke of action potentials. Their contribution was particularly evident under nominally Ca^{2+}-free conditions. Intriguingly, *voltage-gated Na^+ channels were found to be inhibited by Ca^{2+} specifically entering arteriolar myocytes via T-types Ca^{2+} channels, activity of which thus prevents action potential discharge.*

This study nicely illustrates the complex ion nature of electrogenesis in arteriolar smooth muscles, which have intrinsic myogenic tone and respond with membrane depolarization to an increase in intraluminal pressure. Evidently, many complex voltage- and Ca^{2+}-dependent interactions between different types of ion channels producing inward currents, as well as negative and positive feedback controls, exist and need to be further studied.

Intracellular Ca^{2+} Release from the Sarcoplasmic Reticulum Can Significantly Boost Ca^{2+} Signaling in Vascular Myocytes

There are two types of intracellular Ca^{2+}-permeable channels underlying Ca^{2+} release from the sarcoplasmic reticulum (SR) of smooth muscle myocytes, namely RyRs and inositol-1,4,5-trisphospate (IP_3) receptors (IP_3Rs).

Activity of RyRs is rapidly and steeply increased by elevation of $[Ca^{2+}]_i$ in the vicinity of a RyR when Ca^{2+} entries the cell via VGCCs, as well as in a self-regenerative manner due to RyRs openings. This process during the cardiac action potential generation was termed Ca^{2+}-induced Ca^{2+} release (CICR) (Fabiato, 1983). Although it was known for a long time that caffeine, which activates RyRs, induced a transient contraction of smooth muscles, the physiological importance of CICR in smooth muscles, unlike cardiac myocytes, remained questionable. First studies showing that CICR in smooth muscle cells can be induced by voltage dependent Ca^{2+} were published in the early 1990s. In these studies, BK_{Ca} channel activity was used as an excellent indicator of Ca^{2+} concentration near plasmalemma. Various pharmacological interventions, application of Ca^{2+}-free external solution and the use of different voltage-step and ramp protocols revealed that a novel late transient outward that was observed during depolarizing voltage steps of 5 s duration was potassium current via BK_{Ca} channels activated by CICR (Zholos et al. 1991, 1992). However, in contrast to cardiac myocytes in which there is a tight connection between T-tubular and SR membranes, properties of CICR in smooth muscle cells were found to be very unusual. It turned out that the peak of CICR was achieved with a delay of about 1 s after the initiation of membrane depolarization, and, even more intriguingly, that peak voltage-dependent Ca^{2+} current was essentially irrelevant for the initiation of CICR.

Rather, it was the steady influx of Ca^{2+} during membrane depolarization that was sufficient for triggering CICR. Moreover, it turned out that the CICR process in smooth muscle myocytes was both regenerative, as in skeletal muscle, but also graded, as in heart muscle. CICR was somewhat later demonstrated in the guinea-pig coronary artery, this time using quantitative measurements of $[Ca^{2+}]_i$ with Indo-1 (Ganitkevich & Isenberg, 1995). The authors also analyzed the efficacy of peak Ca^{2+} current in triggering CICR and similarly concluded that at physiological $[Ca^{2+}]_o$ a synchronized CICR could not be triggered by peak Ca^{2+} current. This type of interaction between L-type Ca^{2+} channels and RyRs in smooth muscles was later termed "loose coupling" (Kotlikoff, 2003), meaning that activation of RyRs is non-obligate and may occur with a variable delay after activation of L-type channels.

Such graded CICR in vascular myocytes, which is initiated specifically by persistent Ca^{2+} entry (e.g., via the above discussed Ca^{2+} "window current"), rather than by large peak Ca^{2+} currents during strong membrane depolarization, seems to ideally suit requirements for the generation and maintenance of vascular tone.

Apart from the ability of CICR to amplify persistent depolarization-induced Ca^{2+} entry via L-type VGCCs for vascular tone generation/ maintenance, there is another important aspect of CICR's role not to be ignored. With the advancement of laser confocal calcium imaging, it became possible to visualize small, discrete and highly localized Ca^{2+} release events via a cluster of tightly spaced RyRs, which were termed "Ca^{2+} sparks." Such events have actually been initially predicted to occur from recordings of spontaneous transient outward currents, or STOCs, via closely located to RyRs plasmalemmal BK_{Ca} channels (Benham & Bolton, 1986). By combined the whole-cell patch clamp current measurements with simultaneous confocal imaging of $[Ca^{2+}]_i$ using Fluo-3 in voltage-clamped guinea-pig mesenteric artery myocytes it was shown that (i) Ca^{2+} sparks generated by openings of clustered RyRs could occur spontaneously at several frequently discharging Ca^{2+} sites, or FDSs; and (ii) Ca^{2+} sparks could activate either Ca^{2+}-activated Cl^- channels to produce depolarizing spontaneous transient inward currents, or STICs, or BK_{Ca} channels to produce hyperpolarizing STOCs (Gordienko et al. 1999). Evidently, the spontaneous activity of RyRs, which is also enhanced by elevated $[Ca^{2+}]_i$, can be one of the central mechanisms of bidirectional control of membrane potential and hence vascular tone.

IP_3Rs are also abundantly expressed in VSMs. They are activated by IP_3, which is formed by the hydrolysis of phosphatidylinositol 4,5-bisphosphate (PIP_2), along with diacylglycerol (DAG), by the enzyme PLC in consequence to activation of $G_{q/11}$-coupled receptors, of which there are also abundantly expressed multiple subtypes in vascular myocytes. While the key role of IP_3-induced Ca^{2+} release (IICR) in producing receptor agonist-induced contractions is well established, the relation between IICR and vascular tone remains not so clear. For example, inhibition of IP_3Rs with xestospongin C did not affect vascular tone in murine resistance arteries (Mauban et al. 2015).

However, it should be noted that just like RyRs, IP_3Rs can also generate discrete spontaneous Ca^{2+} releases, in this case termed "Ca^{2+} puffs," probably at least in part due to spontaneous activation of G protein-coupled receptors in their ligand-free state (Sadee, 2023). By the same logic as in the case of Ca^{2+} sparks, Ca^{2+} puffs can also locally target plasmalemmal Ca^{2+}-activated channels. Thuse, there are several well-documented cases whereby IICR via IP_3Rs by modulating activity of other types of ion channels, such as TRPM4 or cross-talk with RyRs, can affect vascular tone (Gonzales et al. 2010; Gordienko & Bolton, 2002). There may be even physical coupling between IP_3Rs and other types of ion channels. Most notably, all TRPC channels, the function of which is important for vascular tone (to be discussed in detail later), possess the so-called calmodulin and IP_3R binding domain, or CIRB, at the channels' C-terminus (Tang et al. 2001). Displacement of the inhibitory calmodulin from this site by IP_3R may activate these channels (Chen et al. 2020; Zhang et al. 2001).

Importantly, it was found that an elevation in $[Ca^{2+}]_i$ has both an early potentiating and delayed inhibitory effects on IICR (Zholos et al. 1994). The latter action allows for Ca^{2+} stores refilling and causes a reduction in $[Ca^{2+}]_i$ this way contributing to the cytosolic Ca^{2+} oscillations, which are typically observed in receptor agonist-stimulated myocytes. The elevated $[Ca^{2+}]_i$ implies that some amount of Ca^{2+} will be necessary to extrude from the cell via the action of Ca^{2+} pumps and exchangers. However, in the long term, a tightly regulated balance between Ca^{2+} extrusion and Ca^{2+} entry must be maintained. This leads us to the next import question regarding the relevance of the so-called store dependent Ca^{2+} entry, or SOCE, to the maintenance of vascular tone.

Capacitative Ca^{2+} Entry

The idea that the filling state of intracellular Ca^{2+} stores should somehow signal the activation of some Ca^{2+}-permeable plasma membrane channels was first introduced by J. W. Putney in 1986 (Putney, 1986), but it took many years of research before molecular components of the presumed 'capacitative calcium entry' have been identified (Putney, 2009). It is now well established that STIM1 and STIM2 proteins function as sensors of Ca^{2+} concentration in the endo(sarco)plasmic reticulum, whereby these initiate signalling cascade causing store-operated Ca^{2+}-permeable channels in the plasma membrane to open. Many subtypes of TRP channels have been proposed to serve this purpose (see below) but eventually Orai1, Orai2, and Orai3 channels with little structural similarity to other known cation Ca^{2+}-permeable channels have been identified (Putney, 2009). Expression of Orai and STIM is differentiated, quiescent VSMCs, and their role is likely to be of major importance in phenotypic switching between quiescent and proliferative/migratory myocytes (Ghosh et al. 2017). However, SOCE is well documented in the vasculature, where it an integral part of responses to voltage changes, receptor activation, mechanical stimuli and the filling state of the SR Ca^{2+} stores (X. Liu & Pan, 2021; Y. Wang et al. 2008). We are now witnessing revising the role of TRP channels in SOCE, as it turned out that some TRPs can interact both structurally and functionally with the STIM/Orai machinery (Y. Liao et al. 2008) (see the section on TRP channels below).

Potassium Channels Keep Depolarization-Induced Ca^{2+} Entry in Check

Excessive vascular tone would be obviously detrimental to adequate blood flow. It is now clear that the level of contractility of smooth muscle is determined by membrane potential, which, in turn, largely depends on changes in potassium membrane conductance. There are four main types of potassium channels - potential-dependent K^+ channels (K_V), inwardly rectifying K^+ channels (K_{IR}), ATP-dependent K^+ channels (K_{ATP}) and large-conductance Ca^{2+}-dependent K^+ channels (BK_{Ca} or Maxi-K), which are encoded by the *Slo1* gene (*KNCMA1*). It is through the latter type of channels that a large (up to 80%) part of the outward current flows, which makes it the main modulator of smooth muscle contractile activity under both normal and pathological conditions.

Recent analysis of current drug targets on which 1578 FDA-approved drugs act placed ion channels among the top privileged target families (Santos et al. 2016). In other words, ion channels have represented privileged class of molecular targets for the pharmacological correction of various pathological conditions - currently 19% of all known molecular targets, followed by G protein coupled receptors (GPCRs) – 12%. As the largest number of drugs is acting on GPCRs, this means that there is an important gap to be filled by investigating the exact roles of ion channels in disease states and developing their selective ligands. Maxi-K channel is definitely one of the most promising candidates for such developments, including VSM relaxation in hypertension (Kaczorowski & Garcia, 2016)

Maxi-K channels are under dual control by voltage and $[Ca^{2+}]_i$ since they are allosterically activated by both membrane depolarization and an increase in $[Ca^{2+}]_i$. Moreover, these channels form a unique negative feedback control loop whereby any excessive cell membrane depolarization or abnormally high $[Ca^{2+}]_i$ is efficiently terminated by maxi-K channel openings leading to membrane hyperpolarization and termination of Ca^{2+} influx via depolarization activated Ca^{2+} channels. This restores calcium homeostasis and multiple related functions controlled by Ca^{2+} as universal cellular second messengers. It is thus not surprising that much effort has been already invested in the development of BK_{Ca} channel activators owing to considerable therapeutic perspectives (Bentzen, Olesen, Rønnand, Grunnet, 2014).

Experimental studies of the role of ion channels in vascular dysfunction under different pathological conditions, including ionizing radiation impact (Tishkin, Rekalov, Ivanova, et al, 2007; Soloviev, Tishkin, Ivanova, et al. 2009; Soloviev, Tishkin., Kyrychenko, 2009; Soloviev., Prudnikov., Tsyvkin et al. 2009; Kizub,, Pavlova,, Ivanova., Soloviev, 2010, Kyrychenko, Tishkin., Dosenko, et al. 201), AH (Novokhatska, Tishkin S, Dosenko et al. 2013) and the diabetic angiopathies development (Klymenko, Novokhatska, Kizub et at., 2014; Soloviev, I. Ivanova, M. Melnyk et al. 2019) were performed in our laboratory. All these demonstrated a decrease in the expression level of BK_{Ca} channels and a decrease in the related outward currents carried through potassium channels of high conductivity. Moreover, ыщьу pharmacological interventions, such as the treatment with mesenchymal stem cells (Soloviev, Prudnikov, Tsyvkin et al. 2009), application of liposomal quercetin (Soloviev, Tishkin, Kyrychenko, 2009) and RNA interference technique (Kyrychenko, Tishkin, Dosenko et al. 2012; Novokhatska, Tishkin, Dosenko et al. 2013; Klymenko, Novokhatska, Kizub et at, 2014) aimed at restoring potassium conductivity, were accompanied by visible normalization of vascular tone.

Just recently, we have been fortunate to discover a new, almost exotic way of remote control of BK_{Ca} function and, accordingly, the level of membrane potential using plasmonic gold nanoparticles (Soloviev. Zholos, Ivanova et al, 2015). We will discuss this phenomenon in more detail below.

In this regard, mention should be made of the work of Li, Wang, Sun, Chai et al. (2017) where the authors presented some results of studies of a possible role of Nrf2 signaling in BK_{Ca} regulation. They concluded that BK channel's function, the main ionic trigger of vasodilation, is significantly impaired in diabetes due to oxidative stress development and proteolysis of the auxiliary BK-β1 subunit, which enhances Ca^{2+}-sensitivity of the channel. However, most importantly, they established that the Nrf2 signalling pathway acts as the main regulator of cellular redox status in diabetes. They found that Nrf2 expression was markedly reduced in *db/db* diabetic mouse aortas, and this effect was associated with significant downregulation of the BK-β1 subunit. The authors thus hypothesized that this signaling pathway plays a decisive role in the suppression of BK_{Ca} channel function in diabetic vascular disease. Interestingly, activation of Nrf2 by dimethyl fumarate preserved BK-β1 expression and protected BK_{Ca} channel and vascular function in *db/db* coronary arteries. These studies clearly indicate that Nrf2 should be identified as a novel therapeutic target for pharmacological intervention in diabetic vascular disease. In another study, much reduced Ca^{2+}-sensitivity of the activity of single BK_{Ca} channels from diabetic retinal myocytes due to downregulation of the β1 subunit in diabetes (McGahon et al. 2007).

The heart is by far the most obvious example of autorhythmic activity. Although all cardiomyocytes are initially endowed with pacemaker activity in the early embryonic stages, most cardiac cells eventually differentiate into the working myocardium, which lacks pacemaker properties. While the anatomical structures of the conduction system were identified more than 100 years ago, the molecular mechanisms underlying the cardiac automaticity in pacemaker cells remain controversial. Recently, new data were published on this matter (Weisbord, Khun, Bueno, Peretz, Attali, 2016). The authors presented evidence for the previously unrecognized role of the SK4 ($K_{Ca}3.1$) Ca^{2+}-activated K^+ channel conductance in pacemaker cells. By exquisitely balancing the inward currents during the diastolic depolarization, the SK4 channels appear to play a crucial role in human cardiac automaticity. It is possible that a similar mechanism also exists in SM cells.

With regard to the role of ion channels in smooth muscle and endothelial cells, William F. Jackson has recently published the most comprehensive reviews (Jackson, 2020, 2022). The author states that myogenic tone is a hallmark feature of arterioles in microcirculation. The above-mentioned pressure-induced contractile activation of vascular SM cells significantly contributes to the regulation and maintenance of blood pressure, blood flow, capillary pressure and fluid balance. According to the author, different types of ion channels play an important role in the genesis and maintenance of myogenic tone. Namely, mechanosensitive ion channels such as TRPC6 may serve as one of the sensors of pressure-induced membrane stress, and TRPC6 along with TRPM4 channels are responsible for pressure-induced SM depolarization that may be supported by the activity of Ca^{2+}-activated Cl^- channels and inhibition of voltage-gated K_V channels, inwardly-rectifying K_{IR} channels and ATP-sensitive K_{ATP} channels. Membrane potential depolarization activates voltage-gated Ca^{2+} channels, with $Ca_V1.2$ channels playing a central role. Calcium entry through $Ca_V1.2$ channels, which is amplified by Ca^{2+} release through IP_3Rs in the form of Ca^{2+} waves in some arterioles, provides the major source of the activator calcium responsible for arteriolar myogenic tone. Stabilizing negative feedback comes from depolarization- and Ca^{2+}-induced activation of BK_{Ca} channels and depolarization-induced activation of K_V channels. Myogenic tone also is weakened by the tonic activity of K_{IR} and K_{ATP} channels. In our opinion, all of the above is related to the modulators of the basal tone and is not directly related to the nature of the basal tone.

Of course, in the end, the basal tone is the pure sum of all the effects of the various modulators. At the same time, there must be some main core (a kind of "carrier frequency") intrinsic to smooth muscle cells, on which all possible external modulating influences are superimposed.

In short, the role of potassium and chloride currents in the regulation of vascular tone is as follows. The opening K^+ channels lead to diffusion of K^+ ions out of the cell, membrane hyperpolarization, closure of voltage-gated Ca^{2+} channels, decreased intracellular Ca^{2+}, which leads to vasodilation. The closure of K^+ channels has the opposite effect. The opening of Cl^- channels leads to diffusion of Cl^- ions out of the cell, membrane depolarization, opening of voltage-gated Ca^{2+} channels, increased intracellular Ca^{2+}, which leads to vasoconstriction. Closure of Cl^- channels has the opposite effect.

A special role in the regulation of vascular tone according to Jackson (2020) belongs to calcium-dependent channels with focus on the family of Ca^{2+}-dependent K^+ channels (Ledoux, Werner, Brayden, and Nelson, 2006). The small-conductance (SK) channel and intermediate-conductance (IK) potassium channels, located predominantly in the vascular endothelium, are the first, due to their location, to be included in the chain of events associated with the development of myogenic reactions under the action of autocoids and changes in intravascular pressure and blood flow. The activation of these channels can lead to vasodilation. These channels regulate the membrane potential of endothelial cells and are activated by a rise in $[Ca^{2+}]_i$. Membrane potential hyperpolarization of endothelial cells enhances the driving force for calcium entry, possibly through TRP channels. An increase in $[Ca^{2+}]_i$ would then elevate nitric oxide synthase (NOS) activity and synthesis of NO, as well as production of arachidonic acid metabolites (prostacyclin, PGI_2), epoxyeicosatrienoic acids (EETs), which acting jointly and separately can hyperpolarize and relax the adjacent myocytes (Jackson, 2022).

In turn, endothelial hyperpolarization could also be transmitted through myoendothelial gap junctions (MGJ) to hyperpolarize vascular myocytes, which leads to vasodilation by decreasing calcium entry via VGCCs.

As already noted, increased intravascular pressure leads to membrane depolarization, activation of VGCCs, an increase in $[Ca^{2+}]_i$ and vasoconstriction. This vasoconstriction process is opposed by stimulation of calcium sparks, which activate BK channels in vascular myocytes, membrane hyperpolarization and relaxation of arterial smooth muscle (Nelson et al. 1995). From a practical point of view, it is important because reduced expression of SK channels in the endothelium or inactivation of genes encoding BK_{Ca} proteins inevitably leads to SM membrane depolarization, increased vascular tone, and hypertension development.

Since arterial myocytes are not electrically excitable, we hypothesize that it is the steady-state influx of Ca^{2+} via L-VGCCs due to the existence of the so-called "window current" that may be primarily responsible for maintaining vascular tone and producing HPV in response to relatively small and slow membrane depolarizations. Indeed, it is extensively documented that hypoxia normally inhibits outward K^+ currents in pulmonary artery myocytes, thus causing membrane depolarization (Sweeney, Yuan., 2000), but this effect is lacking in DM (Soloviev, Ivanova, Melnyk et al. 2019).

Voltage-Independent "Leak" Channels Settle the Background Scene for Smooth Muscle Electrogenesis

In electrophysiology, the so-called "leakage" channels have long been known. These are non-operated (independent, "flowing") ion permeable pores in the cell membrane. Of course, this name is conditional and reflects only the basic functional state of such channels. Perhaps, completely independent and uncontrollable ion channels in the membrane simply do not exist, and all of them, one way or another, are regulated. However, the so-called "uncontrolled" channels, as a rule, are in a constantly open state and provide a constant ion current flow through the open pore of the channel both into and out of the cell. The process of moving ions through such channels proceeds passively due to diffusion under the action of chemical forces (along the gradient of their concentration) and/or electric forces (along the electric charge gradient between the inner and outer sides of the membrane). So do, for example, potassium leakage channels (they participate in the formation of nerve cells membrane resting potential), epithelial sodium channels (these provide reuptake of sodium ions in the kidneys, rectum, lungs, sweat glands, etc., and also provide perception of the salt taste with taste buds in the mouth), and anionic channels in erythrocytes (they pass Cl^-, OH^-, HCO^{-3}).

Generally speaking, it is precisely the potassium and chloride channels, with their very close to "ohmic" volt-ampere characteristic, that would seem to be the main candidates for the role of "leakage" channels. But these channels are not constantly open (if that were the case, they could not be identified in single-channel recordings). There must bc a "leak" option through some other type of channel. The 4TM family of K^+ channels, or K_{2P} channels, is one of the most obvious candidates fulfilling the role of background potassium channels in vascular myocytes, similarly to maty other types of cells. These channels are active at potentials that correspond to normal resting potential of vascular myocytes, and they are regulated by various neurotransmitters, second messengers, lipids, pH, temperature, and membrane stretch. Structurally, these channels share a unique design - their pore-forming α-subunit contains two pore (P) loop domains, while the functional channel is formed by two such subunits. Since the activity of these channels is critically important in establishing the resting membrane potential, it is logical to think that the activity of K_{2P} channels is yet another important contributor to vascular tone formation. In vascular physiology, research has mainly focused on several members of the 4TMP family of K^+ channels, namely TWIK-1, TREK-1, and TASK-1(Bryan et al. 2007; Wiedmann et al. 2016a). In rat mesenteric and pulmonary arteries, TASK-1 was implicated in the pH-induced changes in membrane potential (Gardener et al. 2004). Gurney and her co-workers concluded that the activity of TASK-1 channels makes significant contribution to the resting membrane potential of pulmonary artery myocytes (Gurney et al. 2003). In the basilar artery, polyunsaturated fatty acids (PUFA) induced vasodilation specifically via TREK-1 activation (Blondeau et al. 2007). Similarly, in rat cerebral arteries arachidonic acid seems to primarily activate K_{2P} channels, thus producing vasodilation (Bryan et al. 2006). Based on this evidence, K_{2P} channels are currently investigated in terms of their therapeutic significance for the treatment of cardiovascular diseases (Wiedmann et al. 2016b).

Deviation 9. *Some VSM cells are considered to belong to so-called non-excitable tissues (House, Potier, Basalion et al. 2008). This seems to contradict the above-described ion channels that produce inward currents, including even low-voltage-activated T-type Ca^{2+} channels and TTX-sensitive voltage-gated Na^+ channels that underlie pacemaking and action potential generation in other cell types. It is generally accepted that the dominance of outward K^+ currents prevents action potential discharge in vascular myocytes. The question is – can these cells produce an action potential providing that the balance between inward and outward currents is somehow reversed in favor of the inward depolarizing currents? This is exactly the question that Burdyga and his co-workers asked. They performed an elegant study on the rat mesenteric resistance arteries in the presence of TEA, the common blocker of various types of K^+ channels, and BayK 8644, the activator of L-type VGCCs (Borysova et al. 2018). The authors measured, using intact segments of mesenteric arteries, smooth muscle membrane potential with sharp glass microelectrodes together with simultaneous measurement of $[Ca^{2+}]_i$ and force at two ends of the segments of resistance artery. They found that the artificial dominance of L-type channel current triggered action potential discharge, propagating intercellular Ca^{2+} waves and vasoconstriction, which were independent of the endothelium. One novel aspect of this study was the finding that gap junctions are critically important for the spread of electrical activity and vasoconstriction along the entire length of arterial segment.*

Receptor-Operated and Polymodal TRP Channels Are Orchestrating the Function of Other Ion Channels to Enable Appropriate Cell Response to the Changing Environment

In the scheme of the events controlling vascular tone and governed by various types of ion channels discussed thus far the molecular nature of receptor-operated, and in the wider context – chemosensitive Ca^{2+} channels, remained unknown for the longest time. The situation has dramatically changed since the cloning of the first mammalian homologue of the *Drosophila* TRP channel that plays a key role in phototransduction of fruit flies (Minke, 2010). This was done simultaneously by two groups who cloned TRPC1 channel, the human homologue for the *Drosophila trp* gene (Wes et al. 1995; X. Zhu et al. 1995). Other mammalian TRP channels have been cloned in rapid succession, and soon enough their functional characterization, initially in heterologous expression systems and then increasingly in native cells, established a new major class of universal cellular sensors that can respond to a wide variety of chemical (lipids, protons, free radicals, various natural and artificial exogenous compounds etc.) and physical stimuli (membrane voltage, temperature, membrane tension, shear stress etc.) (Clapham, 2003; Numata et al. 2016).

Unlike the previous classification of Ca^{2+}-permeable channels into two main groups, voltage-gated, and ligand-gated channels, the enormous diversity of the gating mechanisms of TRP channels their current classification is based purely on the structural homology of their amino acid sequences. Accordingly, there are six subfamilies of the TRP superfamily in mammalian cells: TRPC, TRPM, TRPV, TRPA, TRPP, and TRPML (Figure 26). An overview of these channels can be found elsewhere (Clapham, 2003; Ramsey et al. 2006; Venkatachalam & Montell, 2007; H. Wang et al. 2020; Wu et al. 2010; Zholos, 2021; M. X. Zhu, 2016). The interested reader can also consult the two volume "Mammalian Transient Receptor Potential (TRP) Cation Channels" that details expression profile, molecular, biophysical and pharmacological properties, as well lessons learned from gene knockout studies for each individual member of this superfamily of TRP channels (Nilius & Flockerzi, 2014). Receptor-operated TRPC4 channel is an excellent example of complex gating diversity of TRP channels. It was most extensively characterized as a molecular counterpart of the cholinergic excitation-contraction coupling in gastrointestinal myocytes, in which the cells current that the channel produces is enormous compared to other TRPs in native cells current, about 1 nA on average. First, TRPC4 activation critically requites co-stimulation of two differentially coupled GPCRs, the M_2 receptor coupled to $G_{i/o}$ proteins and the M_3 receptor coupled to $G_{q/11}$ proteins. Second, TRPC4 is a Ca^{2+}-dependent channel – at abnormally low $[Ca^{2+}]_i$ (e.g. 10 mM BAPTA in the pipette solution) no channel activity could be seen even with strong receptor stimulation. Third, TRPC4 channel is activated by membrane depolarization with a Boltzmann slope factor of about 24 mV, which is a fairly strong voltage dependence. Fourth, TRPC4 activity is controlled by PIP_2 (Zholos, 2006; Zholos et al. 2024). Obviously, such channel gating diversity makes it difficult, even impossible to distinguish between the main and any additional, or modulatory channel activation mechanisms.

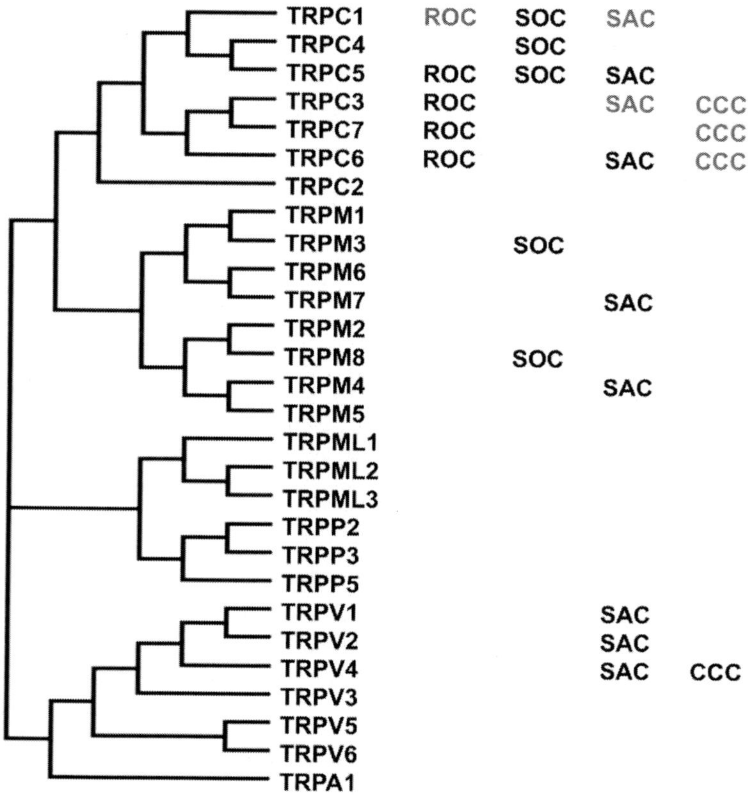

Figure 26. Structural relatedness of mammalian TRP channels. Their established activation mechanisms in the vasculature are denoted: receptor-operated cation channels (ROC), store-operated channels (SOC), stretch-activated cation channels (SAC), and constitutive cation channels (CCC), and sensory cation channels (SCC). These are shown in grey where the evidence is still not compelling.

With this background, we shall now focus on the roles of various TRP subtypes in vascular tone. Due to a number of their features and, above all, their responsiveness to a wide spectrum of chemical and physical factors and diversity of their regulation, TRPs are most suitable for the role of modulators, a kind of adjusters of basal tone (Figure 26).

Various cation TRP channels, most of which are Ca^{2+}-permeable channels, are expressed in the vasculature, both in vascular myocytes (Alonso-Carbajo et al. 2017; Beech et al. 2004; Di & Malik, 2010; Gonzalez-Cobos & Trebak, 2010; Guibert et al. 2011; Zholos et al. 2011) and in the endothelium (Earley & Brayden, 2015; Kwan et al. 2007; Thakore & Earley, 2019; Wong

& Yao, 2011). When activated these channels produce two major effects: (i) membrane depolarization causing Ca^{2+} via TRPs themselves, as well as via VGCCs, and (2) an increase in $[Ca^{2+}]_i$. Notably, the latter can be induced by intracellular located (e.g. in the SR membranes) TRP channels, which can thus support Ca^{2+} release from the SR. In this connection, there is increasing interest to the function of TRP channels in other intracellular organelles, including the mitochondria and lysosomes (Zhang et al. 2018; Zhao & Tsang, 2017). Consequently, the impact of TRP channels on intracellular Ca^{2+} homeostasis was linked to diverse vascular functions, including receptor-activated contractility, myogenic tone, endothelial permeability, responses to oxidative stress, cell proliferation, migration, phenotypic changes, and thermoregulation of vascular tone.

Comprehensive analysis of the diverse signal transduction pathways and gating mechanisms of native TRP channels in vascular myocytes led W. A. Large and his colleagues to propose an operational classification of these channels into four main types: receptor-operated cation channels (ROCs), store-operated channels (SOCs), stretch-activated cation channels (SACs), and constitutive cation channels (CCCs) (Albert & Large, 2006).

ROCs

The best characterized TRP ROC channel is TRPC6, which underlines norepinephrine-induced membrane depolarization and contraction of vascular myocytes. This current was initially investigated in rabbit portal vein myocytes (Byrne & Large, 1988), eventually culminating in the identification of TRPC6 as its molecular counterpart in 2001 (Inoue et al. 2001). In vascular myocytes, TRPC6 is primarily activated by DAG produced by activation of $G_{q/11}$ G-proteins and PLC. Surprisingly, mice deficient in TRPC6 instead of the expected loss of vascular tone and hypotension showed a higher agonist-induced contractility in isolated aortic rings, as well as an elevated systemic blood pressure (Dietrich et al. 2005)/ This was explained by upregulation of TRPC3, which is the closely related, but constitutively active member of the DAG activated TRPC3/6/7 group of the TRPC subfamily. TRPC3 mediates pyrimidine receptor-induced depolarization of cerebral arteries. These channels also contribute to basal tone, but do not appear to be involved in the myogenic response (Dietrich et al. 2006; Reading et al. 2005). One important level of complexity regarding studies of TRP channels in vascular myocytes, as well as in other cell types, is formation of heterotetramers, which show altered gating mechanisms and functional properties. TRPC3 and TRPC6 channels can heteromultimerize. This is of clinical relevance as an increased contribution of TRPC3 to TRPC3/C6 heteromultimeric assembly was found to promote membrane depolarization and contractility of mesenteric artery myocytes in essential hypertension (Álvarez-Miguel et al. 2017).

Other receptor agonists, such as angiotensin II and endothelin-1, can activate TRPC6, as well as TRPC1, TRPC3, TRPC5 and TRPC7 channels, in smooth muscles of different blood vessels (Peppiatt-Wildman et al. 2007; Saleh et al. 2006, 2009a)

SOCs

It has been known for a long time that depletion of intracellular Ca^{2+} stores in vascular myocytes increases the uptake of the radioactive isotope ^{45}Ca (Casteels & Droogmans, 1981). In patch-clamp experiments, agents that are known to cause Ca^{2+} store depletion, such as thapsigargin and cyclopiazonic acid, activated inward currents, and especially clear-cut evidence was obtained in single channel recordings (Albert & Large, 2003). Consequently, TRPC1 has received much attention in vascular physiology as a putative SOC channel, already beginning from the early studies of the SOCE phenomenon (Golovina et al. 2001; Saleh et al. 2009b; Sweeney et al. 2002; Takahashi et al. 2007; Xu & Beech, 2001). In endothelial cells, TRPC4 functions as an SOC channel, and its knockout significantly impairs agonist-induced vasorelaxation (Freichel et al. 2001).

SACs

Multiple TRP isoforms have been implicated in the control of arterial myogenic tone, including TRPC6, TRPM4, and TRPV1 (Brayden et al. 2008; Earley & Brayden, 2015; Jackson, 2020; McGahon et al. 2016; Watanabe et al. 2008; Zholos et al. 2011). There are other mechanosensitive TRPs, but their involvement in the myogenic response is less well established. Overall, regarding the role of various TRPs in the myogenic response, the picture becomes rather blurred. There are simply too many different candidates for this role, which makes it difficult to be certain whether or not this is due to imperfectly selective channel modulators used in different studies, compensatory upregulation of other TRPs in gene knockouts, technical difficulties in reproducing myogenic response in single cells, differences between vascular beds examined, the already mentioned issue of hetero-multimerization of different TRP subtypes, or even some other yet unknown factors.

The role of the stretch-activated TRPV2 in the myogenic constriction of retinal arterioles is most interesting. The retina is considered to be one of the most metabolically active tissues, yet the retinal microcirculation lacks an autonomic nerve supply. Therefore, retinal blood flow is predominantly controlled by local signaling mechanisms, most importantly by autoregulation via a myogenic mechanism (Barabas et al. 2020). Surprisingly, T.M. Curtis and his co-workers found that a number of putative mechanosensitive TRPs were expressed in VSMs in retinal arterioles, including TRPC1, TRPM7, TRPP1, TRPV1, and TRPV4, but only TRPV2 specifically mediated hypotonic stretch-induced Ca^{2+} influx and cation currents in these cells. In the cell-attached configuration of the patch-clamp techniques, application of negative pressure to the pipette interior induced bursts of single channel openings, which were blocked by the TRPV2 inhibitor tranilast and TRPV2 pore-blocking antibodies when these were added to the pipette solution (McGahon et al. 2016).

CCCs

Constitutively active Ca^{2+}-permeable cation channels are undoubtedly important in the regulation of membrane resting potential, but their definition is rather vague. In principle, any type of ion channel can open spontaneously. Even the classical depolarization-activated ion channels can show rare openings at very negative potentials in single-channel recordings, if these are long enough. This is because the Boltzmann-type equation that describes the relation between channel open probability and voltage approximates zero level asymptotically, never reaching absolute zero open probability.

The real question is whether or not such spontaneous channel openings are functionally relevant. In rabbit ear artery myocytes, spontaneous openings of cation channels with conductances of 15, 25 and 40 pS were observed in outside-out patches (Albert et al. 2003). These channels had similar, but not identical properties compared to TRPC6 in portal vein. They were thus suggested to belong to the TRPC3/6/7 subgroup of TRP channels (Albert & Large, 2006). Other TRPs detected in vascular myocytes and implicated in mechanotransduction include TRPC1, TRPC5, TRPM4, TRPM7, TRPV1, TRPV2, and TRPV4 (Zholos & Curtis, 2013).

The discussed functional roles of vascular TRPs are denoted in Figure C. It is evident that different members of the TRPC subfamily have been largely implicated in vascular functions where they can fulfil the various discussed roles. However, significant complexity is also evident as the same channel type, depending of course on the experimental conditions but, most likely, on physiological conditions as well, can assume different roles. Indeed, it is now well appreciated that different TRPs can be activated, often in synergy, by multiple signals. Another level of complexity arises when one includes into consideration endothelial TRPs. In endothelial cells, activation of Ca^{2+}-permeable ion channels causes the production of various vasoactive substances, most of which evoke vasodilation, thus opposing generally vasoconstrictive roles of TRPs expressed in vascular myocytes. Endothelial TRPs have been comprehensively reviewed elsewhere (Thakore & Earley, 2019; Watanabe et al. 2008; Wong & Yao, 2011; Yao & Garland, 2005; Zholos & Curtis, 2013).

It should be noted that survey of functional expression of vanilloid channels showed that TRPV4, which is mechano-, osmo- and temperature sensitive channel, was the most abundantly expressed TRPV subtype in pulmonary arterial and aortic smooth muscle, followed by TRPV2 (X. R. Yang et al. 2006). This stimulated our interest in this particular vascular TRP channel.

Deviation 10. *We investigated TRPV4's role in vascular tone of pulmonary arteries (Dryn et al. 2016). TRPV4 is a multifunctional channel that can interact with numerous other proteins and that is active at temperatures over 30°C. In addition, it is activated by osmotic and mechanical stimuli, the endocannabinoid anandamide (via its metabolites arachidonic acid and 5,6-EET) and it is upregulated under hypoxic conditions (Garcia-Elias et al. 2014). This rather unique set of properties makes TRPV4 an important vascular TRPV4 channel. Indeed, there are now more than 400 papers published on the role of TRPV4 in vascular function and disease!*

In our research, we found that activation of TRPV4 by its selective agonist GSK1016790A in the presence of PE caused a biphasic contractile response, whereby the initial vasorelaxation (by about 65% of PE-induced contraction) was followed by strong contraction (to about 140% of PE-induced contraction). These reactions remained after de-endothelialization of the rat pulmonary arteries, and they were completely abolished by the selective blocker of TRPV4, HC-067047, confirming the specific involvement of

TRPV4 (D. Dryn et al. 2016). A more recent study addressed the evident complexity of the underlying ion channel mechanisms of these biphasic contractile responses. Using selective blockers of BK_{Ca} and L-type VGCCs, the authors showed that the relaxation was caused by STOCs, which are known to be activated by Ca^{2+} sparks and BK_{Ca} channel activation as explained above (Gordienko et al. 1999), while the secondary TRPV4-mediated membrane depolarization induced Ca^{2+} entry via L-type VGCCs and thus VSM contraction (Dryn, Melnyk, Melanaphy, et al. 2023). To explain these observations, as well as their similar findings regarding the role of the menthol and cold receptor TRPM8 in rat tail artery myocytes, the authors proposed that both types of TRP channels can functionally interact via Ca^{2+} signaling and membrane depolarization with RyRs and L-type VGCCs to cause such complex vascular responses. Namely, they suggested the existence of a TRP (TRPV4 or TRPM8)/RyR/BK_{Ca}/L-type VGCC functional signaloplex in vascular myocytes, whereby (i) local Ca^{2+} signaling (Ca^{2+} sparks) activate STOCs to produce membrane hyperpolarization via the TRP-RyR-BK_{Ca} coupling to deactivate L-type VGCCs for vasorelaxation, while (ii) simultaneously globally engaging, via TRP-induced depolarization, L-type VGCCs to produce Ca^{2+} entry, likely amplified by CICR in the form of global Ca^{2+} waves, for vasoconstriction. Such global Ca^{2+} waves in smooth muscle myocytes are known to recruit Ca^{2+} sparks as their "building blocks," as Ca^{2+} sparks typically proceed the development of a propagating Ca^{2+} wave (Gordienko et al. 1999; Gordienko & Zholos, 2004). Such intracellular Ca^{2+} waves in rat tail artery myocytes in response to menthol application were directly visualized using fast laser confocal imaging of the fluo-4 fluorescence signal intensity (Melanaphy et al. 2016).

Of course, the concept that local Ca^{2+} signaling (Ca^{2+} sparks) by activating STOCs and thus evoking membrane hyperpolarization can lead to vasorelaxation is not new. It was initially proposed by M.T. Nelson and his co-workers in 1995 (Nelson et al. 1995) and since then it found much experimental support in different blood vessels (Fan et al. 2019; Jaggar et al. 1998; Knot et al. 1998; Tykocki et al. 2017; Q. Y. Zhao et al. 2017).

What is new in the above scheme of events proposed by A.V. Zholos and his co-workers (Dryn et al. 2023) is that TRP channels can bi-directionally fine-tune vascular contractility (Figure 27). Through parallel membrane potential changes, as well as local and global Ca^{2+} signaling, the latter generally causes vasoconstriction.

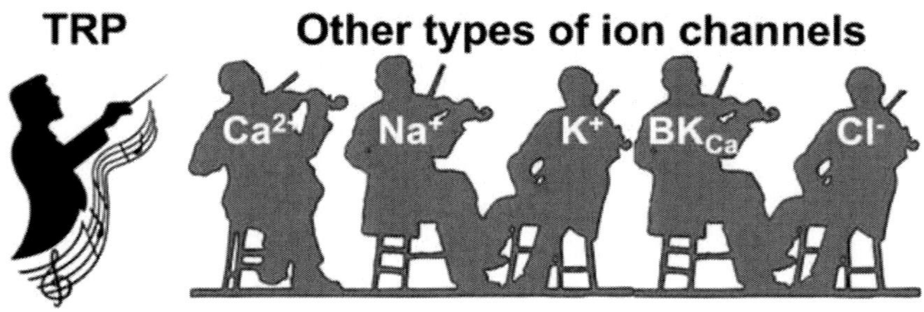

Figure 27. In vascular smooth muscles, various TRP channels can act as a "molecular conductor" of the whole orchestra composed of other "musicians" – ion channels activation or deactivation of which regulate vascular contractility. Bidirectional control of vascular tone by the activation of TRP channels, which act.

Some studies suggest that Ca^{2+}influx through TRP channels themselves can also directly initiate myocyte contraction (Earley, Brayden, 2015). The connection between oxidative stress and the activation of TRPs is also notable. Several TRP channels, namely TRPA1 and TRPM2, are redox-sensitive and play important roles in physiological and pathophysiological changes in cell function that involve redox signaling. Thus, TRPA1 and TRPM2 could be proposed as a promising pharmacological target for the therapy of redox-related vascular diseases (Kashio, and Tominaga, 2017). Moreover, TRP channels on their own are directly involved in the development of oxidative stress. Some data indicate that the TRPC sub-family serves as a necessary link between cellular redox state and intracellular Ca^{2+} homeostasis. This way, pharmacological modulation of these cellular redox sensors may be used as unique opportunities for relevant therapy (Groschner, Rosker, and Lukas. 2004; Song, Makino, and Yuan, 2011). Taken together, these data on the role of TRP channels in the implementation of oxidative stress allow us to conclude that ROS-sensitive TRP channels must have an extremely important role in the cell life or death, and related data may be the fundamental basis for new anti-ROS therapeutic agents' development (Öz, Çelik, Bejarano et al. 2017).

TRP channels present in endothelial cells also contribute to endothelium-dependent vasodilation, regulation of vascular permeability, and angiogenesis. TRP channels in other cell types, such as perivascular neurons and parenchymal astrocytes, are also important in the regulation of vascular function, primarily through the control of vascular tone. The primary regulatory paradigm for most of these functions is the control of global $[Ca^{2+}]_i$ or the propagation of subcellular Ca^{2+} signaling events that modulate cellular activity. These effects can result directly from TRP channel-mediated Ca^{2+}

influx; can be secondary to cation influx-induced membrane depolarization or activation of GPCRs; or can be caused by CICR from internal sources. Compelling evidence supports substantial roles for TRP channels in vascular disease states such as hypertension, neointimal injury, oxidative stress response, neurogenic inflammation, and pulmonary edema. These disease mechanisms involve increased expression or activation of TRP channels leading to elevated contractility, vascular hypertrophy, hyperplasia, or other forms of remodeling within the vascular wall. In light of these findings, selective pharmacological blockers of TRP channels may present exciting opportunities for the development of new therapies to prevent and treat vascular-related diseases. Our above-described findings regarding their ability to bidirectionally affect vascular tone pave the way for the development of novel drugs that can normalize vascular tone depending on its level and current functional requirements, that is increase vascular tone when it is abnormally low, and vice versa. This could be useful for vascular abnormalities, such as Raynaud's disease.

However, considerable work is needed to more fully understand the structural, functional, and mechanistic aspects of vascular TRP channel biology. In particular, important features of the organization and interactions between closely related, colocalized TRP channels and other signaling modalities in vascular cells remain largely unknown. Several recent studies have highlighted the importance of such signaling networks in native smooth muscle and endothelial cells, and further advances in this area will greatly enrich our understanding of vascular function. Proteomic analyses and super-resolution imaging approaches may be useful in providing a more complete understanding of the interactions between TRP channels and cellular elements, such as the cytoskeleton and membrane phospholipids.

Resolving the controversy surrounding the relative Ca^{2+} fractional composition of TRP currents *in vivo* will require additional efforts to record TRP currents from native vascular cells under physiological ion gradients. Such experiments can help resolve such disputes and disagreements. Successful completion of these studies will likely require the development of a more extensive array of selective pharmacological tools for modifying TRP channel activity, such as those that are currently available for probing TRPV4 channel function. There has been recent remarkable progress in the development of small-molecule potent and selective TRPC1/4/5 modulators (D. O. Dryn, Melnyk, Bon, et al. 2023; Minard et al. 2018). In addition, little is currently known about how TRP channel gene expression is regulated under normal conditions, during development, or disease.

Finally, advanced genetic approaches, including the development of cell-specific, conditional knockouts targeted to the vasculature, genetically encoded indicators, and the application of optogenetic techniques to modulate channel activity in specifically targeted locations, are needed to address deeper questions regarding the physiological significance of TRP channels. These new approaches will allow a more comprehensive appreciation of the molecular and cellular complexity of TRP channels in the vasculature, providing substantial insight into fundamental mechanisms of vascular physiology and pathophysiology (Earley and Brayden, 2015).

Jackson WF (2022) argues that myogenic tone is a hallmark feature of resistance arteries and arterioles. This pressure-induced contractile activity of VSMCs sets the resting diameter of resistance arteries and arterioles such that they can dilate or constrict to regulate their hydraulic resistance controlling blood flow to and within the body's tissues and organs, thus maintaining homeostasis. Despite the fundamental importance of myogenic tone to the physiology of the cardiovascular system in health and disease, our understanding of the mechanisms responsible for myogenic tone remains incomplete. Phan, Ton, Gulyás et al. (2022) presented recently interesting data and concluded that TRPV1 channels contribute to changes in a rapid myogenic tone of arteries. They postulated that arterioles maintain blood flow by adjusting their diameter in response to changes in intravascular pressure. In this process called the myogenic response, a VSM mechanosensor controls tone predominantly by altering the membrane potential. In general, myogenic responses occur relatively slowly (minutes). However, in the heart and skeletal muscle tone is activated rapidly (tens of seconds) and terminated by brief (100 ms) arterial constrictions. Only renal afferent arterioles, which show high autoregulatory speed and efficiency that maintain renal blood flow and glomerular filtration rate, can compete with them (Carlstrom et al. 2015).

These authors identified extensive expression of TRPV1 in the smooth muscle of arterioles supplying skeletal muscle, heart, and fat and revealed a critical role for TRPV1 in the rapid myogenic tone of these tissues. TRPV1 antagonists dilated skeletal muscle arterioles *in vitro* and *in vivo*, increased coronary flow in isolated hearts, and transiently decreased blood pressure. All of these pharmacologic effects were abolished by genetic disruption of TRPV1.

The stretch of isolated VSMCs or raised intravascular pressure in arteries triggered Ca^{2+} signaling and vasoconstriction. The majority of these stretch responses were TRPV1-mediated, with the remaining tone being inhibited by the TRPM4 antagonist, 9-phenanthrol.

Notably, tone developed more quickly in arteries from wild-type compared with TRPV1-null mice. Furthermore, the immediate vasodilation following brief constriction of arterioles depended on TRPV1, consistent with a rapid deactivation of TRPV1. Pharmacologic experiments revealed that membrane stretch activates PLC/PKC signaling combined with heat to activate TRPV1, and in turn, L-type Ca^{2+} channels. The authors supposed that these results suggest a critical role for TRPV1 in the dynamic regulation of myogenic tone and blood flow in the heart and skeletal muscle.

It will also be interesting to determine how TRPV1 channels interact with other ion channels that have been implicated in myogenic tone (Jackson, 2021). For example, IP_3Rs produce pressure-induced Ca^{2+} signals (Ca^{2+} waves) that contribute to myogenic tone in skeletal muscle resistance arteries and arterioles (Jackson, 2021). Does Ca^{2+} influx through TRPV1 channels directly contribute to the activation of IP_3Rs and then give rise to Ca^{2+} waves? Does Ca^{2+} influx through TRPV1 channels directly activate other Ca^{2+}-activated ion channels such as Ca^{2+}-activated Cl– channels (a positive feedback signal, amplifying membrane depolarization) or large-conductance Ca^{2+}-activated K^+ channels (a negative feedback signal that dampens membrane depolarization) (Jackson, 2021)? All these questions are still waiting to be answered. This issue may not be relevant here or it may come up later, but some recent evidence suggests that the trans-activation of angiotensin II type-1 receptors (ATR-1) is involved in the myogenic response (Hong et al. 2016; Cui et al. 2022).

Defining the precise role played by PKC in TRPs activity and vascular myogenic tone will also require further study. PKC isoforms are well established to increase the activity of CaV1.2 voltage-dependent calcium channels and inhibit several K^+ channels, all of which contribute to myogenic tone in resistance arteries (Jackson, 2021). PKC can also inhibit myosin light-chain phosphatase, producing Ca^{2+} sensitization of the contractile machinery and promoting remodeling of the actin cytoskeleton, which may contribute to myogenic tone (Jackson, 2021). How do these other PKC targets integrate with the function of TRPV1 channels concerning determining myogenic tone?

Answering these and other questions that arise from the findings of Phan et al. (2022) will require additional research. It is necessary to use multiple methods, including patch clamp recording of membrane currents, biochemical assessment of protein phosphorylation and protein-protein interactions, microelectrode or optical recording of membrane potential, high-speed Ca^{2+} imaging, pressure myography and intravital imaging of resistance arteries and arterioles that develop myogenic tone in vascular beds around the body. These studies will help to place the findings reported by Phan et al. (2022) regarding TRPV1 channels in context with the growing body of evidence indicating that an expanding list of ion channels and signaling pathways contribute to the myogenic response, myogenic tone, and their modulation in the resistance vasculature.

A note of caution - the development of drugs affecting TRP channels for the treatment of vascular disease may be problematic. Unlike, for example, the serotonin receptor, of which multiple variants have been identified thereby enabling the development of more specific antagonists, there is no evidence of similar success being likely in the context of TRP channels. With much recent interest in the multifunctional TRPV4 channel in the vasculature, a more selective blocking of identified delinquent variants of TRPV4 is not yet possible. However, another alternative may be to attempt to confine the antagonist to the locale of pathological interest by attaching it to another molecule that can be restricted to that locale. The practical utility of a drug that can inhibit TRPV4 is demonstrated by the use of butamben (n-butyl-p-aminobenzoic acid) as a local anesthetic that provides analgesia. TRPV4 and TRPA1 are blocked by micromolar butamben (although butamben also activates TRPA1 at millimolar concentrations). Butamben attenuates acute animal pain behaviors in a TRPA1- or TRPV4-dependent manner and its efficacy in accessing its target receptors through the skin can be considerably enhanced by using liposomal gel formulations, compared to plain gel formulations. While a complete identification of the extent of the functional importance of TRPV4 remains to be elucidated, sufficient is known at this juncture to justify the application of resources to develop the capacity for effective pharmacological management of this ion channel for prophylactic and therapeutic purposes in humans.

Our overview of ion channels, which are the most important in the regulation of vascular tone, would be incomplete without mentioning that fine-tuning of their pore-forming proteins involves their interactions with the so-called ancillary subunits that interact with α-subunit proteins of ion channels, this way regulating their expression, trafficking, membrane insertion, and biophysical properties. These interactions enhance the diversity of ion channel mechanisms acting in different vascular beds and under different physiological and pathological conditions. There is currently much hope that more selective pharmacological interventions may be developed along these lines (Jepps, 2017).

Chapter 14

Why Do We Need Water Channels in the Cell Membrane?

Again, about the role of water in cellular function. More precisely, about the channels of the cell membrane that selectively transport water. No matter how trite it sounds, the basis of life is water, which makes up approximately 70% of the mass of most living organisms. All biochemical reactions of the body occur in the aquatic environment. However, the water content inside and outside the cell differs, because of which the cell is forced to strictly regulate the flow of this "universal" solvent. It turns out that the regulation of the water balance inside the cells affects their ability to perform a specific, vital function for the whole organism. By regulating the flow of water and thereby their volume, nerve cells, for example, affect the state of their own ion channels that generate nerve impulses and finally our mental activity. However, back to blood vessels.

The concentration of salts, fats, proteins and carbohydrates inside the cell usually exceeds that outside, which means that the relative amount of water in it is less than in tissue fluids. The cell experiences constant both osmotic and hydrostatic water pressure, which must resist for the rest of your life. It has long been clear to researchers that water cannot overcome the cell membrane only by diffusion, since the speed and intensity of such water exchange is clearly insufficient. It was suggested that, apparently, for the rapid transport of water in the cell, there are special membrane channels with a special mechanism for regulating water flows, which, moreover, must be very specific so that harmful water-soluble (hydrophilic) compounds do not penetrate along with the water molecule, capable of damaging DNA and cellular proteins or blocking intracellular reactions.

The presence of this mechanism was found in special transmembrane channels that ensure the rapid transport of water through biological membranes. In 2003, molecular biologist Peter Agre and biochemist Roderick MacKinnon were awarded the Nobel Prize in Chemistry for the discovery of a system of special proteins called aquaporins (AQP), proteins that regulate intracellular water transport in tissues. In 1993, P. Agre proposed a name for a family of allosterically regulated proteins that form channels of the cytoplasmic membrane, which selectively let water molecules into the cytoplasm, but prevent the flow of ions of other substances. They were called "aquaporins," from Latin "aqua" – water and Greek "poros" – passage (Rainaz, Preston, Guggino and Agre, 1995).

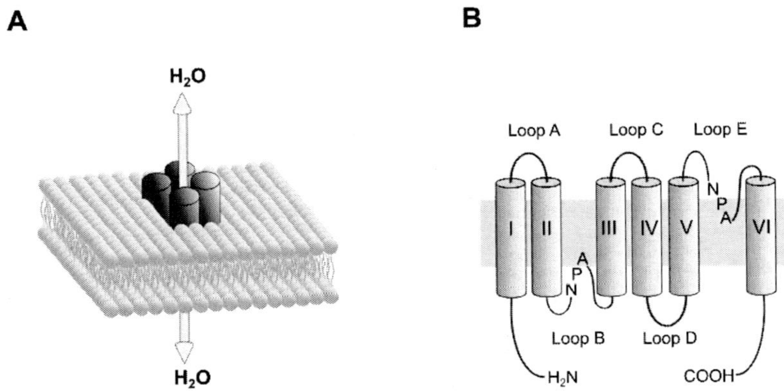

Figure 28. Topology, organization and functioning of the aquaporin water channel molecule. A: Each AQP monomer consist of six transmembrane domains (I-VI) connected by five loops (a-e) with two enclose the strictly conserved three-amino acid motif (asparagine-proline-alanine,NPA) boxes shaping the water pore, and the amino and carboxyl termini oriented toward the cytoplasm; B: Aquaporins are arranged in tetramers. The water pore does not reside in the center of the molecule but is formed by connecting loops b and e in each subunit that functions as a unique water pore allowing bidirectional water movement; C: The hourglass model for aquaporin structure. The channel consists of an extracellular and intracellular vestibule containing water in bulk solution joined in the center by a central constriction 20 Å in length where water molecules pass in single file. The a/R constriction delimited by arginine in the position 195 (R195) and histidine in the position 180 (H180) provides fixed positive charges which prevent proton passage. Two asparagine residues bound the second constriction from the highly conserved NPA motif. The single water molecule passes through the constriction with no resistance as it forms transient hydrogen bonds with the nearby asparagines. Adapted from Lehmann, Larocca, Soria, Marinelli, 2008.

Thus, AQP are a family of membrane channels that are selective for water in many tissues and cell types (Figure 28). AQP1 was the first member of the AQP family to be identified. Aquaporins are a homotetramer in which each monomer consists of six membrane-penetrating domains with cytoplasmic C- and N-termini. Loops B and E connecting the second and third, and the fifth and sixth domains, respectively, are also partly hydrophobic and are required for the formation of a single pore. According to the "hourglass" hypothesis (Figure 28), loops B and E overlap and form a permanently open narrow pore for water molecules. For instance, the structure of aquaporin-1 was firmly established by X-ray crystallography: the length and position of all helical fragments and the loops connecting them, the angle at which neighboring helices deviate from each other were determined. The segments of the polypeptide chain crossing the membrane were identified; the role of conserved amino acid residues and the effect of their individual side groups on the stability and operation of the channel has been elucidated. The architecture of the channel is such (a narrow gap in the center and expansions at opposite ends) that water can only penetrate in the form of a thin chain of molecules connected by hydrogen bonds. As a result, we now know in detail what a channel looks like that selectively passes water, but not ions.

Although aquaporins are not directly involved in the formation of transmembrane ion currents, they play an important role in providing the osmotic pressure of the cell. Aquaporins are involved in water reabsorption in the kidneys, secretion and reabsorption of cerebrospinal fluid, formation of respiratory secretions, lacrimation, and many other physiological processes. Aquaporins are easily permeable to water, but not to ions (Agre, Bonhivers, Borgnia, 1998). The plasma membrane of all mammalian cells is permeable to water, but to varying degrees. 10 types of aquaporins have been identified, each of which has its own distribution in the kidneys, lungs, retina, and brain. The first functional group of mammalians aquaporins includes AQP0, AQP1, AQP2, AQP4, and AQP5, which are only permeable to water. The second group (recently designated as aquaglyceroporins) includes AQP3, AQP7 and AQP8. These channels are highly permeable to water, glycerol, and even bulkier solutes.

The first of the open proteins that form a transmembrane channel for active water transport was named "aquaporin-1" (AQP-1) (Figure 28). Following the first molecule, other proteins of the aquaporin family were discovered: AQP-2, AQP-3, AQP-4, etc. To date, 13 aquaporins have been described in mammals, but it is assumed that this is not all. Aquaporin genes have been found and cloned. Then, the most interesting thing began - finding out their physiological role in the body. Aquaporins are the biochemical foundation for the normal functioning of the "metabolic boiler" of all organs and tissues. They are able to conduct 3 billion water molecules per 1 s per each monomer, and are present in all living cells without exception. First, the localization of aquaporin was studied in the kidneys, since in the functional unit of the kidney, the nephron, blood is filtered, forming the primary urine, which is then concentrated by reabsorption of water. Aquaporins provide water reabsorption in the urinary tubules and urinary ducts of the kidneys. Six different aquaporins work in the kidneys. Mutation of one of them leads to the disease - diabetes insipidus. In such patients, the urine in the kidneys does not concentrate, because of which their body removes a lot of fluid, the body is dehydrated, and they are constantly thirsty. Aquaporin-4 is present in the cells of the cornea of the eye and brain, and aquaporin-5 is present in the cells of the secretory glands that produce tears, sweat, and saliva. Aquaporin-3 is contained in epithelial cells and protects the skin from dehydration, which is of particular interest to cosmetologists. The same protein is found in erythrocytes. P. Agre, who at one time headed the Johns Hopkins Institute for the Study of Malaria, as well as his colleagues, paid great attention to studying the role of aquaporins in brain erythrocytes in malaria, when erythrocytes burst and cerebral edema develops. Aquaporins-7 and ¬9, belonging to the class of glycerol aquaporins, are present in adipose tissue cells, participate in fat metabolism and are activated during starvation. Aquaporin-9 is found in the liver, where it takes part in detoxification.

Aquaporins are ubiquitous, found in insects and bacteria, as well as in plants, which are necessary, since plants are dependent on the presence of water and cannot move in search of it. The nature of many diseases is associated with aquaporins. First, these are kidney diseases, visual impairment, damage and swelling of the brain, obesity, hyperthermia, malaria, and various intoxications. It should be noted that the study of aquaporins is at the stage of intensive development, so the list of diseases associated with aquaporins may expand substantially over time. For example, recently researchers from the University of Linköping (Sweden) determined that cells are able to move due to the power of water. In general, the ability of cells to move and change shape is important for many biological processes. White blood cells, for example, collect at "hot spots" such as inflammation or infection.

The stem cells of the embryo move in different directions to form organs. One of the unwanted movements is the movement of tumor cells, which leads to cancer metastasis. Cancer cells have distinct margins (leading margin and posterior margin) and move by wide, thin membrane protrusions that are thrown forward and pull the cells up. Small, finger-shaped filopodia may also protrude from the protrusion, probably a type of cell antennae that senses an external chemical stimulus. But what governs this ability to move? Water - say Swedish researchers led by Tommi Karlsson (Karlsson, Bolshakova,

Magalhães, et al. 2013), who set out their hypotheses in pLoS ONE. It turned out that AQP-9 increases the ability to move white blood cells, accumulating in the cell membrane and leading to the formation of protrusions. Data on the decisive role of aquaporin in this process opens the way to new strategies to prevent the spread of cancerous tumors.

Aquaporins can be located not only on plasma membranes. Thus, AQP6 was first identified as an intracellular water channel colocalized with H+-ATPase in intracellular vesicles. This indicates that low pH may be a natural activator of AQP6. The water permeability of activated AQP6 contributes to vesicle swelling and membrane fusion during exocytosis, as well as other cellular processes (Venero, Vizuete, Machado, Cano, 2001). Of the known cloned aquaporins, only two are localized in the brain: AQP1 is localized in adult animals in the choroid plexus, and AQP4 is the dominant membrane protein that allows water to pass into the CNS.

In the CNS, aquaporins play an important role in maintaining homeostasis of water and potassium ions, which is essential during high-frequency activity of neurons and in the postnatal period, starting from the second week, when neuronal proliferation and growth are accompanied by a decrease in extracellular space. AQP4 are involved in the regulation of osmotic balance and are possible osmosensors in the neurosecretory cells of the supraoptic nuclei of the hypothalamus, which regulate diuresis by releasing vasopressin. Aquaporins are involved in the production of cerebrospinal fluid and play a key role in the development of cerebral edema.

Are there currently any drugs that target aquaporins? P. Agre, the discoverer of aquaporins himself, believes that aquaporins are targets for pharmacological preparations of the future. In this regard, I would like to mention one important aspect of the use of aquaporins in the clinic, associated with the treatment of patients with hyperplasia and prostate cancer. Sophiris developed the drug pRX302 (topsalysin), which is a recombinant protein that, when introduced into the gland tissue, is able to bind to glycerol phosphatidyl inositol and, thus, "anchor" in the plasma membrane. Under the action of prostate tissue-specific enzymes (prostate-specific antigen - PSA), pRX302 forms water channels in the membrane. Uncontrolled entry of water leads to the destruction of glandular tissue without damaging the surrounding tissues (Agre, King, Yasui, Guggino, Ottersen, Fujiyoshi, Engel and Nielsen, 2002).

What is the role of aquaporins in the vascular tone regulation still little studied, although some data have already appeared? For instance, it has been shown that the gene for aquaporin-1 (AQP-1) is expressed in rats, aortic VSMCs implying a specific role for AQP-1 in vascular function. In this study the expression of AQP-1 in human arteries were documented and mRNA and protein were found in normal endothelial and SM cells of human arteries and capillaries and in a subset of SM cells in human atherosclerotic plaques. Secondly, the authors examined the regulation of AQP-1 gene expression during vascular development and following vascular injury. Studies in the rat demonstrated that AQP-1 mRNA is induced in the neonatal aorta at week 2 of postnatal development and that the protein is present in neointimal SM cells following balloon injury. Finally, they measured the rate of change in cell size induced by changes in external osmolarity and demonstrated that water transport can be inhibited with mercuric chloride. It is clear that AQP-1 is responsible for water transport across human vascular SM cells membranes. Thus, this study provides evidence for a hitherto unrecognized role for aquaporins in mediating rapid water transport across human vascular SM cells membranes. By analogy with other tissues, these data argue for an important role for AQP-1 in regulating transcellular fluid flow and tissue hydration (Shanahan, Connolly, Tyson et al 1999).

It is known that hypoxic pulmonary hypertension (HPH) is characterized by proliferative vascular remodeling. Abnormal pulmonary artery smooth muscle cells proliferation and endothelial dysfunction are the primary cellular bases of vascular remodeling. AQP1 (aquaporin-1) is regulated by oxygen level and has been observed to play a role in the proliferation and migration of pulmonary artery smooth muscle cells. It is likely that AQP1 plays an important role in the pathogenesis of HPH and its possible involvement in HPH development was confirmed using Aqp1 knockout mice (Liu, Liu, Pei et al. 2019). It was determined that AQP1 expression was upregulated by chronic hypoxia exposure, both in pulmonary artery endothelium and medial smooth muscle layer of mice. Aqp1 deficiency attenuated the elevation of right ventricular systolic pressures and mitigated pulmonary vascular structure remodeling. AQP1 deletion reduced abnormal cell proliferation in pulmonary arteries and was accompanied by accumulation of HIF (hypoxia-inducible factor). In vitro, Aqp1 deletion reduced hypoxia-induced proliferation, apoptosis resistance, and migration ability of primary cultured pulmonary artery smooth muscle cells and repressed HIF-1α protein stability. Furthermore, Aqp1 deficiency protected lung endothelial cells from apoptosis in response to hypoxic injury. The data obtained showed that Aqp1 deficiency could attenuate hypoxia-induced vascular remodeling in the development of HPH. Thus, AQP1 may be a potential target for pulmonary hypertension treatment.

Deviation 11. *To be fair, it should still be remembered that this class of proteins was first discovered by a group of Romanian researchers (Cluj-Napoca, Romania) led by Gheorghe Benga. In 1985, in experiments with human erythrocytes, they discovered a protein that forms the basis of the water channel. They named it water channel protein, or WCP, which is currently called aquaporin 1. For its identification and isolation, the authors used labeled mercury (203Hg) in the form of p-chloro mercuri benzenesulfonate (PCMBS), which blocked the channel and allowed it to be separated from the rest of the erythrocyte proteins. The results of the work were first published in 1986 in Biochemistry and Eur. J. Cell Biol. Currently, many researchers recognize the priority of the discovery of aquaporins by George Benga.*

Interestingly, progesterone reduces the expression of aquaporin AQP4 in cultured rat astrocytes in an ischemia-reperfusion model, which depends on the PKC signaling pathway. This effect explains the ability of progesterone to increase the survival of astrocytes in ischemia and cerebral edema. Aquaporin-9 (AQP9), or aquaglyceroporin, is expressed in brain astrocytes, in ventricular ependymal cells, in tanycytes of the mediobasal hypothalamus, in cerebral vascular endothelial cells, in catecholaminergic neurons, in the organ of Corti, in hepatocytes, in goblet cells of the digestive tract, in testicular Leydig cells, epididymis cells, placenta, leukocytes, vascular endothelium, vascular SMCs, and cardiomyocytes.

Glutamate is known to induce cerebral edema. It is believed that the basis is an increase in the permeability of astrocytes to water under the influence of glutamate, which, acting on metabotropic receptors, increases the concentration of Ca^{2+} *ions in astrocytes, which enhances the translocation of AQP4 from the cytosol to the surface membrane. A similar situation occurs with cerebral ischemia, which is accompanied by the development of ischemic and postischemic cerebral edema. Therefore, it is important to search for substances that block the translocation of aquaporins from the cytosol to the plasma membrane, or reduce the expression of aquaporins, or directly block the ability of aquaporins to transport water. Attempts to find effective aquaporin inhibitors that would be safe for the body continue to the present, but so far, they have been of little success. It is possible that such a substance is oxytocin, which increases the stability of the erythrocyte in a hypoosmotic environment.*

Thus, the prospect of further study of the involvement of aquaporins in the pathogenesis of various human diseases is obvious, as well as the development of substances that inhibit or, conversely, activate the activity of aquaporins. It is believed that the most promising is the search for inhibitors and activators of aquaporins among low molecular weight substances. They can be widely used in the prevention of cerebral and pulmonary edema, in the regulation of intraocular pressure, in the treatment of tumor processes and heart disease. The importance of such a search is demonstrated by the clinical picture of the Covid-19 coronavirus infection pandemic, which is characterized by pulmonary edema, leading to mortality in the elderly.

And finally, the observation that some membranes are CO_2 impermeable led to the discovery of a gas molecule moving through a channel; namely, CO_2 diffusion through aquaporin-1 (AQP1). At least in some cells, CO_2-permeable proteins could provide important pathways for transmembrane CO2 movements. Such pathways could be amenable to cellular regulation and could become valuable drug targets. (Michenkova, Taki, Blosser, Hwang, Kowatz et al, 2021).

Chapter 15

Living Cell Behavior in an Electromagnetic Field

"The visible world is neither matter nor spirit,
but the invisible organization of energy."
Pagels, 1982

All living organisms - plants, fungi, unicellular and multicellular animals, humans - along with geocosmic sources are generators of electromagnetic fields (EMF) and have their own electromagnetic frequency characteristics.

The following field parameters have been established for the human body: electrostatic field strength - up to 80 V/m (15±2.0 V/m); surface density of electric charges - 10^{-5}-10^{-8} C/cm^2; the potential of the electrostatic field relative to the Earth at a distance of 10 cm from the surface of the body - from 2-3 to 300 mV.

Below are some options of constant and alternating magnetic field (MF) for humans. MF of the heart - 0.05-0.07 mT (10^{-6} T); MP of the brain - 0.1–0.07 nT (10^{-9} T); MF near the human head is about 0.01–0.1 pT and is identified as MF of the α-rhythm; EMF of nerve action potentials - about 150 μV at a distance of 12 mm from the trunk; MF of muscles - about 0.1 mT. Macroscopic loop ion currents with an amplitude of up to 12 μA, varying according to muscle tone, were detected in human legs. Photon emission intensity on the body surface is <10-16 W/cm^2 with a maximum on the face. Hands and feet, with the highest intensity in the blue and red parts of the optical range, and an intensity area in the ultraviolet part of the spectrum; in the area of biologically active points, there is a sharp increase in the EMF potential.

How did it happen? How did this electromagnetic environment of our body form? Jirı Pokorny et al. (Pokorny Jin, Pokorny Jan and Kobilkova, 2013) explain it like this. A living organism transforms chemical energy into a form suitable for entering biological processes. Chemical bonds (including covalent, ionic, hydrogen, and van der Waals type) were commonly assumed to be dominant for biological organization and activity. However, these bonds represent the forces of a short-range nature in the nm region. Biological systems maintain order at every level of dimensions and display even a macroscopic long-range order and interactions. The biological order is discussed in general terms of energy supply and the release of heat from cells. Long-range forces of physical origin and adequate high capacity of information transfer may explain order.

The exceptional electrical polarity of biological objects suggests a fundamental role of endogenous electromagnetic fields in biological activity. Since the majority of proteins and protein structures are electrically polar, any oscillation generates an electromagnetic field. Therefore, biological activity should be based not only on biochemical–genetic processes but also on biophysical mechanisms of the electromagnetic field. Research on electromagnetic activity of biological systems was initiated by a hypothesis presented by H. Frohlich at the First Versailles Conference on Theoretical Physics and Biology in 1967. Frohlich assumed strong excitation of one or a few modes of motion, stabilized due to low emission and friction losses, phases correlated over macroscopic regions, and superimposed on random thermal fluctuations. He recognized that the strong polarity of biological objects suggests longitudinal electric oscillations as stabilizing modes.

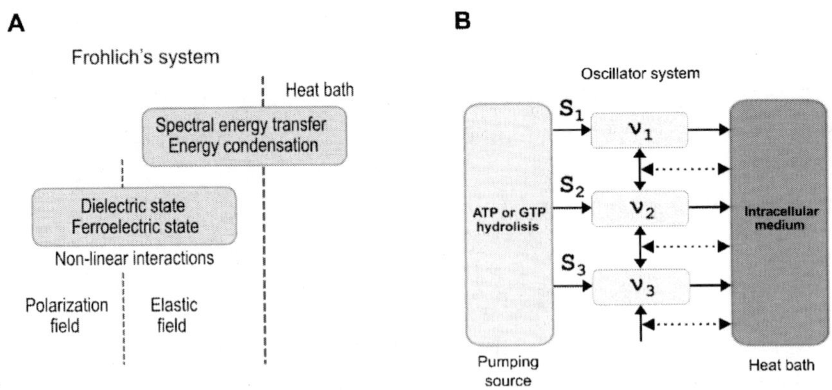

Figure 29. An abstract physical model of Frohlich's hypothesis for generation of an electromagnetic field in different biological systems (see explanation in the text below).

In accordance with Frohlich (1967, 1968), a schematic presentation of the generation process includes mechanisms based on longitudinal elastic and polarization oscillations, and energy transfer from the source to the oscillation systems and from them to the heat bath. The term mode is used for oscillation at a distinct frequency and energy equivalent to a harmonic oscillator. The source and the heat bath are any parts of the model system supplying and accepting energy from the oscillating modes, respectively. (A) Non-linear interaction between the polarization field and the longitudinal elastic field and spectral energy transfer between oscillating modes along the frequency scale are essential mechanisms. (B) Energy comes from the source to particular modes with different frequencies. Energy flow from the modes to the heat bath causes losses (horizontal solid arrows). Due to non-linear coupling between the modes with different frequencies and the heat bath, energy is then transferred between modes (the transfers are denoted by vertical solid arrows and horizontal dashed arrows). Energy can be transferred between any two modes but only transfer between neighbouring modes is denoted. Energy condenses in the lowest frequency mode (Figure 29).

As a result, the author of the hypothesis formulated six main postulates:

- *Postulate I.* It is likely that all eukaryotic living cells generate an endogenous electromagnetic field and the field is coherent.
- *Postulate II.* Cell microtubules are non-linear oscillating structures generating an electromagnetic field.
- *Postulate III.* Mitochondria create conditions for generation of the electromagnetic field.
- *Postulate IV.* Synchronization of activity, interactions between elements of the system, mass and information transfer are functions of the electromagnetic field.
- *Postulate V.* Consciousness, instinct of self-preservation, and the central control function of the brain and less developed structures depend on quantum electrodynamic processes.
- *Postulate VI.* Disturbances of the energy processing system and the coherent electrodynamic state far from thermodynamic equilibrium produce pathological states, in particular cancer

We are most interested in the postulates II, IV and partially, VI, i.e. nonlinear structures, synchronization and mention of thermodynamic disturbance violation as a disease state. In other words, an oscillation trigger and a mechanism that allows them to be synchronized.

Frohlich assumed generating structures in the plasma membrane. But microtubules, due to their non-linearity to a greater degree, suit the role of trigger for oscillatory activity. Pokorny´ et al. (2013) proposed the generation of electromagnetic fields by microtubules based on Frohlich's mechanism of electric polar vibrations. In subsequent years, this idea was supported by a measurement of electric oscillations at the plasma membrane of living cells in the M phase, which displays enhanced electric activity in some periods coinciding with mitotic spindle formation and its specific developmental features. Microtubule electromagnetic activity in heterodimer attachment was also suggested to occur by disruption of microtubule polymerization in cells by an external electromagnetic field at the frequency of 0.1–0.3 MHz. Resonant frequencies of microtubules in the frequency range of 10–30 MHz and 100–200 MHz were later reported. Their research and its outstanding results deserve at least a short description. The resonant frequencies were obtained by measurement of dc conductivity after application of an oscillating electromagnetic signal and from transmittance and reflectance of microtubules with and without compensation of parasitic reactance in the frequency range of 1 kHz – 1.3 GHz. These experiments showed that the resonant frequencies do not depend on the length of the microtubule. The resonant peaks were not observed after the release of water from the microtubule cavity.

Thus, the living cell represents itself as an electrical system. The cell membrane is electrically charged. There is a potential difference between the inner and outer surfaces of the plasma membrane. If the cell is at rest, its membrane potential has a negative and a stable value. It is commonly referred to as the resting membrane potential. The resting membrane potential of cells of various tissues ranges from -55 mV to -100 mV. Given the thickness of the membrane, the electric field strength in the membrane must be very high. As a result, at a transmembrane potential of -70 mV and a membrane thickness of 8 nm, the intrinsic electric field strength of the membrane is 7x106 V/m. It is indeed a very large value that is quite capable of capturing the imagination of any technical specialist who is not familiar with biology. Under normal conditions, such voltage cannot be obtained in air - a spark discharge will occur between the electrodes at potential differences that are 2-3 times smaller. Biological membranes function normally in living cells just in the "pre-breakdown" mode: an increase in the potential difference by 30-40% above the physiological level can already cause an electrical breakdown of the membrane and cell death.

The existence of a membrane potential is an indispensable condition for the existence of any living cell. Each cell converts some of its metabolic energy into electrostatic energy. The source of the electric field of the cell is the plasma membrane and the mitochondrial membranes. From an energy point of view, the membrane potential is a kind of energy reservoir, the energy of which can be used to perform certain work. According to the arrangement of negatively charged ions in the cytosol and positively charged ones on the outer side of the membrane, the cell resembles an electric capacitor or battery, that is, a device capable of storing electrical energy and serving as its source. Energy is released in the form of ions migrating in the direction of their electrochemical gradient and can be used in the processes of transport of other ions or metabolites against the concentration gradient.

It would not be too much of an exaggeration to say that we all live in a huge slow-cooling microwave oven. In other words, we are electrically charged objects, which live in an electromagnetic field. What is this field? In addition, here you cannot do without great science.

Everyone imagines beauty in different ways, but there is an opinion that there is nothing more beautiful than Maxwell's equations. No, it would probably be more correct to say this - Few things in this world can compare in beauty with Maxwell's equations (at least for a scientist).

Deviation 12. *Maxwell's equations connect the quantities that characterize the electromagnetic field with its sources, that is, with the distribution of electric charges and currents in space. In a vacuum, an electromagnetic field is characterized by two vector quantities that depend on spatial coordinates and time: the electric field strength (E) and magnetic induction (B). These quantities determine the forces acting from the field on charges and currents, the distribution of which in space is given by the charge density (r, the charge in unit volume) and current density (j, the charge transferred per unit time through a unit area perpendicular to the direction of charge movement). To describe electromagnetic processes in a material environment (in matter), in addition to the vectors (E) and (B), auxiliary vector quantities are introduced that depend on the state and properties of the medium: electric induction (D) and magnetic field strength (H). Maxwell's equations make it possible to determine the main characteristics of the field (E, B, D and H) at each point in space at any time, if the sources of the field j and r are known as functions of coordinates and time. They can be written in integral or differential form (below they are given in the absolute system of Gaussian units).*

For instance, the first Maxwell's Equation is a generalization to variable fields of the empirical Ampère's law on the excitation of a magnetic field by electric currents. Maxwell hypothesized that the magnetic field is generated not only by currents flowing in conductors, but also by alternating electric fields in dielectrics or vacuum. Maxwell the displacement called the value proportional to the rate of change of the electric field in time current. The displacement current excites the magnetic field according to the same law as the conduction current (later this was confirmed experimentally). The total current, equal to the sum of the conduction current and the displacement current, is always closed.

As is often the case, Maxwell's equations were not understood for a long time. This is indeed not an easy task. Especially if you have not taken a course in electrodynamics at one time. It will be clearer for biologists if we give the floor to a specialist.

Nobel laureate Wilczek FA (2016) wrote that Maxwell took as the basis of his concept four laws discovered by several scientists earlier: two laws of Gauss, Ampère's law and Faraday's law of induction. Maxwell expressed these laws in Faraday's language of electrical and magnetic fluids, which he made precise and mathematical in his even earlier work.

Maxwell also added his own law, dual to Faraday's law. This supplement was not based on experiments. Maxwell originally came to postulate this law by working with the implications of his absurd model. In a new interpretation, he showed that a new law was necessary to make the old laws consistent!

Everyone, in regard to Maxwell's equations, now knows this system of four equations, combining four already known laws with a new addition. There are five laws hidden in the four equations, because one of the equations sums up two physical phenomena. Up until now, they remain the best fundamental description of electromagnetism and light.

Gauss' electric law expresses the equality between the flow of an electric field leaving a certain volume and the electric charge inside this volume. He says that electric charges are the points of origin of electric lines of force (or the points of their completion). They are where electrical power lines can start or end. Its association with fluid flow most easily understands the definition of flow. The electric field, as we have already discussed, is a quantity that at each point has a numerical value and direction. The velocity field in a flowing fluid has the same character. Given a volume and a velocity field, we can calculate how fast the fluid leaves that volume. This, by definition, is the flow of fluid leaving a given volume. If we perform the same mathematical operations on the electric field that we just performed on the fluid velocity field to calculate its flux, we get (by definition) the flux of an electric field.

Gauss' magnetic law states that the flux of a magnetic field emanating from any volume is zero. The magnetic law of Gauss, of course, is very similar to the electrical law of Gauss, but with an additional simplification - after all, there can be no magnetic charge! He says that magnetic fields have no sources - magnetic lines of force can never end, but must instead go on forever or close on themselves.

Faraday's law is especially interesting because it includes time. The law establishes the relationship between electric fields and the rate of change of magnetic fields. The law says that when magnetic fields change over time, they create electric fields that swirl around magnetic fields.

To formulate Faraday's law exactly, imagine a curve that forms the boundary of a certain surface. Faraday's law states that the circulation of the electric field along this contour (with a negative sign) is equal to the rate of change of the magnetic flux through the surface. Circulation, like flow, is most easily understood through association with the velocity field in the fluid flow. Let's mentally expand our curve, turning it into a narrow tube, and calculate the amount of fluid passing through this tube per unit time. This will be the circulation of the fluid flow. If we perform the same mathematical operations on the electric field that we performed on the fluid velocity field, then we get (by definition) the circulation of the electric field.

Finally, to be perfectly accurate, we must resolve the ambiguity with direction: when defining a circulation, in which direction should we move around the curve? When defining flow, in which direction should we move through the surface? To get a certain ratio, we must establish a correspondence between the existing choices. The standard way is the so-called right-hand rule: if we move along a curve in the direction indicated by the four fingers of the right hand, then we should consider the flow towards the thumb.

Ampère's law establishes the relationship between magnetic fields and electric currents. It says that electric currents generate magnetic fields that swirl around them. To formulate Ampère's law exactly, let us again imagine a curve that forms the boundary of the surface. Ampère's law states the equality between the circulation of a magnetic field along a curve and the flow of an electric current through a surface.

It is worth noting that the same concepts of flow and circulation are repeated several times in these laws. Flow and circulation are the two main definitions necessary in order to truly comprehend and understand the physical meaning and essence of the field concept. They contain, respectively, lines of force, rushing away in a straight line and curling into loops. Their prominence in physical laws is the gift of Matter to Mind.

However, when Maxwell put all these four laws together, he found a contradiction! Maxwell's fifth law corrects it. The problem arises if you are trying to apply Ampère's law in a situation where the electrical current is interrupted. Imagine an electric current flowing into and out of a pair of plates separated by a gap (something like a capacitor). According to Ampère, the magnetic circulation along a circuit is equal to the current flow through any surface it delimits. However, here we will get different values for the flow depending on which surface we take! If we take the disk inside the gap between the plates, we get zero. If we take a hemisphere that intersects the wire, we get the full flow. What to do? To deal with this contradiction, we need something new. Through earlier work with his model, Maxwell had an answer ready.

Maxwell's law, something like the inverse statement to Faraday's law with the replacement of the roles of electric and magnetic fields. It says that when electric fields change over time, they give rise to magnetic fields swirling around them! Thus, the contradiction disappears. After the addition of Maxwell's law, the complete system of Maxwell's equations becomes consistent. In this capacity - as a tidying up version of the "Dynamic Electrodynamic Field Theory" - Maxwell's law has acquired a new status. (Wilczek Frank Anthony, 2016).

$\nabla \cdot \boldsymbol{D} = \rho$ **(1) Gauss' Law**
$\nabla \cdot \boldsymbol{B} = 0$ **(2) Gauss' Law for magnetism**
$\nabla \cdot \boldsymbol{E} = -\frac{\delta \boldsymbol{B}}{\delta t}$ **(3) Faraday' s Law**
$\nabla \cdot \boldsymbol{H} = \frac{\delta \boldsymbol{D}}{\delta t} + \boldsymbol{J}$ **(4) Ampère-Maxwell Law** (12)

These are Maxwell's equations! Equations of classical electrodynamics describing the dynamics of the electromagnetic field and its connection with charges and currents.

Electrical law of Gauss:

$\nabla \cdot \mathrm{D} = \rho$ Electric charge is the source of electrical induction (13)

Gauss' law for a magnetic field:

$\nabla \cdot \mathrm{B} = 0$ (No magnetic charges detected) (14)

Faraday's law of induction:

$$\nabla \times E = -\partial B / \partial t \qquad (15)$$

The change in magnetic induction generates a vortex electric field.

Magnetic field circulation theorem

$$\nabla \times H = j + \partial D / \partial t \qquad (16)$$

Electric current and change in electric induction generate a vortex magnetic field, where:

ρ - volumetric density of a third-party electric charge (in SI units – C/m^3);

j - electric current density (A / m^2); in the simplest case - the case of a current generated by one type of charge carriers, it is expressed simply as j =u ρ1, where u is the (average) speed of movement of these carriers in the vicinity of a given point, ρ1 is the charge density of this type of carriers. c is the speed of light in vacuum (299,792,458 m/s);

E is the electric field strength (V/m);

H - magnetic field strength (A / m); D - electrical induction (C / m^2);

B - magnetic induction (Tl, Wb / m^2, \ kg•s-2•A-1);

∇ is the nabla differential operator, where: ∇ · E ≡ r o t E means the curl of the vector E, and ∇ · E ≡ d i v E means the divergence of the vector E.

Note. The above equations of Maxwell do not constitute a complete system of electromagnetic field equations, since they do not contain the properties of the medium in which the electromagnetic field is excited. The relations connecting the quantities E, B, D, H and j and taking into account the individual properties of the medium are called constitutive equations.

Fields are an abstract concept, far from the familiar world of things and forces. Maxwell's equations that describe them cannot be expressed in simple terms, such as, for example, Newton's laws of motion. At the same time, along with Newton's laws and the principles of thermodynamics, these equations are the basis of modern science.

However, all above mentioned is for an advanced reader. For myself, for the rest of my life I remembered a clear definition of the field, heard at a lecture at Moscow State Lomonosov University in 1966 - a field is a region of space, each point of which can be associated with a number or a vector. In my opinion, this definition is universal and applicable to any kind of field.

An electric field is a specific physical field that surrounds each electric charge and exerts a force on all other charges, attracting or repelling them. Electric fields arise from electric charges or time-varying magnetic fields.

Electric and magnetic fields should be considered as manifestations of a more general reality - the electromagnetic field, which is responsible for one of the most important and fundamental interactions in nature (along with, for example, the gravitational field).

An electromagnetic field is a fundamental physical field that interacts with electrically charged bodies, as well as with bodies that have their own dipole and multipole electric and magnetic moments. It is a combination of electric and magnetic fields, which can, under certain conditions, give rise to each other, but in fact, they are one entity, formalized through the electromagnetic field tensor.

In other words, electric and magnetic fields are considered manifestations of a more general reality - the electromagnetic field, responsible for one of the fundamental interactions of nature (along with gravitational, strong and weak). Every physiologist who has worked with smooth muscles knows what electrical field stimulation is. Each charged object forms an electric field in the surrounding space. An electric field is a kind of matter through which charged objects interact with each other. In fact, we are talking about how an external electromagnetic field affects the field of a smooth muscle cell, i.e. one field overlaps another.

Electric Field Strength

Every electric charge generates an electric field around itself. If another charge q is introduced into this field, then a force F proportional to q and the electric field strength E will act on it:

$$\vec{F} = q\,E \tag{17}$$

The electric field strength E (or simply strength) at any point is defined as the electric force F, which acts on a positive charge q placed at that point:

$$\vec{E} = \vec{F}/q \tag{18}$$

E is a vector quantity, that is, it has both magnitude and direction. The unit of tension is volt per meter [V/m].

The electric field strength is a negative gradient of the electric potential - an indicator of potential change with distance x: $\mathbf{\vec{E} = -\,d\varphi/dx}$. With the help of instruments, you can measure the potential difference, but not the field strength. The latter can be calculated using the relationship between **E→** and **Δφ**, where **Δφ = E•I** is the distance between two electric field currents.

Electric fields are a normal factor in the functioning of most biological membranes. Above, we have already noted how high the electric field strength of the membrane is at rest. The impact of an external electric field of high intensity causes qualitatively new phenomena in the cell. In particular, it was found that hyperpolarization of the algae cell membrane to a certain critical potential value causes a sharp increase in the transmembrane current - a phenomenon similar to the electrical breakdown of dielectrics. However, in the case of cell membranes, the breakdown can be completely reversible: upon repolarization of the cell, the low conductivity of the membrane is restored, and the phenomenon of electrical breakdown itself can be observed repeatedly.

Under the action of high-intensity, pulsed electric fields on cell suspensions (pulses lasting from several microseconds to several milliseconds at a field strength of several kV/cm), cell membrane permeability disturbances and cell death were noted. Electrically stimulated cell lysis has been demonstrated for bacteria, yeast, erythrocytes and protoplasts. Violation of the barrier properties of the membrane is due to the induction of a transmembrane potential up to 1 V in the electric field as it has been shown in molecular genetics and biotechnological research. Along with membrane poration, electric fields can induce cell fusion, which can be used to obtain heterokaryons and hybrids. In addition, exposure *to electric fields can activate the function of membrane proteins*, stimulate cellular processes, and cause morphological changes, such as the formation of cell outgrowths or local spherical swellings of membranes (blebs) on the cell surface.

The effects caused by the action of electric fields on cell membranes can be classified as follows: 1) electroporation, 2) electrofusion, 3) movements in an electric field (electrophoresis, dielectrophoresis and electrorotation), 4) membrane deformation, 5) electrotransfection, 6) electro activation membrane proteins. Below is a short description of each of them.

Electroporation

After exposure to an electrical impulse, leading to the formation of pores in the membrane, permeable to ions and sucrose, the cells, as a rule, swell in a few seconds to several minutes. After electroporation, due to the appearance of through pores in the membrane, the concentrations of salts and sucrose in the cell and in the medium quickly level off. However, the cell membrane remains impermeable to cytoplasmic macromolecules, which maintain excess osmotic pressure in the cell. Due to this, water moves into the cell, accompanied by swelling. Thus, swelling of cells after electroporation has a colloid osmotic nature. Additionally, electroporation is used to load molecules (siRNA, oligonucleotides, small peptides, etc.) into cells.

Membrane Electrofusion

The phenomena of cell electrofusion seem to be closely related to membrane electroporation. There are hypotheses based on relatively simple physicochemical models and the theory of colloid stability. The fusion of the membranes of contacting cells can be likened to the coagulation of hydrophobic colloidal particles. The modern theory of stability considers the sticking process as the result of the combined action of attractive van der Waals forces and electrostatic repulsive forces between particles carrying a surface charge. Depending on the balance of forces in a thin film of water separating the particles, either a positive pressure arises, which prevents the particles from joining, or a negative one, leading to the thinning of the water layer and the formation of contact between the particles.

At the first stage of fusion, the membranes converge and the thickness of the water layer decreases; then, due to thermal fluctuations of the membranes, the barrier preventing the connection of the membranes is overcome, and a membrane partition is formed. Subsequently, as the result of thermal fluctuations, a pore of a relatively large radius appears in the septum, leading to rupture of the membrane septum and complete cell fusion.

When studying the fusion of whole cells, it was found that the probability of fusion increases in the presence of certain lipids (saturated carboxylic acids with 10-14 carbon atoms) that induce colloidal osmotic swelling of cells. Swelling accompanied by fusion was also observed when erythrocytes were heated to 50°C.

The electrofusion procedure usually includes a preliminary step of bringing the cells into contact. Such contact can be achieved by exposing the cell suspension to an alternating electric field: as the result of dielectrophoresis, the cells line up in chains. Centrifugation, bringing cultured cell monolayers together under pressure, and other methods are also used to bring cells into contact. After bringing the cells into contact, they are treated with a short pulse of an electric field, which causes the formation of pores and the induction of fusion. At the next stage, swelling of the cells and an increase in the cross section of the membrane tube connecting the cells occur.

The electrofusion mechanism is presented as follows. Under the action of an external electric field in the contact zone of cell membranes, coaxial pores are formed, through which the current passes. The lines of force of the electric field are distributed in such a way that pressure arises that brings the membranes together and closes the edges of the pores. When the edges of the pores of the contact membranes are closed, a membrane tube is formed that connects the cytoplasm of the merging cells. Cell swelling caused by electroporation causes membrane tension, due to which an increase in the intercellular bridge parameter and complete mixing of the cell cytoplasm occurs.

Cell Movement

There are two types of cell movement in electric fields. A constant field causes the movement of cells with a surface charge - the phenomenon of electrophoresis. When cell suspensions are exposed to an alternating inhomogeneous field, cell movement is observed, called dielectrophoresis. In dielectrophoresis, the surface charge of cells does not play a significant role; the mechanism of motion consists in the interaction of the induced dipole moment with the external field.

The difference in the directions of the dielectrophoretic force at low (kilohertz) and high (megahertz) frequencies is due to the different orientation of the induced dipole moment with respect to the external electric field. From the courses on electricity, it is known how the dipole moments of poorly conducting dielectric particles in a conducting medium and well-conducting particle surrounded by a low-conducting medium are oriented. In the case of exposure to a low-frequency field, the membrane is a good insulator and the current bypasses the cell through a conducting medium. The induced charges increase the field strength inside the particle. This distribution of induced charges corresponds to the antiparallel orientation of the dipole moment of the particle with respect to the external field.

When exposed to a high-frequency field, the conductivity of the membrane is high; and since the electrical conductivity of the intracellular medium is higher than the electrical conductivity of the salt-free extracellular medium, the current flows predominantly through the cell. Under these conditions, the distribution of induced charges on the particle surface corresponds to the parallel orientation of the dipole moment with respect to the external field.

Membrane Deformation

The phenomena of dielectrophoresis and electrorotation of cells are closely related to the action of forces on the cell surface, called Maxwellian stresses. The magnitude and direction of the force acting on cell membranes in an electric field are determined by the relation:

$$T = \varepsilon\varepsilon o[E[En]-(E^2/2) \cdot n], \tag{19}$$

where T is the force, E is the electric field strength, n is the normal vector to the surface, ε is the relative permittivity of the dielectric, εo - 8.85-10 ‘12 F/m is the absolute permittivity of the vacuum.

When a cell is exposed to a low-frequency field, the lines of force bypass the cell, i.e., the field is directed tangentially to the surface. In the case of exposure to a high-frequency field, the lines of force pass through the cell, i.e., the field is directed perpendicular to the membrane at both ends of the cell facing the electrodes.

Deformation of cells in alternating electric fields is observed experimentally and contains information about the viscoelastic characteristics of the cell. In addition to reversible deformations that disappear after turning off the field, irreversible changes in cell morphology were also found, caused by exposure to alternating fields. It has been shown that the application of an electric field leads to the formation of processes in fibroblasts, which are similar in their morphology to processes that form under physiological conditions, for example, when cells spread on a substrate.

The forces acting on cell membranes in an electric field play an important role in the convergence of membranes during electrically induced cell fusion. According to one hypothesis, electrofusion begins with the formation of coaxial pores in the contact membranes of adjacent cells. In the area of coaxial pore formation, the field lines are located tangentially to the membrane surface and create a force that forces the membrane sections near the pore to approach each other. Because of the action of these forces, the probability of closing the edges of the pores increases. After the formation of a through pore, the field directed tangentially to the edge of the pore tends to stretch the pore, which leads to complete cell fusion.

Electrotransfection

Electrotransfection and electrotransformation are understood as the introduction of foreign DNA into cells. For penetration through the DNA membrane, two factors are important: the formation of pores in the membrane under the action of the field (electroporation) and the presence of a charge on the DNA molecule, which ensures the electrophoretic movement of DNA at the moment the pulse is applied. Electro Treatment of cells in the presence of DNA leads to a stronger increase in membrane permeability compared to similar treatment without DNA. Based on these data, it was suggested that the interaction of DNA with the membrane during electroporation leads to an increase in the effective diameter of pores or an increase in their lifetime.

Electrical Activation of Proteins

An example of electrical activation of membrane enzymes is the activation of Na-K-ATPase in human erythrocytes under the action of an alternating electric field with an amplitude of 20 V/cm and a frequency of 1 kHz. It is essential that electric fields of such low intensity do not have a damaging effect on cell functions and their morphology. Weak low-frequency fields (60 V/cm, 10 Hz) also stimulate ATP synthesis by mitochondrial ATPase. It is assumed that electro activation is due to the influence of the field on protein conformation. The theoretical analysis of the model of facilitated membrane transport with the participation of a carrier (a model with four states of the transport system) indicates the interaction of the transport system with an alternating field. As a result of such interaction, the field energy can be used by the transport system and converted into the chemical bond energy of ATP.

Weak constant fields can cause the movement of free cells (electrophoresis), as well as the lateral movement of charged receptors along the surface of the cell membrane in immobilized cells. The phenomenon of membrane receptor electrophoresis is used as a tool to study the mobility of proteins in the plasma membrane.

Interaction of Cell Membranes

Under normal physiological conditions, the fusion of cell membranes is an important biological process underlying such phenomena as the exocytosis of hormones, enzymes, neurotransmitters, as well as the formation of giant cells in inflammatory processes, the introduction of enveloped viruses into host cells (AIDS virus). The above mechanisms of action of electric fields on bilayer membranes and cells give an idea of the physicochemical factors that affect the interaction of cell membranes, which lead to their fusion. However, the specific molecular mechanisms of this biological phenomenon are much more complex. Their main feature is the active participation of special membrane proteins in the fusion process.

How can an electromagnetic field act on the contractility of smooth muscle cells? What will be the severity and direction (constriction or relaxation) of this effect?

For instance, in the work of Victor Martynyuk et al. (Martynyuk, Melnyk, Artemenko, 2016) influence of electromagnetic fields (EMFs) with rectangular pulse frequencies of 8 and 50 Hz and flux density of 25 μT on contraction, nitric oxide/nitrite synthesis, and intracellular calcium concentration in the gastric smooth muscles of rats was investigated. An approximately 8-Hz field reduced the fast component of contraction induced by KCl depolarization and slowed down the time to reach the maximum of the slow component of contraction, whereas the 50-Hz field increased the fast and slow components and accelerated the time to reach the maximum of the slow component of contraction. After turning off the EMF, the force and character of contraction returned to the control values. In addition, the 8-Hz field increased nitric oxide/nitrite synthesis in the excited smooth muscle tissue with KCl depolarization, while the 50-Hz field had no significant effect. 8- and 50-Hz fields had no significant effects on nitric oxide/nitrite production in non-stimulated tissue. However, the 50-Hz field significantly increased the basic intracellular calcium concentration in smooth muscle cells (SMC) in a time-dependent manner, whereas the 8-Hz field only slightly increased calcium levels. Thus, the data obtained demonstrated that responses of gastric smooth muscles to EMFs are clearly expressed and pulse-frequency dependent.

The question arises. Is it possible to regulate the function of the ion channel with the help of electromagnetic fields? Then a surprising discovery awaited us.

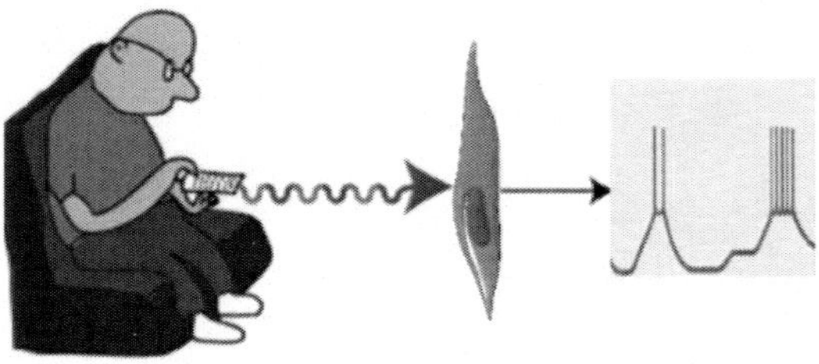

Figure 30. This cute old man in the picture, most likely, does not think about how the signal from the remote control interacts with his TV. For him, the main thing is that the channels switch and the volume could be changed. We have a more difficult task for us. We definitely need to know exactly how our potential drug molecule or physical; factor interacts with its pharmacological target.

Do plasmon gold nanoparticles really capable of remotely opening ion channels? Is it fact or fancy? (Figure 30).

It is well known that ion channels (IChs) are proteins that form pores in cell membranes and regulate the flux of ions between the intracellular and extracellular spaces of cells. They are involved in the control of many fundamental physiological processes in various tissues including neurotransmitter/hormone release, activation of gene transcription, and muscle contraction. An alteration in their functions give rise to a wide range of life-threatening diseases ranging from cardiovascular diseases to neurological and psychiatric disorders and even cancer development including widely distributed cardiovascular disorders such as diabetic vascular disease, hypertension and cardiac arrhythmias etc. There are also about 60 different inherited ICh diseases, known as 'channelopathies', that have been identified across cardiovascular, neuronal, muscular, metabolic and respiratory systems, and this number is expected to grow as knowledge about ICh functions is continuously increased.

Consequently, IChs represent a rich vein of future therapeutic targets, especially in view of extreme "druggability" of these proteins because of their location at the cell surface, and are currently the second most important class of drug targets. However, to realize their potential is proving harder than first imagined. The most challenging aspect is the identification of an appropriate drug lead with desirable selectivity that is difficult to realize within the traditional pharmacological targeting based on small molecules. In this case, ICh protein binds chemically, more or less specifically/tightly, to the drug directly leading to a desirable therapeutic effect due to ICh activation or inhibition. But such effects can be controlled only by varying the dose of the drug, while current demands for personalized medicine are beyond the realms of this strategy.

Deviation 13. *The following possible interactions of the main types of cellular receptors (including pharmacological targets) with the ligands are well known: (A) Intracellular receptors bind to small or lipophilic molecules that can cross the cell membrane. The resulting ligand-receptor complexes may travel to the nucleus and thereby affecting expression of specific genes; (B) Ion-channel receptors, which selectively allow the passage of specific ions, thereby effecting changes in the membrane potential; (C) Receptors with an intracellular region containing an enzymatic domain. This group includes receptor tyrosine kinases involved in the response to many growth factors; (D) G-protein-coupled receptors that associate with cytosolic or membrane-bound proteins with enzymatic activity for signaling; (E) Adhesion receptors involved in binding with other cells or with the extracellular matrix.*

Please note that in all above-mentioned cases direct interaction of the ligand with the target molecules is necessary.

The current millennium has been enriched by promising scientific and technological trends in the study of living systems, in which light very often is a key factor. Why light? Analysis of cell functions in normal and pathological conditions is carried out at many levels, from molecular and cellular to behavioral. To investigate the principles of organization and functioning of the living system properly, effectively identify molecular and cellular structures, selectively control the activity of neuron cells, and record changes in the concentrations of ions and many important intracellular components, methods are needed that provide noninvasive, remote and rapid control of biological molecules. It turned out that electromagnetic radiation, close to the wavelength range of visible light, could serve as an ideal tool for management of biological systems due to a number of important qualities:

- provides high temporal and spatial resolution;
- allows for remote, noninvasive control of molecules;
- makes it possible to regulate with high accuracy the intensity and length of light impacts;
- does not change the properties of proteins and membranes of biological organisms at moderate intensities and durations of light signals.

These unique properties, as well as the success of molecular biology and modern technologies, provided the emergence of three main areas in which light is the main tool are optogenetics, optopharmacology, and optosensorics (Bregestovski, Zefirov, 2019). It is becoming clear that light can modulate the conductivity and kinetics of ion channels (Gorostiza, Isacoff, 2008; Miesenböck, 2011; Szymański et al, 2013).

We propose to change the approach to ICh control, which shifts the main paradigm of pharmacology based on the latest advances in nanotechnology. There is good reason to believe that it is possible to remotely control the activity of the ion channel group, which is able to open when the membrane potential changes and is of great interest to the pharmaceutical industry. This is done through the physical interactions of ICh proteins with metal nanocrystals located in close proximity to the cell membrane, which are able to amplify the electromagnetic field when external visible light falls on their surface. The combination of nano- and photonic influences into a single approach creates a unique synergy to open up prospects for fundamentally new technological opportunities.

How did we come to this conclusion? That all started when we decided to modify the American patent No.: US 2012/0295969 A1. Pub. Date: Nov. 22, 2012 "Novel muscle relaxant using negative charge gold nanoparticles with choline" using phosphatidylcholine with the aim to use it for smooth muscle control.

Deviation 14. *Briefly, about the patent No. US 2012/0295969 A1. The authors of patent supposed that a drug having a skeletal muscle relaxing effect can be prepared by binding negatively charged gold nanoparticles having a size of 1.4 nm fitted to synaptic clefts to choline through ionic bonds, thereby inducing gold-sulfur bonds in the Cys loop of an acetylcholine receptor in neuromuscular junction, and thus blocking the electric current induced in signal transduction from a nerve to a muscle, thereby blocking neuromuscular transmission chemically and physically. When the reverse is administered after surgery, the gold-sulfur bonds are broken due to the re-flow of the electric current, and thus the gold nanoparticles are again released and metabolized into neuromuscular junctions. Further, such muscle relaxing effects can be applied as an anticonvulsant.*

The combination we used, i.e., phosphatidylcholine liposomes and gold nanoparticles, did not have an expected effect on smooth muscle, but while studying the individual components of the construct, i.e., gold nanoparticles per se and liposomes, the first one demonstrated an unexpected and surprising influence on smooth muscle tone. Nanoparticles of a certain size have shown the surprising ability to relax smooth muscles, which no one expected from them.

Deviation 15. *It is important to note that we have tested a number of AuNPs different both in their size and stabilizer used but only AuNPs in core size of* $\approx$ *5 nm stabilized with ascorbate demonstrated clearly expressed ability to relax thoracic aorta SM. By the way it is considered that the origin of properties on the nanoscale is different for metal nanoparticles than the semiconductor nanoparticles, i.e., a simple change in semiconductor size alters the optical properties of the nanoparticles while when metal (gold) nanoparticles are enlarged their optical properties change only slightly. It turned out that this is not always the case.*

Deviation 16. *Gold (Au) is a chemical element of group 1 of the periodic table with an atomic mass of 196.9665. Pure gold is a chemically stable (noble) metal, which is due to the abnormally high value of the first ionization potential (890 kJ / mol). Gold is the most inert metal, standing in the series of voltages to the right of other metals; under normal conditions, it does not react with most acids and does not form oxides, due to which it belongs to noble metals, unlike ordinary metals, which are easily destroyed by the environment. In the Middle Ages, gold was used in the treatment of severe infections: tuberculosis, syphilis. Modern medicine uses gold ions as an effective remedy in the treatment of rheumatoid diseases, arthritis, lupus erythematosus, dermatitis associated with collagen synthesis. Organic compounds of gold (drugs chrysanol and auranofin) are used in medicine in the treatment of autoimmune diseases, in particular rheumatoid arthritis. The radioactive isotope* ^{198}Au *(half-life 2.967 days) is used in the treatment of tumors with radiotherapy. It has also been found that gold inhibits some viruses, including AIDS and infectious hepatitis. Experimental data on the anti-cancer effect of gold are of particular interest. In preliminary experiments, gold preparations inhibited the growth of malignant cells, which can be used to prevent postoperative metastases and to prevent cancer. Nano gold attracts special attention. It turned out that it is sufficiently biologically active. Methods and variants of interaction of nanogold particles with biomolecules maybe different: (A) hydrophobic binding, (B) electrostatic binding, (C) simple covalent binding, (D) coordination binding, (E) oligonucleotide hybridization, and (F) photolabile bonds.*

Below we provide some experimental evidence for our hypothesis.

Contractile Recordings

Colloidal gold nanoparticles (AuNPs) having plasmon resonance of 532 nm were synthesized via reduction of sodium tetrachloroaurate by sodium ascorbate in aqueous solutions at room temperature as it was described before (Soloviev, Ivanova, Novokhatska et al. 2013; Soloviev, Zholos, Ivanova et al. 2015). Then prepared colloids were neutralized to pH 6-7 by acetic acid. A dynamic light scattering study of colloidal Au solutions (200 mg/L, i.e., ~10-3 M or 6.02 x 10^{20} particles/L) showed that the average hydrodynamic size of gold nanoparticles was around 5 nm. The surface of Au nanoparticles stabilized by ascorbate anions supposed to be negatively charged (Zeta-potential of -35 mV). The colloidal solutions were stable for months and did not show any appreciable temporal changes in the size and size distribution of Au nanoparticles.

The word plasmon is the key in this paragraph, since it is with the existence of plasmon on the gold nanoparticles surface that we connect their ability to relax smooth muscles. The terms “plasmon” and “surface plasmon resonance” designates collective charge density oscillation at the metal interface, propagating in a waveguide fashion along the surface within the distance of the order 1 μM (Jacak, Popko, Hendrikowski, Zielony, Gwodz et al. 2016).

Figure 31 shows the dose-response curves to AuNPs for rat thoracic aorta SM pre constricted with norepinephrine (NE, 10^{-6} M). It is clear that AuNPs in a range of concentration 10^{-6} - 3x10^{-4} M possess the ability to decrease the amplitude of NE-induced contraction significantly (pD2 = 4.2±03, Emax = 55 ± 4%), i.e., AuNPs demonstrated clearly expressed vasorelaxant activity. Endothelial disruption was without significant effect on AuNPs-induced SM relaxation.

It is interesting that the dose-response curve shows that AuNPs-induced SM relaxation takes place in a manner similar to so-called all-or-nothing fashion, i.e., threshold concentration of AuNPs required evoking significant relaxation. There was no change in smooth muscle tone in the 10-6-10-5 M concentration range, i.e., the concentration of nanoparticles must reach such a concentration that the total strength of the plasmon field reaches a certain critical value.

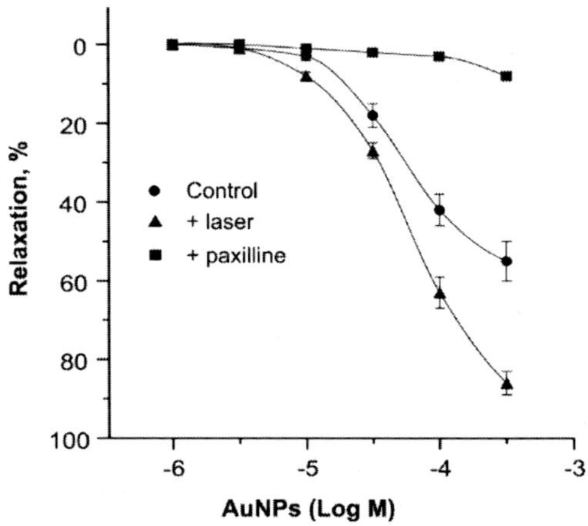

Figure 31. Cumulative concentration-relaxation curves for AuNPs ≈ 5nm core size and for AuNPs combined with 5 W/532 nm green laser irradiation (AuNPs+laser) obtained in intact and endothelium denuded rat thoracic aorta rings preactivated with 10-6 M norepinephrine before and after paxilline (500 nM) action.

It is important to note that stabilizer (a basic solution in which nanoparticles are suspended) per se had no effect on the tone of thoracic aorta SM pre constricted with NE.

It was difficult to explain this relaxation, since, at first glance, there seems to be no obvious target for gold in a smooth muscle cell. Is that the sensor of the potential of ionic potential-dependent channels, which could somehow react to the intensity of the electromagnetic field (plasmon) existing on the surface of gold nanoparticles? It seemed like a fantasy.

To facilitate possible plasmon resonance, we irradiated tissue organ bath using 5 mW/532 nm green laser during all periods of AuNPs-induced relaxation. That was the decisive moment. In this case AuNPs application led to significantly increased amplitude of maximal AuNPs-induced relaxation from 55 ± 4% to 85±5.0% ($n = 10$, $P < 0.05$). At the same time the sensitivity of SM to AuNPs had not increased, mean value of pD2 was 4.2 ± 0.013, ($n = 10$, $P > 0.05$). It is important to note that the temperature of Krebs solution in organ bath was without significant changes under laser irradiation. In the presence of paxilline, potent BK_{Ca} channels blocker, AuNPs lost their vasorelaxant activity in isolated SM aorta segments almost completely (Figure 31).

Similar results, when green laser illuminated AuNPs, were obtained in pulmonary artery rings: Emax = 89 ± 5% ($n = 8$, $P < 0.05$), pD2 = 4.2 ± 0.1 ($n = 8$, $P > 0.05$), respectively.

A significant increase in the relaxation amplitude upon the combination of the action of gold and a green laser has supported our assumption about the important role of plasmon in this process.

Deviation 17. *An electromagnetic field is a region of space, at each point of which a vector is given, which is a function of coordinates and characterizes the force interaction of the field and any charged body. Including the sensor of the potential in ion channels. A plasmon is a density wave in an electron gas. It is analogous to a sound wave, which is a density wave in a gas consisting of molecules. Plasmons exist mainly in metals, where electrons are weakly bound to the atoms and free to roam. The free electron gas model provides a good approximation (also known as jellium model). The electrons in a metal can wobble like a piece of jelly, pulled back by the attraction of the positive metal ions that they leave behind. In contrast to the single electron wave function, a plasmon is a collective wave where billions of electrons oscillate in sync. When a nanoparticle is much smaller than the wavelength of light, coherent oscillation of the conduction band electrons is induced by interaction with an electromagnetic field. This resonance is called Surface Plasmon Resonance (SPR). Excited surface plasmons with a variable dipole moment, in turn, emit an electromagnetic wave. The quantum yield of radiation shows how much of the power lost by radiation goes to scattering. The smaller the particle diameter, the less it is. The enhancement of the electric field near the metal surface, caused by the surface plasmon, opens up new possibilities for influencing the ion channel.*

Thus, one plausible explanation for AuNPs interaction with potassium channels may be related to plasmon resonance phenomenon, i.e., the excitation of surface plasmons on the AuNPs surface that may be increased due to light irradiation. It is known that AuNPs, as noble nanometer-sized structures, are inherent in their own distinctive feature that collective electron charge oscillation associated with the surface plasmon resonance give rise to induced local electrical fields near the nanoparticle surface. In case of laser irradiation, this local electrical field is significantly enhanced due to local plasmon resonance that, in turn, interacts with ionic channel voltage sensors and increases outward currents leading to SM relaxation. In the absence of external irradiation, such plasmon may be excited by natural tissue chemiluminescence in the presence of nonlinear effects on AuNPs surface. The strength of the electrical field at the cell membrane depends on the concentration of AuNPs, and K^+ channels activation can be reached when threshold AuNPs concentration takes place.

Electrophysiological Evidence

The next series of experiments were performed to study outward K^+ channel activity in control thoracic aorta SM cells. Enzymatically isolated thoracic aorta cells from healthy rats were held at the resting potential of -60 mV, and then stimulated with an increasing depolarizing voltage step. The original traces and current-voltage (I-V) relationship are shown in Figure 32 A. The total outward current density amplitude (IK) in intact SMC was an average of 32 ± 2 pA/pF (n = 12) at +70 mV. All cells demonstrated clearly expressed tail currents suggesting that the currents measured were carried mainly due to activation of outward potassium channels (IK). Spontaneous current oscillation on the plateau of I_K appears to be due to the spontaneous transient outward currents (STOCs) superimposed onto the total current indicating BK_{Ca} activation (Figure 32 B).

Figure 32 A, B show that both original traces of IK and I-V relation curves obtained for SM cells treated with AuNPs (10-4 M) demonstrated a significant increase in outward K^+ current density amplitude from 32 ± 2 pA/pF to 59 ± 5 pA/pF at +70 mV, respectively ($P < 0.05$, n = 10). External green laser irradiation increased AuNps-induced increment in IK from 59 ± pA/pF to 74 ± 1 pA/pF (n = 10, $P < 0.05$).

Current-voltage (I-V) relation curves are measured also in isolated pulmonary artery SM cells in control and in the presence of AuNPs. At maximum depolarization of +70 mV the net outward K^+ (I_K) current density was 49.7 ± 4.9 pA/pF (n = 10). Application of AuNPs (10^{-4} M) produced a significant enhancement of I_K density (to 130.2 ± 5.7 pA/pF). GLI in the presence of AuNPs further increased I_K density to 205.3 ± 7.6 pA/pF (n = 10, $P < 0.05$).

After that, we identified the different components of total potassium current activated under AuNPs action (Figure 41C, D). It is clear that total outward current in rat thoracic aorta SM cells is mainly due to activation of the current carried through paxilline-sensitive BK_{Ca} channels. This conclusion is based on the next evidence. Paxilline (500 nM), added to the external bathing solution, significantly decreased (from 32±2 to 6±1pA/pF, n = 10, P < 0.05) outward current in non-treated SM cells from rat thoracic aorta. An additional tetraethylammonium (10 mM) application led to decrease of outward current up to 3 ± 1pA/pF (n = 10, P < 0.05). Paxilline (as well as TEA) application abolished AuNPs-induced increment in IK.

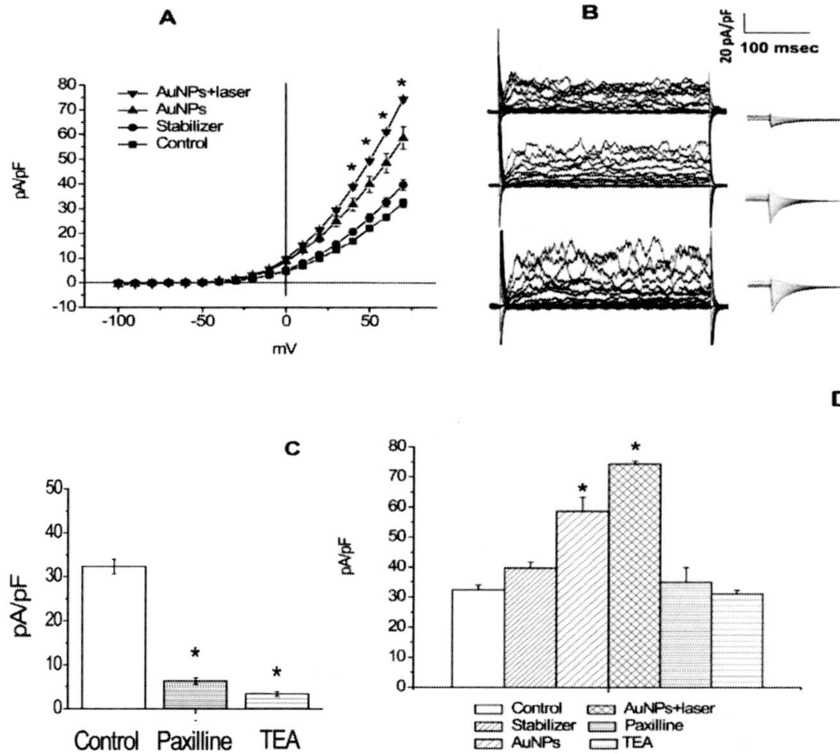

Figure 32. I -V relationships (A) and original traces (B) of outward currents recorded in isolated rat thoracic aorta smooth muscle cells in control and after treatment with AuNPs (10-4 M) and AuNPs combined with 5W/532 nm green laser irradiation. C, D – effects of potassium channels blockers (paxilline, 500 nm and tetraethylammonium, 10 mM) on outward potassium channel in non-treated (C) and treated with AuNPs (D) aortic SM cells. Currents were elicited by 10 mV step pulses with 300 ms duration between -100 and +70 mV from a holding potential of -60 mV. Data shown are mean ±SEM (n = 8). * - P < 0.05 vs AuNPs combined with laser irradiation.

It is known that the Boltzmann relation describes the voltage-dependence of channel gating. So, the standard Boltzmann equation can be used to evaluate statistically the effects of AuNPs on Ik in aortic SM cells before and after AuNPs application. Plotting the conductance against the voltage gives a curve that reflects the nature of channel gating, namely, the movement of charges in the voltage-sensitive region of the channel protein in the membrane voltage field. Plots of mean steady-state activation were fitted with a Boltzmann distribution giving voltage for half-maximal activation, i.e., significant increasing in V1/2 values under AuNPs and AuNPs plus green laser treatment, ($V_{1/2}$ = 8.5 ± 0.5 and 14 ± 0.8 mV, for control and AuNPs, respectively, n =10, P < 0.05). Laser irradiation further enhanced this effect ($V_{1/2}$ = 16 + 0.8 mV, n = 10, P < 0.05), suggesting that this conductance is most likely related to the changes of unitary conductance or single channel open time. The data indicate a significant conductance increase due to K^+ channel activation above -50 mV.

To describe the voltage-dependence of voltage-activated channels, we are normally interested to know the way in which voltage affects channel gating, independent of its effect on the electrochemical driving force. One possible way to extract the effect of voltage channel gating alone is to measure instantaneous current at a fixed voltage, so that the driving force is constant.

It is known that the current density amplitude (or membrane conductance) depends on the number of channels available in the plasma membrane, the single channel conductance and the open channel probability that, in turn, is a function of time and membrane potential. It has been established that the main outward current in aortic smooth muscle under AuNPs treatment is carried through BK_{Ca} channels. Conduction-voltage relationship studies demonstrated that the potential-dependent open probability of potassium channels appeared to be increased under AuNPs action.

Nevertheless, the question remains what is the manner in which AuNPs do it? It is likely that AuNPs as well as AuNPs combined with 5W/532 nm green laser irradiation act primarily by increasing unitary channel conductance. Unfortunately, these parameters cannot be determined from the analysis of total currents amplitudes obtained in whole-cell modification of patch-clamp technique. Now we can postulate the opening of potassium channels under AuNPs treatment. Unfortunately, there is little data to suggest precisely how this opening came about. The single-channels voltage clamp experiments are required to solve this problem properly.

Analysis of AuNPs and Combined AuNPs/ Green Laser Irradiation Effects at the Single-Channel Level

To investigate the phenomenon further, we have performed experiments using single channel recordings using on-cell patches formed on rat aorta, pulmonary artery, and mouse ileal myocytes. In on-cell patches formed on rat aortic myocytes, activity of 3-5 BK_{Ca} channels was usually observed at potentials from -20 to 40 mV. Depending on the extent of channel activity in each individual membrane fragment, the most appropriate holding potential was set within this range in order to have the initial channel activity (commonly expressed as NPo) not too high, e.g. about 0.05-0.1. Application of AuNPs to the bath potentiated BK_{Ca} activity with a delay of 1-2 min (Figure 33A), as was seen initially by more frequent channel openings followed by the progressive appearance of additional open levels corresponding to multiple openings of channels with identical single-channel current amplitudes (Figure 33A, middle panel). Eventually, after 10-15 min in the presence of AuNPs and especially when combined with the green laser illumination, there was a massive increase in channel activity with >10 channels evident (e.g., Figure 33 B, top trace at about 35 min of the recording). Precise measurement of NPo at such high channel activity became even problematic because of the noisy appearance of the trace, but as an estimate, a 5-10-fold increase in NPo values was observed in all 3 patches recorded.

A, BK_{Ca} channel activity was recorded at -20 mV (top) before and after AuNPs application at 10^{-5} M, as indicated by horizontal line (top). Two 10 s duration segments of the current trace are illustrated on the expanded time scale in the middle panel, taken at time points marked as a and b on the whole time-course trace (top panel). Up to 11 active channels were evident in this membrane fragment at full activation, as evident from multiple openings shown by the horizontal dotted lines. Bottom panel shows NPo measured over consecutive 5 s time intervals.

B, in a different patch held at 40 mV AuNPs were applied initially at 10^{-5} M, followed by 10^{-4} M, as indicated by the thinner horizontal lines, while green laser illumination was additionally used (thicker horizontal lines). Otherwise, the data were analyzed and illustrated similar to panel A.

Similar results were obtained for BK_{Ca} channels expressed in rat pulmonary artery and mouse ileal myocytes (Figure 34, 35) indicating that AuNPs act as BK_{Ca} "openers" both in vascular and visceral smooth muscles.

Thus, our single channel recordings provided a direct confirmation of BK_{Ca} activation by AuNPs at the single-channel level. Green laser irradiation acted as an additional potentiating factor in the presence of Au nanoparticles, but was inefficient by itself. Regarding the possible mechanism of AuNPs action, several observations in these experiments seem to be very pertinent.

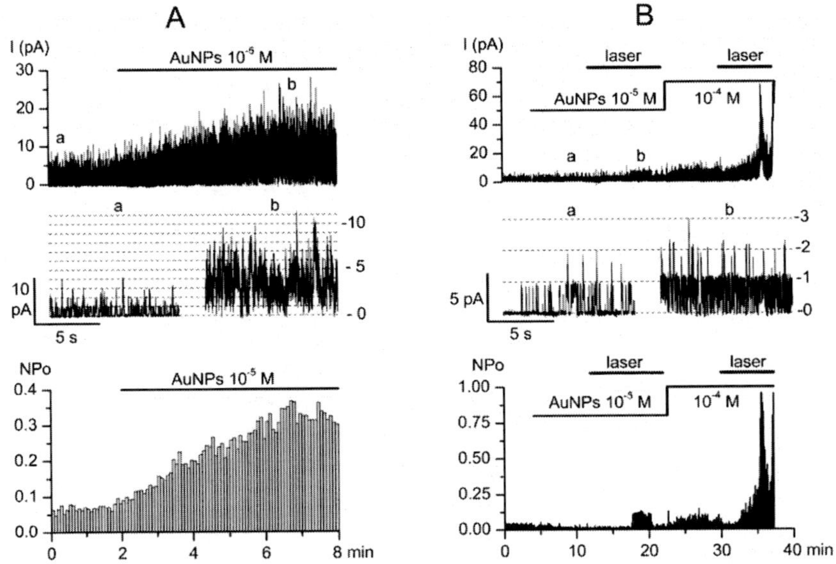

Figure 33. Potentiating effect of AuNPs on single BK_{Ca} channel activity in rat aortic myocytes.

First, the effect of AuNPs was observed in the cell-attached configuration, whereby the exterior of the membrane is not directly accessible to the bath solution. For example, it is known that even small neurotransmitter molecules cannot act on ligand-gated ion channels, when they are isolated from the bath by the tight gigaseal. This indicates that either AuNPs can cross the membrane and act on the intracellular site of the channel, or that they somehow alter membrane properties in such way, that this signal (most likely surface Plasmon resonance energy) can be transduced within the membrane plane by at least 1 mkm distance. The slow onset of AuNPs action seems to favor the first hypothesis, while the additional activation induced by laser illumination may work either way.

Second, single-channel current amplitude during AuNPs application remained constant indicating that these nanoparticles do not interfere with the ion conductance pathway, or channel pore. Instead, or additionally, activation of the whole-cell currents at the single-channel level can be explained by the significant NPo increase as the main determinant (see Figure 33).

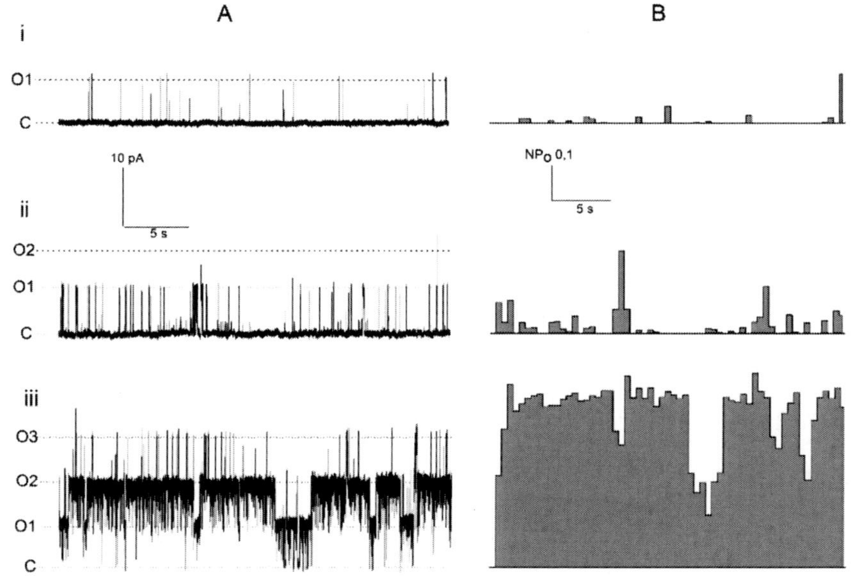

Figure 34. AuNPs activate single BK_{Ca} channels in rat pulmonary artery myocytes. A, representative single-channel recording of BK_{Ca} channel activity in a cell-attached membrane patch held at 60 mV (n=3). The periods of AuNPs application (10-4 M) followed by 5 mW/532 nm laser irradiation are indicated by the horizontal bars. B, expended segments of the trace shown in A with the dashed horizontal lines indicating closed (C) and open (O) levels. Simultaneous openings of up to 4 channels (denoted O1-O4) of identical conductance were observed when BK_{Ca} channels were strongly activated by AuNPs irradiated by green laser. C, time course of BK_{Ca} channel activity expressed as NPo measured in consecutive segments of 5 s duration. Time scale is the same as in panel A.

Third, although we could not analyse open and closed times, as multiple channels were present in all patches, at early times NPo increase by AuNPs seemed to be due to more frequent channel openings, rather than increase in channel open times (e.g. Figure 33 B, compare 2 traces shown in the middle panel). Understanding of the exact mechanism of channel activation requires additional experiments, but it seems to be due to AuNPs may modulate BK_{Ca} channels one by one, with variable time delays, which is different from the action of most other channel modulators. This effect is evident in Figure 33 **B**, middle panel, where one channel becomes already very active, yet double and triple openings remain rare, clearly showing that other channels in this patch have not been yet potentiated at this point in time. With time, as AuNPs activated more and more channels, a massive increase in NPo occurred in all experiments (Figure 33 A, B, top panels).

These experiments have revealed that the potentiating effects of AuNPs were due to a significant increase in channel open probability (NPo), while unitary current amplitude at the same test potential remained constant.

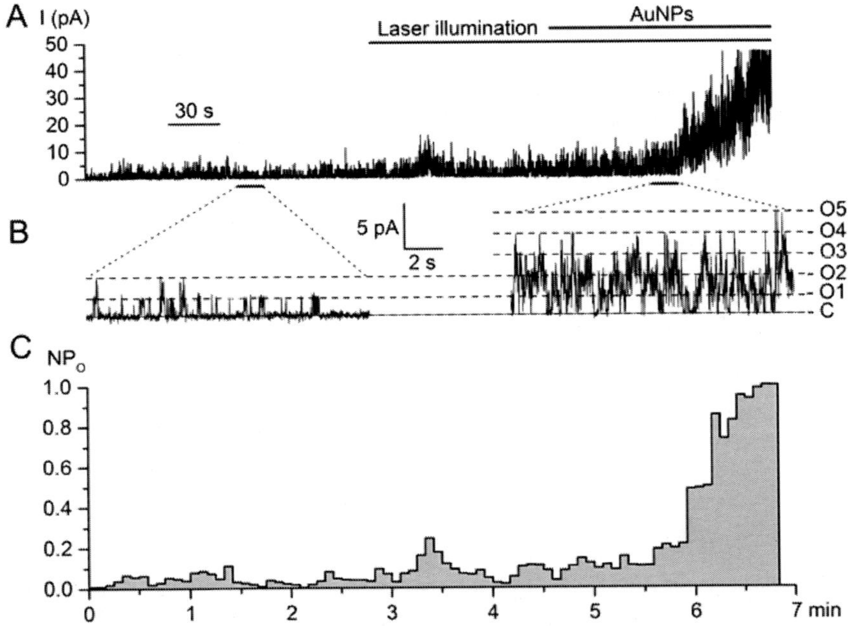

Figure 35. AuNPs activate single BK_{Ca} channels in mouse ileal myocytes. A, representative single-channel recording of BK_{Ca} channel activity in a cell-attached membrane patch held at 0 mV (n=4). The periods of 5 mW/532 nm laser irradiation followed by application of AuNPs (10-4 M) are indicated by the horizontal bars. B, expended segments of the trace shown in A with the dashed horizontal lines indicating closed (C) and open (O) levels. Simultaneous openings of up to 5 channels (denoted O1-O5) of identical conductance were observed when BK_{Ca} channels were strongly activated by AuNPs irradiated by green laser. C, time course of BK_{Ca} channel activity expressed as NPo measured in consecutive segments of 5 s duration. Time scale is the same as in panel A.

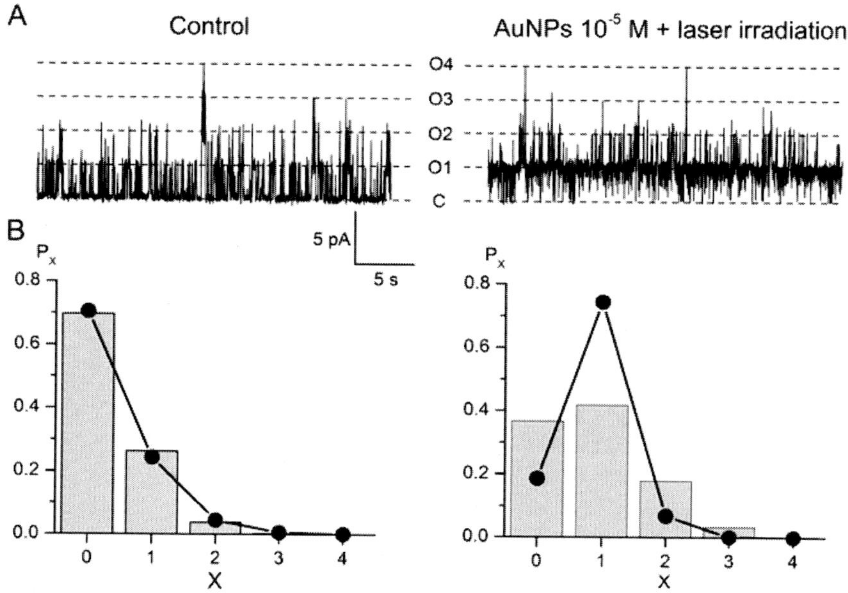

Figure 36. AuNPs-induced BK_{Ca} channel activation is associated with deviation from the principle of independent ion channel gating. A, simultaneous openings of up to 4 BK_{Ca} channels were observed in a membrane patch both in control and with AuNPs/GLI. These current levels are denoted O1-O4, corresponding to probabilities PX = 1, PX = 2, PX = 3 and PX = 4 in panel B, while C denotes closed level, e.g., all channels are closed (PX = 0). B, experimentally found PX values (closed circles) and those predicted by binomial distribution (columns) assuming N = 4, P_O = 0.086 in control and N = 4, PO = 0.222 in the presence of AuNPs/GLI. The P_O values were obtained from the measured NPO values, 0.345 and 0.887 in control and with AuNPs/GLI, respectively.

It is conceivable that AuNPs and the energy of their plasmonic resonance do not directly interfere with the ion conductance pathway, or channel pore, rather they act as gating modifiers that affect kinetics of transitions between closed and open states of the channel and, ultimately, channel open probability. Such mechanism of regulation is common for most pharmacological modulators of ion channels. However, in sharp contrast to other drugs, which typically access and similarly modulate the activity of all channels present, we have occasionally observed an unusual channel behavior during AuNPs/GLI, as illustrated in Figure 36. This phenomenon could be described as a deviation from the principle of independent channel gating. Briefly, when multiple channels (N - their total number) are present in a membrane patch all having similar open probability PO, the probability of seeing all channels closed or 1, 2, 3…X channels simultaneously open (PX) is given by the binomial distribution:

$$PX = \{N! / X! (N-X)!\} POX (1-PO) N-X \tag{20}$$

In control, all channels are gated independently as confirmed by closely similar measures and calculated according to the binomial distribution PX values (Figure 35). With AuNPs/GLI the probability of seeing one channel open was unusually high (right panel) as if only one out of four channels were activated. Indeed, the experimentally observed probabilities of seeing all channels closed or 1, 2, 3 or 4 channels simultaneously open did not confirm the principle of independent channel gating. The deviation was especially clear for PX=0, PX=1 and PX=2.

Role of Intracellular Ca^{2+} in AuNPs-Induced Maxi-K Facilitation and Following Relaxation

In rat pulmonary artery myocytes, we tested the hypothesis that plasmonic gold nanoparticles are able to modulate the function of calcium-dependent ion channels by co,5mparing the effects of AuNPs and AuNPs/GLI, under strong buffering of intracellular calcium by BAPTA chelator. 100 μM gold nanoparticles induced an increase in the average amplitude of the whole-cell outward current with 56±5 pA/pF to 115±6 pA/pF at 70 mV). External green laser irradiation (5 mW/532 nm) caused a further increase in the AuNPs-induced rise in current amplitude to 160±8 pA/pF (Figure 37 A). Under conditions of strong calcium buffering (10 mM EGTA/4.6 mM Ca^{2+} intrapipette solution mixture; $[Ca^{2+}]_i$ = 150 nM), no effect of AuNPs on outgoing current amplitude was observed. Moreover, laser irradiation did not induce any additional effects, suggesting that this phenomenon is strongly calcium-dependent (Figure 37 B).

Recording the activity of individual Maxi-K channels expressed in rat aortic myocytes, rat pulmonary arteries, and mouse ileum clearly demonstrated that AuNPs exert their action as BKCa "openers" in both vascular and visceral smooth muscles. However, this phenomenon is calcium-dependent, because the potentiating effect of AuNPs could be completely abolished by fixing the intracellular Ca2+ concentration at 150 nM. To clarify this effect, we more precisely studied the processes of changes in intracellular calcium concentration upon AuNPs-induced activation of Maxi - K channels by measuring $[Ca^{2+}]_i$ with confocal microscopy.

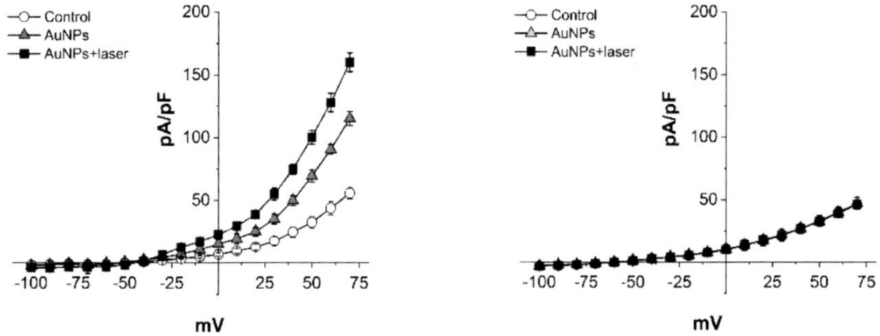

Figure 37. Effects of AuNPs alone and in combination with green laser irradiation on whole-cell outward potassium currents in isolated rat pulmonary artery smooth muscle cells under conditions of strong intracellular Ca^{2+} buffering with BAPTA (free $[Ca^{2+}]_I$=150 nM). A) Mean I-V relationships of outward whole-cell currents under control conditions, in the presence of 100 μM AuNPs, and after AuNPs were illuminated with a 5 mW/532 nm green laser, as indicated. B) The current-voltage relationships were recorded under the same conditions as in (A), but with 10 mM EGTA/4.6 mM Ca^{2+} in the pipette solution.

Thus, we next compared the Ca^{2+} store load intact and AuNPs treated SMCs of PA using applications of 5 mM caffeine. Whether this is a sufficient concentration to assess the sarcoplasmic reticulum (SR) Ca^{2+} load in PA myocytes was examined in separate experiments. The myocytes were stimulated with 3-sec caffeine pulses applied at 30-s interval, and use-dependent changes in the amplitude of the fluo-3 responses were analyzed in control conditions and following 10^{-4} M AuNPs application.

To test this hypothesis further and to clarify whether AuNPs influence the change in $[Ca^{2+}]_i$, SMCs freshly isolated from PA, were preloaded with the high affinity Ca^{2+} indicator fluo-3 and bathed in modified Krebs solution. Intact cells were tested with an application of 5 mM caffeine. After being washed with the modified Krebs solution, 10^{-4} M AuNPs were added to the pulmonary artery cell suspension. Spatio-temporal patterns of AuNPs-induced $[Ca^{2+}]_i$ oscillations are illustrated in Figure 38 showing the results obtained in 3 different cells. Depending on the cell, 3-5 min after application of 10^{-4} M AuNPs, we observed an appearance of $[Ca^{2+}]_i$ oscillations with a certain periodicity. Each subsequent oscillation was of a smaller amplitude, i.e., progressively decreased in amplitude, which probably corresponded to a decrease in the Ca^{2+} content of the SR. It thus seems to be related to the SR Ca^{2+} release, whereas activation of Ca^{2+} entry across the plasma membrane efficiently re-stores Ca^{2+} transients, which indicates effective Ca^{2+} store refilling. Thus, it seems likely that the effect of AuNPs is calcium-dependent but precise mechanisms of the genesis of AuNPs-induced $[Ca^{2+}]$ i oscillations in vascular myocytes await further investigations (Soloviev, Melnyk, Ivanova, Dryn, Zholos, 2016).

This work confirms that this effect is not restricted to Maxi-K channels in rat thoracic aorta SM cells only and could be realized in other types of SM. We can now postulate the opening of Maxi-K channels under AuNPs treatment as a prototypical mode of regulation of voltage-gated ion channels, and other types of voltage-gated ICh could likely demonstrate this effect. We suppose that AuNPs-induced vasorelaxation is due to Maxi-K channels activation, which, in turn, is realized via interaction of its voltage sensor domain and surface plasmons on the AuNPs surface that may be increased due to green laser irradiation.

Taken together, we conclude that AuNPs may be considered a novel and potent K^+ opener because of their chemical stability and biocompatibility combined with their unique optical properties. Nevertheless, therapeutic usage of AuNPs as an effective potassium channel opener will become possible only when the manner in which it functions, as well as AuNPs toxicity, will be investigated more precisely. At this stage, it is clear that AuNPs-based control of voltage-dependent ICh remains a new, evolving technology for novel therapeutics. It remains an open question whether its activity can be realized in in vivo conditions or if it is just one more tool of a restricted experimental utility. In any case, it may have a profound impact on non-invasive control of excitable tissues such as vascular and neural activity.

It is likely that the strength of the electrical field at the cell membrane depends on the concentration of AuNPs, and K^+ channel activation can be evoked when threshold AuNPs concentration takes place. It has been recently established that the plasmon excitations in metallic nanoparticles can be propagated within the distance of the order of 1 mkm (Jacak, Popko, Hendrikowski, Zielony, Gwodz et al. 2016).

Our single channel recordings using SM cells from different tissues provided a direct confirmation of Maxi-K activation by AuNPs at the single-channel level. GLI acted as an additional potentiating factor in the presence of

AuNPs, but was inefficient by itself. Regarding the possible mechanism of AuNPs action, several observations in these experiments seem to be very pertinent.

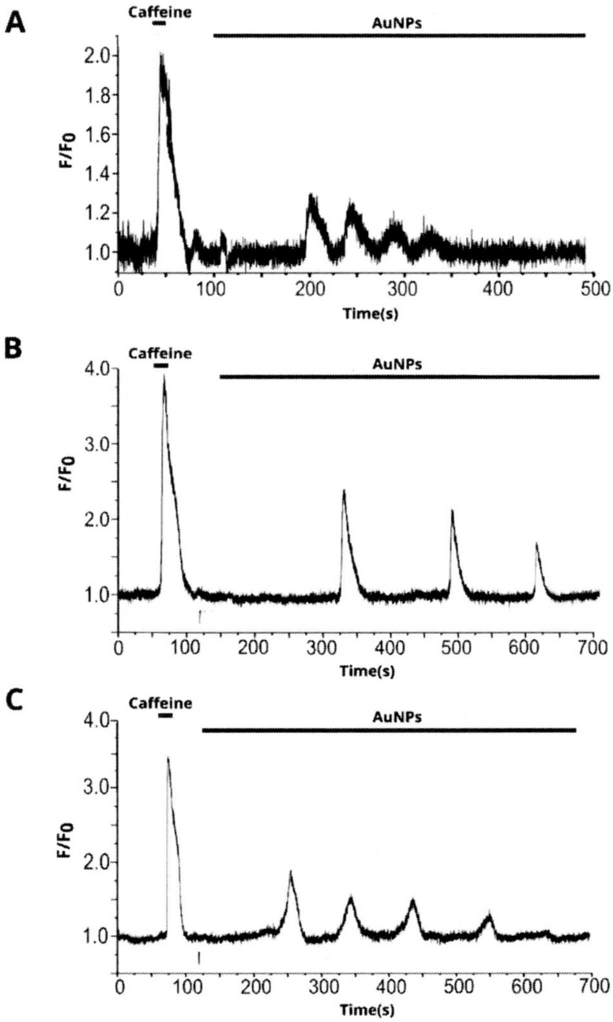

Figure 38. Spatio-temporal patterns of AuNPs-induced $[Ca^{2+}]_i$ oscillations after control caffeine application recorded in 3 different representative cells to illustrate similarities (e.g., oscillatory nature) and variability (e.g., amplitude and frequency of $[Ca^{2+}]_i$ rises) of the responses. For each cell (A-C), the time course plot of the normalized fluo-3 fluorescence intensity was averaged within the total optical slice of the SM cells, where Ca^{2+} waves induced by 10-4 M AuNPs occurred.

Thus, AuNPs were effective in the cell-attached configuration, whereby the exterior of the membrane is not directly accessible to any molecules in the bath solution. It means that either AuNPs can penetrate the membrane and act on the intracellular part of the channel, or surface plasmon resonance energy can be transduced within the membrane plane by at least 1 mkm distance. The slow onset of AuNPs action seems to favor the former hypothesis, while the additional activation induced by laser illumination may work either way. Moreover, it is possible that AuNPs affect BK_{Ca} channels not directly, but instead they somehow alter channel interaction with the membrane lipids. Such a scenario could also easily account for the distant regulation of the channel protein contained in the cell-attached membrane patch that is without any drug access to its extracellular domains.

Importantly, single-channel current amplitude during AuNPs application remained constant, indicating that these nanoparticles do not interfere with the ion conductance pathway, or channel pore. Instead, activation of the whole-cell currents at the single-channel level can be explained by the significant NPO increase as the main determinant.

Maxi-K channels are both Ca^{2+} and voltage-sensitive, hence we compared the effects of AuNPs on Maxi-K channel activity under weak (0.3 mM EGTA) or strong Ca^{2+} buffering (10 mM BAPTA/4.6 mM Ca^{2+}) to "clamp" the intracellular Ca^{2+} concentration at 100 nM. With weak Ca^{2+} buffering, Maxi-K current density was significantly increased by AuNCs and further increased by GLI while under conditions of strong intracellular Ca^{2+} buffering no effect of AuNCs on current density was observed. It became clear that these processes are calcium-dependent, as the potentiating effect of AuNCs could be completely abolished by "clamping" the intracellular Ca^{2+} concentration at 100 nM.

Third, although we could not analyze open and closed times, as multiple channels were present in all patches, at early times NPO increase by AuNPs seemed to be due to more frequent channel openings, rather than increase in channel open time. Understanding the exact mechanism of channel activation requires additional experiments, but it seems that AuNPs may modulate BK_{Ca} channels one by one and with variable time delays, which is different from the action of most other known channel chemical modulators. Such an effect is evident when one channel becomes very active, yet double and triple openings remain rare, clearly showing that other channels in this patch have not been yet potentiated at this point in time. Indeed, measuring open probability for levels 1, 2, 3 and 4 (e.g., 1, 2, 3 or 4 simultaneously open channels) and comparing these values to those expected from the binomial distribution, which describes the discrete probability distribution for N independent events, confirmed that channels gated independently before, but not after AuNPs application. With time, as AuNPs activated more and more channels, a significant increase in NPO occurred in all experiments. Within the technical limitations we encountered in single-channel recordings, the effect of AuNPs appears to be concentration-dependent.

For this effect to be of any practical usability, the real question concerns the delivery of light irradiation to a biological target. The depth of light penetration usually does not exceed several hundred micrometers. It is enough for isolated single cells and smooth muscle preparations in vitro, but is it plausible for some internal organs, for instance, the heart or blood vessels? One approach consists of using pulse nanosecond irradiation in contrast to a continued one, which enables irradiation energy to be enhanced while avoiding its side effects. Another possible approach proposes fiber-optic devices for endoscopic or intra-tissue delivery of radiation. There is also an intriguing possibility that natural tissue chemiluminescence could be used to mediate AuNPs-induced activation of BK_{Ca} channels. This is a very attractive hypothesis to be tested since enhanced reactive oxygen species production associated with diseases such as diabetes mellitus could enhance tissue chemiluminescence thus facilitating BK_{Ca} activation and self-correcting blood flow (by relaxing blood vessels) in the affected tissues. In this connection it is important to note that Dykman and Klebtsov (Dykman, Klebtsov, 2012) postulated that AuNPs are being used with diagnostic aims and for cell photothermolysis mainly but rather seldomly used directly for therapeutic purposes. Namely, they were used for the treatment of rheumatoid arthritis due to AuNPs anti-angiogenic activity and as a vector for the delivery of tumor necrosis factor to solid tumors in rats. However, they were never used as a therapeutic agent for cardiovascular system treatment.

It should be noted that similar results, but with a different charge carrier, were obtained by American scientists. The data presented by the group from the University of Washington demonstrate that so called quantum dots (i.e., very small amounts of semiconductor nanoparticles) possess the ability to stimulate cells and to trigger neuron firing with light (Lugo, Miao, Rieke, Lin, 2012). When quantum dots excite light shining on it, it becomes polarized that one part of the material is more positive, and the other is more negative. This, in turn, sets up an electric field, which can interact with a neuron of another cell of interest. How strong that interaction depends on how close the polarized quantum dots are to the cell.

Thus, the relaxant effect of AuNPs of core size of 5 nm and its ability to open Maxi-K channels in a remote-control manner in smooth muscle cells is now evident from a series of our studies. To the best of our knowledge this is the first evidence that AuNPs possess the ability to control ion channel gating at a distance and this way it is likely to possess the ability to restore normal vascular contractility in a number of disease states related to the development of vascular SM hypercontractility.

This work confirms that this effect is not restricted to BK_{Ca} channels in rat thoracic aorta SM cells only and could be realized in other types of SM. We can now postulate the opening of Maxi-K channels under AuNPs treatment as a prototype mode of similar remote control of opening in other types of voltage-gated ICh. We suppose that AuNPs-induced vasorelaxation is due to BK_{Ca} channel activation, which, in turn, is realized via interaction of its voltage sensor domain and surface plasmons on the AuNPs surface that may be significantly increased due to green laser irradiation.

The new finding of this study is that AuNPs-induced ion channel activation appears to be very sensitive to Ca^{2+} homeostasis suggesting intimate calcium involvement in this process.

AuNPs may be considered as the potential K^+ opener because of their chemical stability and biocompatibility combined with their unique optical properties. Nevertheless, therapeutic usage of AuNPs as an effective potassium channel opener will become possible when the manner in which it functions as well as AuNPs toxicity are additionally and more precisely investigated. At this stage, it is clear that AuNPs-based control of voltage-dependent ICh remains a new, evolving technology for novel therapeutics. It remains an open question whether its activity can be realized in *in vivo* conditions or if it is just one more tool of a narrow experimental utility. In any case, it may have a profound impact on non-invasive control of excitable tissues functioning such as vascular and neural activity.

Later, we compared the effect of 5 nm gold nanoparticles on BKCa channels and associated calcium signaling in freshly isolated rat pulmonary artery SM cells and cultured hippocampal neurons. Outward potassium currents were recorded using patch-clamp techniques. Briefly, in pulmonary artery SM cells, AuNPs increased the amplitude of currents via BKCa channels, which was potentiated by green laser irradiation near plasmon resonance wavelength (532 nm). As in our previous studies, buffering of intracellular free calcium with EGTA abolished these effects. Furthermore, using confocal laser microscopy it was found that the application of gold nanoparticles caused oscillations of intracellular calcium concentration that were decreasing in amplitude with time. In cultured hippocampal neurons gold nanoparticles inhibit the effect of EGTA partially restoring the amplitude of the slow after hyperpolarizing (AHP) currents.

In the current-clamp configuration, approximately 80% of neurons identified morphologically as pyramidal cells exhibited the afterhyperpolarization (AHP) following the action potential train generated by 1 nA inward current injection step (Figure 39A). It has been suggested that several types of voltage-gated calcium channels (L-, N-, and P-types) modulate the slow AHP current. Calcium-binding proteins may also underlie the sensitivity of sAHP to intracellular calcium. (Abel, Lee, Callawa, Foehring, 2004; Tzingounis, Kobayashi, Takamatsu, Nicoll, 2007).

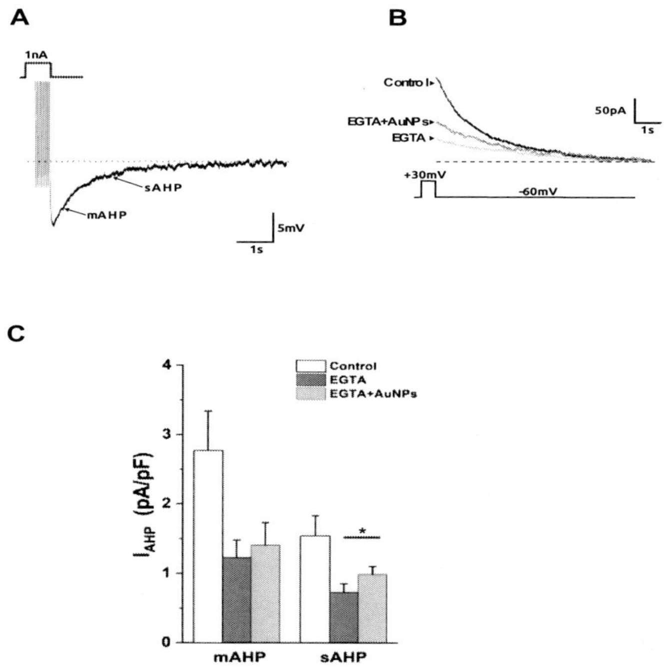

Figure 39. Effects of gold nanoparticles on medium (I_mAHP) and slow (I_sAHP) AHP currents in hippocampal pyramidal neurons. (A) AHPs following spike trains elicited by 1 nA 4 s current step in the current-clamp mode. (B) I_mAHP and I_sAHP generated by a voltage step from -60 mV to 30 mV in the voltage-clamp mode with intracellular perfusion of 200 µM EGTA. Control trace recorded at zero time, "EGTA" after 2-3 minutes with buffer perfusion and "EGTA+AuNPs" following external application 100 µM AuNPs. (C) AuNPs did not affect I_mAHP amplitude, but partially recovered the I_sAHP amplitude.

Thus, we concluded that fluctuations in intracellular calcium can modulate plasmonic gold nanoparticles-induced gating of BK_{Ca} channels in smooth muscle cells and in neurons through an indirect mechanism, probably involving the interaction of plasmon resonance with calcium-permeable ion channels, which leads to a change in intracellular calcium level (Soloviev, Ivanova, Sydorenko et al, 2023).

Chapter 16

Reactive Oxygen Species (ROS) and Vascular Tone

Two Faces of Reactive Oxygen Species: Are They Good or Bad?

According to the famous evolutionary biologist Theodosius Dobzhansky "Nothing in Biology makes sense except in the light of evolution" (Dobzhansky, 1973). Until about 2.5 billion years ago, there was no oxygen in the atmosphere, but then the so-called "Great Oxidation Event" happened due to significant accumulation of oxygen produced by the photosynthetic Cyanobacteria. In the short term, this oxygen nearly eliminated other life forms, for most of which were toxic. However, in the long term, the surviving and evolving organism's oxygen opened access to the entirely new form of energy (Kump, 2008; Blaustein, 2016).

It is clear that the production of so-called reactive oxygen species (ROS) is an unavoidable consequence of aerobic metabolism and, therefore, life. Generation of mitochondrial ROS mainly takes place at the electron transport chain located on the inner mitochondrial membrane during the process of oxidative phosphorylation Leakage of electrons at complex I and complex III from electron transport chains leads to partial reduction of oxygen to form superoxide. Subsequently, superoxide is quickly dismutated to hydrogen peroxide by two dismutases including superoxide dismutase 2 (SOD2) in the mitochondrial matrix and superoxide dismutase 1 (SOD1) in the mitochondrial intermembrane space. Collectively, both superoxide and hydrogen peroxide generated in this process are considered mitochondrial ROS.

Another source of ROS in living cells is a family of NADPH oxidases (NOX). NOX is an enzyme complex on the cell membrane that generates superoxide by transferring electrons NADPH across the cell membrane to oxygen molecules. Xanthine oxidase (XO is a source of ROS during ischemic attack. Other intracellular enzymes that catalyze the ROS production are cyclooxygenase (COX), lipoxygenases (LOX and cytochrome P450 enzymes (Li and Yang, 2016).

Based on all this it became clear that this phenomenon cannot be avoided, and it is a normal manifestation of the vital activity of the organism. ROS overproduction due to ionized irradiation impact is an example of external oxidative stress, which can and should be avoided.

It is interesting to note that disparate antioxidants demonstrate very often a positive effect in experimental conditions; they failed in clinical trials. There may be a reason precisely in their critical need for the course of life processes.

Cardiovascular problems are common side effects that happen during cancer therapy, and the heart and blood vessels are the major organs that are involved in potential damage following radiation exposure impact. The most visible radiation-mediated cell death derives from the overproduction of free radicals, which initiate oxidative stress. Reactive oxygen species (ROS) are generally accepted as a hallmark in cardiovascular diseases, mainly because of its sometimes-unwanted interplay with nitric oxide (NO) leading to peroxynitrite (ONOO-) production.

NO provides cardioprotection against ROS-induced damage, although this in turn limits the beneficial effects of NO itself. In addition, radiation causes adaptive morphological changes in the vasculature, leading to dysfunction of the coronary vessels. It has been suggested that an increase in ROS content contributes to long-term damage to the heart after radiation exposure.

Histological analysis indicated a loss of cardiac tissue in irradiated animals suggesting not only functional but anatomical remodeling. Confocal microscopy studies showed an increase in intracellular ROS in irradiated tissue, but no significant difference was observed in NO production. Different NOS isoforms evaluation showed elevated iNOS protein expression in irradiated animals.

In conclusion, gamma radiation stimulates sustained ROS production in heart tissue and activation of iNOS might be a mechanism for counterbalancing the disruption in the heart antioxidant system (de Oliveira, Somasekhar, Mitra, et al. 2019).

An article with a similar title was published just recently (Patel, et al. 2018). The role of ROS as a trigger of a number of pathological conditions is more often emphasized, including such severe and well-known pathologies as diabetes, AH, and cancer. At the same time, ROS are an integral component of many vital pathological processes. For instance, ROS are required to maintain normal redox homeostasis and normal functioning of the immune system. They modulate the normal growth of vascular cells, proliferation and apoptosis, and are an essential link in a number of signaling pathways. RNS, in particular peroxynitrite, is used by macrophages to fight pathogenic bacteria.

The problem lies in the fact that for the normal functioning of the body in its internal environments, an optimal balance of oxidative components and antioxidants must be maintained. The same principle is true for all other biologically active compounds and molecules such as nitric oxide, carbon monoxide, hydrogen sulfide, etc.

Plasmalemmal Na^+/K^+ ATPase as Unexpected but Important ROS Amplifier

The role of the Na^+/K^+-ATPase in the formation and maintenance of membrane potential has long been well known. Currently, new and rather unexpected properties of these ATPases are becoming known. It is becoming clear that the pharmacological fight against excess ROS can be effective only if somehow it is possible to activate the signaling pathways of the cell that control the expression of genes, which, in turn, are involved in the processes of detoxification and removal of ROS and/or activation of antioxidant systems. It is known that transcriptional response to oxidative stress is mediated via so-called ARE (antioxidant response elements). In turn, activation of transcription with ARE is realized with the help of Nrf2, the nuclear factor erythroid 2–related factor 2 (Nguyen, Nioi, Pickett, 2009).

Nrf2 is a potent regulator of cellular resistance to stress produced by ROS and RNS. Nrf2 controls both the basal and induced expression of a number of ARE–dependent genes to regulate or eliminate the physiological and pathophysiological effects of oxidant exposure. Nrf2 mRNA is expressed broadly and independently of inducers, suggesting a post-transcriptional mechanism(s) for Nrf2 activation (Ma, 2013).

Recently, unexpected data have appeared on the new role of Na/K ATPase in the regulation of cellular functions. It is well known that Na/K-ATPase is related to ion pumping function but it signaling function represents a surprising discovery. This signaling function requires the generation of reactive oxygen species (ROS) which, in turn, requires the activation of Src and the transactivation of the epithelial growth factor receptor (EGFR). These new data suggest that the Na/K-ATPase may be used as a receptor for some kind of ROS and in this way operates as an amplifier of oxidant signalling (Maxwell, Shah and Shapiro, 2015). The authors summarized that the data obtained would suggest that any pathway, which involves ROS capable of carbonylation (e.g., O_{2-}, H_2O_2), may become amplified by the Na/K - ATPase-Src-ROS signal cascade. If this is the case, the Na/K-ATPase may prove to be a useful therapeutic target in a variety of disease states associated with excessive oxidation."

The data shows that Nrf2 is activated in many types of cancer (Jung, Yoo, Shin, Park, Jeon, 2018). If so, then Nrf2 inhibition may be a prospective pharmacological intervention for cancer therapy and maybe other important diseases.

Chapter 17

Vascular Smooth Muscle and Ionized Irradiation: Consequences of Interaction

The data obtained clearly indicate that ionized irradiation represents itself as genotoxic oxidative stress. When the Chernobyl nuclear reactor in Ukraine blew up in 1986, radioactive contamination spread over a wide area and up to three million people are thought to have suffered ill health as a result of the accident.

The Chernobyl catastrophe really created many health problems for the civil Ukrainian population and adjoined territory of Russia and Republic of Belarus. At the same time, it gave us very important health information. The first surprising discovery was the fact that the most common health problem in the Ukrainian population exposed to radiation was diseases of the cardiovascular system, and hypertension especially. Although hypertension is common in the normal population, it seems to have an ever-higher incidence in survivors of the tragedy. In 2001 the prevalence of cardiovascular diseases was ranked third, in the general population of Ukraine, but it was ranked highest among Chernobyl emergency workers (Bennett et al. 2006). It is important to note that the same phenomenon was also found in survivors of the Nagasaki and Hiroshima atomic bombs (Wong et al. 1993).

Thus, the results of clinical observations clearly indicated that the frequency of hypertension development in the population within the contaminated areas in Ukraine and Republic of Belarus has increased. People who were engaged in clean-up of the Chernobyl disaster consequences demonstrated the increased level of arterial blood pressure, but underlying mechanisms are unknown, and this has complicated the treatment of hypertension. It was a surprising discovery for us that experimental rats being irradiated at both early and prolonged terms of post-irradiated period also demonstrated a high level of blood pressure as compared to non-irradiated animals. We discovered the similarity in mechanisms of vascular damage in irradiated rats and rats with genetically determined hypertension. It seems that endothelium damage contributes to the increased vascular tone in both cases.

Taken together, these data gave powerful impetus to studies with the aim to clarify the intrinsic mechanisms of radiation-induced vascular malfunction and to find possible pharmacological interventions that could normalise vascular tone increased due to ionized irradiation.

Not every electromagnetic field act on the body as favorably as the green region of the visible light spectrum. Gamma radiation is also a flow of photons. However, this stream of photons has much more energy (more than 105 eV) and a very short wavelength, less than 0.1 nm. Gamma radiation is emitted by excited atomic nuclei during radioactive transformations and nuclear reactions (explosions), as well as arising from the deceleration of charged particles in matter, their decay, during the annihilation of particle-antiparticle pairs. For comparison, the energy of a green light quantum is about 2.4 eV. Due to its extremely high penetrating power, gamma rays easily penetrate living cells, causing damage. When interacting with the cells of the body, there is a sharp excitation of atoms, their ionization, because of which the structure of molecules begins to change, various pathologies and diseases arise. Unfortunately, the likelihood of a person colliding with this type of electromagnetic waves has recently become more and more likely and the result of such an interaction will usually not be in favor of a person. Unless, of course, we exclude cases of using gamma rays in the clinic. Ionization is the process of formation of ions by emitting electrons from atoms and molecules after exposure to high temperatures, electrical discharges, or electromagnetic and nuclear radiation. Ionized radiation (IR) can be divided into electromagnetic radiation (X-rays and γ-rays) and particle radiation, including neutrons.

IR can affect biological targets via direct and indirect mechanisms. The indirect mechanism involves production of free radicals that consequently cause cell damage. The direct effect theory or target theory proposes that IR may act by direct hits on atoms in cells. All atoms and molecules in the cells, such as enzymatic and structural proteins and RNA, are very vulnerable to radiation effects. The principal target of IR is DNA, in which radiation produces single- or double-stranded chromosomal breaks. The theory of indirect effect proposes that IR has an effect through the radiolysis of cellular water, forming free radicals. These free radicals interact with atoms and molecules inside the cells, and especially with DNA, to produce chemical modifications and, therefore, harmful effects in the cells. When ionizing rays interact with water, the presence of an excess of oxygen when cells are irradiated allows additional free radicals to be formed. About two thirds of the biological damage caused by radiation with low linear energy transfer (LET) is due to the indirect effect (Elgazzar, Kazem, 2006).

Let us consider some consequences of the influence of radiation on blood vessels, limiting ourselves, for obvious reasons, to the role of BK_{Ca} channels.

Effect of IR on BK_{Ca} Channels in Endothelial Cells

The initial ECs response to most stimuli is an increase in the concentration of intracellular free calcium $[Ca^{2+}]_i$. This increase in $[Ca^{2+}]_i$ is mainly due to the influx of extracellular Ca^{2+}. The sustained influx of Ca^{2+} is required by the production of NO by ECs (Moncada, Higgs, 2002). Therefore, one of the potential mechanisms of IR-induced decrease in NO production can be alterations in Ca^{2+} signaling. K^+ channels, including the large conductance Ca^{2+}-activated K^+ channels (BK_{Ca}), small conductance Ca^{2+}-activated K^+ channels (SK_{Ca}), intermediate conductance Ca^{2+}-activated K^+ channels (IK_{Ca}), inward rectifying K^+ channels (IRK), and voltage-gated K^+ channels (IKv), are the major classes of ion channels involved in setting ECs membrane potential (Edwards et al. 2010; Coleman et al. 2004). BK_{Ca} channels are important targets for regulating the entry of Ca^{2+} into the ECs and, therefore, activation of Ca^{2+}-dependent ECs functions. (Félétou, Vanhoutte, 2009) and have been shown to be involved in endothelium-dependent vasodilatation (Coleman et al. 2004). Activation of the BK_{Ca} channels leads to vasodilation by several mechanisms. The outward K^+ current hyperpolarizes the membrane of endothelial cells, thereby increasing the driving force for Ca^{2+} entry, which will lead to an increase in the formation of vasodilator mediators NO and prostacyclin. Alternatively, an increase in the cytosolic Ca^{2+} in ECs can stimulate the formation and subsequent release of EDHF. The release of EDHF will lead to vasodilation by hyperpolarizing the membrane of the vascular SMCs and reducing Ca^{2+} entry into the cells (Félétou, 2009). Another possible scenario is passage of hyperpolarizing current from ECs to smooth muscle cells via myo-endothelial gap-junctions (Garland, Dora,2021).

In addition, the increased K^+ current can lead to an increase in K^+ concentration in the endothelial cell, which itself can act like EDHF by hyperpolarizing the SMCs membrane through activating the inward rectifying K^+ current or the Na^+/K^+-ATPase (Busse et al. 2002). It is known that the BK_{Ca} channels can indirectly modulate the production of NO and, because of this modulation, are important in endothelium-dependent vasodilatation (Nilius, G. Droogman, 2001). The open probability of BK_{Ca} channels is regulated by intracellular Ca^{2+} levels in such a way that the increase in endothelial $[Ca^{2+}]_i$ increases the probability of opening BK_{Ca} channels and vice versa.

Therefore, the K^+ channels and, in particular, the BK_{Ca} channels, are important for controlling the driving force for Ca^{2+} entry and, therefore, for regulating NO synthesis. The isotypes of BK_{Ca} channels that are expressed in ECs varies by species and vascular network, and may also depend on the culturing conditions (Kohler et al. 2000). It likely that BK_{Ca} channels are clearly expressed in endothelial cells isolate intact isolated from rat coronary arteries (Tihkin, Rekalov, Ivanova et al. 2007) and coronary artery hypertensive rats (Briones, Padilha, Cogolludo et al. 2009).

It has been shown in coronary artery ECs of rats subjected to a dose of 6 Gy from a 60Co source, that outward K^+ currents on the 9th day after irradiation are suppressed or even completely abolished. The reversal potential for these currents in the cells was shifted to more positive values, and selective inhibition of BK_{Ca} channels with paxilline did not have or only slightly affected irradiated cells (Tishkin et al. 2007).

Experiments on isolated rat aorta showed that both paxilline and γ-radiation significantly shifted the ACh dose–response curve to the right. In aorta of control rats paxilline shifted the dose-response curve for Ach-induced relaxation to the right to a degree similar to that induced by γirradiation, and did not affect the aorta from irradiated animals (Tishkin et al. 2007), indicating that paxilline mimics the effects of irradiation. Inhibition of BK_{Ca} channels may allow expression of a non-selective cationic and/or Cl− conductance, which leads to depolarization of the ECs membrane to more positive potentials. This leads to a significant reduction in the driving force for Ca^{2+} entry, resulting in a decrease in NO synthesis and the formation of blunted endothelium-dependent vasodilatation.

Therefore, nonfatal γ-irradiation of the whole body suppresses the endothelial BK_{Ca} channels, which control the driving force for the entry of Ca^{2+} and, therefore, Ca^{2+}-dependent synthesis of NO in the ECs. This may contribute to radiation-induced endothelial dysfunction and an increase in blood pressure. In Figure 43, we illustrated the main pathways of BK_{Ca} channels involvement in inhibition of NO-mediated vasodilatation under IR impact.

BK_{Ca} Channels In Smooth Muscle Cells Under Ionized Irradiation

BK_{Ca} channels are known the predominant types of K^+ channels in the SMCs of most arteries that play an important role in vascular function due to its participation in changes in the polarization of vascular SMCs membrane (Hill, Yang, Yella et al, 2010). BK_{Ca} channels are different from all other K^+ channels because of their high sensitivity to both $[Ca^{2+}]_i$ and voltage. Inhibition of BK_{Ca} channels causes membrane depolarization and vasoconstriction, and their dysfunction plays an important role in the pathogenesis of vascular diseases (Berkefeld et al, 2010). BK_{Ca} channels open in response to depolarization and intracellular Ca^{2+}, and are associated with auxiliary β1-subunits that responsible for Ca^{2+} sensitivity of the channel and its activation directly counteracts vasoconstriction, making myocyte membrane potential more negative and, as a result, inhibiting voltage-dependent Ca^{2+} influx into SMCs (Ghatta et al. 2006). It is important to note that the BK_{Ca} channels have low sensitivity to Ca^{2+} that renders them silent under resting conditions even in arterioles with a significant resting tone (Berkefeld et al, 2010). BK_{Ca} channels are also very sensitive to ROS and oxidative stress (Braklemeier, Eishler, Knorr et al, 2004; Tishkin et al. 2007).

It has been found that the whole-body ionizing irradiation of rats at 6 Gy dose from a ^{60}Co source significantly inhibits whole-cell outward K^+ current in aortic SMCs at 9th and 30th days after irradiation, moreover this inhibition was increased throughout the post-irradiation period. It has also been determined that the main component of K^+ current in SMCs of rat aorta is BK_{Ca} current which was significantly suppressed on the 30th day after animals' irradiation and this effect was comparable to siRNA - induced KCNMA1 gene silencing (Soloviev, Tishkin, Ivanova et al, 2009; Kizub et al. 2010; Kyrychenko, Tishkin, Dosenko et al, 2012). This mechanism may contribute to hypercontractility of vascular SMCs and to development of AH evoked by IR (Figure 40).

Vascular SMCs membrane depolarization leads to an activation of voltage-gated calcium channels, consequently causing the elevation in $[Ca^{2+}]_i$ and vasoconstriction. Vasoconstriction can be opposed by stimulation of calcium sparks that activate BK_{Ca} channels in vascular SMCs. Additionally, the ablation of the genes for the α- or β1 subunits of the BK_{Ca} channels finally leads to a vascular SMCs membrane depolarisation increasing the vascular tone contributing to the development of the AH (Soloviev, Tishkin, Ivanova et al. 2009). A number of studies have shown that inhibition of the BK_{Ca} channel is involved in mechanisms of AH development (Chang, Gao, Zuo et al, 2005; Novokhatska, Tishkin, Dosenko et al. 2013).

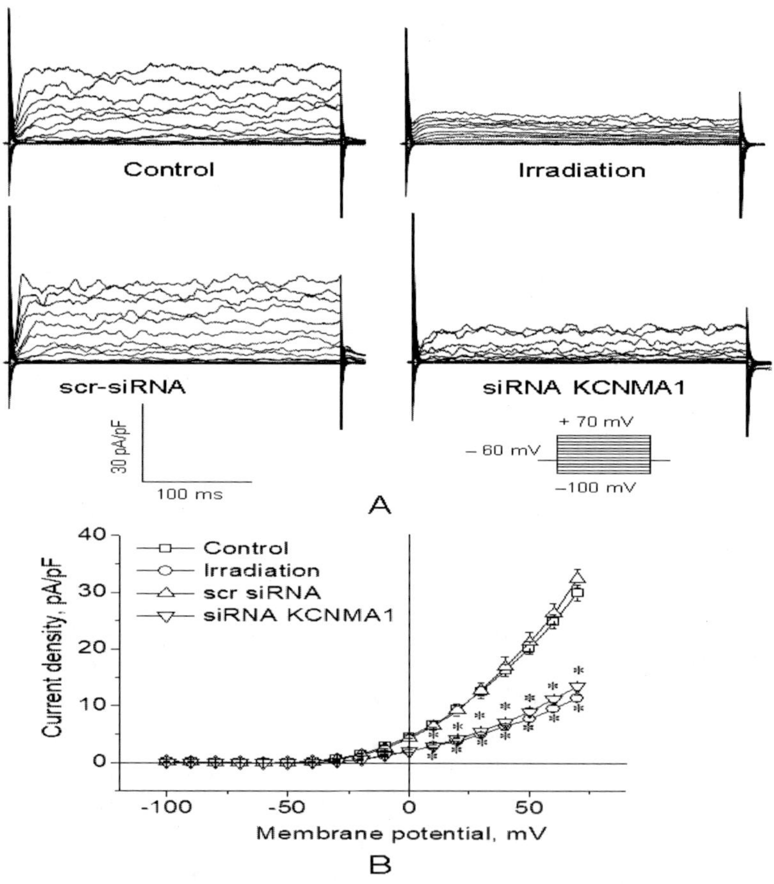

Figure 40. Effects of siRNA - induced KCNMA1 gene silencing on total outward currents in VSMC in comparison to non-fatal whole-body irradiation. Outward membrane currents were elicited by a series of 10 mV pulses with 300 ms duration from -100 mV to +70 mV from a holding potential of -60 mV. A – original traces, B – current-voltage relationship of total currents recorded in isolated rat thoracic aorta SMC obtained before and after irradiation impact and siRNA treatment. Data shown are mean ± SEM; experiments were carried out on 24 cells from 12 control rats, 17 cells from 12 irradiated animals, 12 cells from 6 rats after scr siRNA and 15 cells from 7 rats after siRNA KCNMA1 injection. The asterisks indicate statistical significance as compared to control tissues and scrRNA ($P < 0.05$).

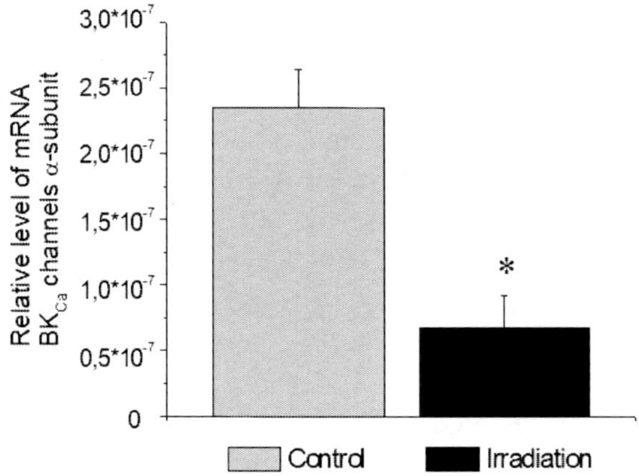

A

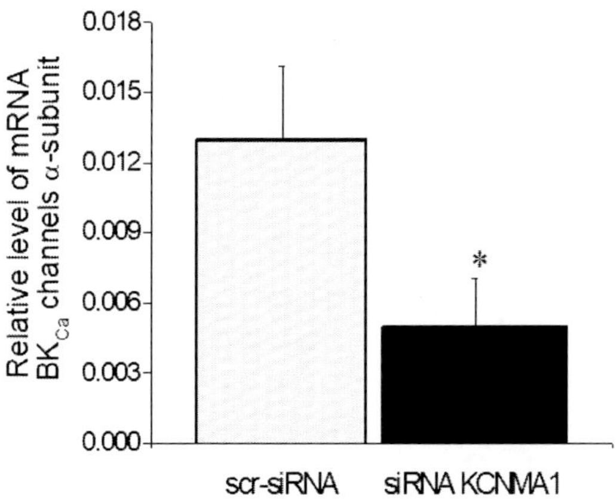

B

Figure 41. Expression of mRNA BK_{Ca} channels α-subunit in rat thoracic aorta smooth muscle after irradiation (A) and KCNMA1 gene silencing (B). A, aortic total RNA was isolated from 5 control rats and 6 rats on 30th days after irradiation impact. β actin were used as internal control; B, aortic total RNA was isolated from 6 control rats (scrRNA) and 7 rats on 7th day following siRNAs injection. 18S RNAs were used as internal control. The asterisks indicate the statistical significance as compared to control and scrRNA ($P < 0.05$).

BK_{Ca} channels consist of at least two different integral membrane subunits: the pore-forming (ion-conducting) α-subunit (KCNMA1) and the regulatory β-subunit (KCNMB1-4), which is responsible for the sensitivity of the channel to Ca^{2+} (Hill, Yang, Ella et al, 2010). The α-subunit is the minimum component for the activity of the BK_{Ca} channels, and functional channels are formed with four α-subunits. The channel α-subunit of the mammalian BK_{Ca} channels is encoded by KCNMA1 gene, formerly known as Slowpoke, Slo or Slo1 (Berkefeld et al, 2010). Four family members of the β-subunit have been identified in different tissues. The β1-subunit is expressed predominantly in arterial SM cells (Cox, Aldrich, 2000). γ-Radiation has been shown to reduce BK_{Ca} α- and β1-subunit mRNA levels in rat aortic SM cells (Soloviev, Tishkin, Ivanova et al. 2009). This could be evidence of the ability of these channels to decrease K^+ outward current and diminishing the dilatation in blood vessels exposed to IR.

Kyrychenko et al. (2012) have compared the results of small interfering RNAs (siRNAs)-induced KCNMA1 gene silencing and effect of γ-radiation in rat aorta SM cells on the 30th day after the whole-body irradiation (6 Gy). They have found that the expression profile of BK_{Ca} mRNA transcripts in vascular SM has been decreased in siRNAs treated rats in a manner similar to SM cells from vessels of γ-irradiated animals. In contrast, the mRNA levels of Kv and KATP in irradiated tissue have been increased while L-VDCC mRNA transcripts demonstrate a tendency to increment (Figure 41, 42)).

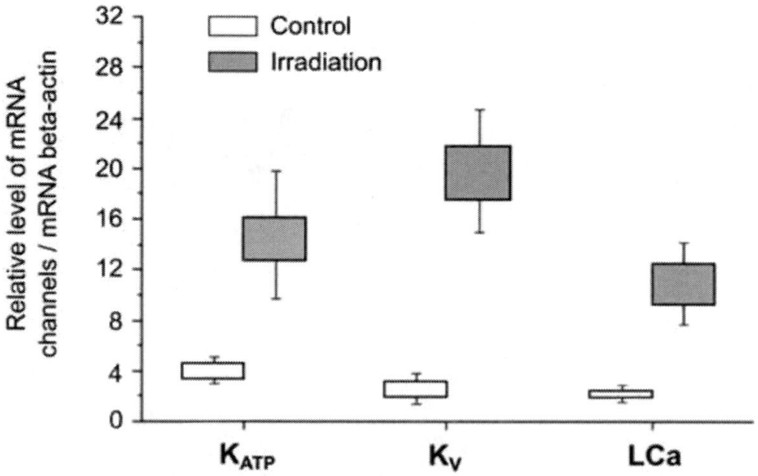

Figure 42. mRNA expression of Kv, KATP and LCa channelsin aortic SM cells with silencing KCNMA1 gene vascular tissues from healthy and irradiated rats. A, aortic total RNA was isolated from 5 control rats and 6 rats on 30th days after irradiation impact. β actin was used as internal control; B, aortic total RNA was isolated from 6 control rats (scrRNA) and 12 rats on the 7th day following siRNAs injection. β actin was used as internal control. The asterisks indicate the statistical significance as compared to control ($P < 0.05$).

Silencing of KCNMA1 gene also led to a decrease in ACh-induced endothelium-dependent dilatation in γirradiated rat aorta and accompanied with elevated contractility in denuded arteries to norepinephrine in a radiation-like manner. Thus, γ-radiation can change the shape and function of the BK_{Ca} channels, and this type of channelopathy can contribute to the occurrence of associated vascular anomalies.

Taken together, the results of longitudinal studies of humans exposed to IR and the data obtained in studies on animal models support the hypothesis of a direct and consistent relationship between IR exposure and vascular anomalies development. A large amount of evidence clearly shows that blood vessels can be one of the main targets for IR. In our studies, we demonstrated that IR evokes clearly expressed vascular tone abnormalities contributing to the development of AH. To our mind the main question we need to address in radiation medicine is how to prevent/restore vascular function damaged by IR impact and how cellular function can be preserved during radiation impact. The solution is associated with the precise identification of the main pharmacological targets for the therapy along with establishing the intracellular structures and mechanisms involved in vascular wall damage by IR. External-beam radiation therapy is commonly used as a primary and adjuvant therapeutic modality in patients with neoplasm, however, despite the improvement in technology, it affects normal tissues, including the vasculature. The effects of IR manifest in blunted vasodilatation and vasospasm development and led to significant cardio-vascular complications (stroke, myocardial infarction, hypertension, etc.) with negative impact on the course and treatment of the primary disease. IR-induced locally occurring and generalized vasospastic conditions represent a real health hazard for patients with neoplasm treated with external beam irradiation as well as for any person who was exposed to IR impact.

The existing data demonstrate that non-lethal doses of IR evoke depression of endothelium-dependent NO-mediated vasodilatation and increase vessels' sensitivity to vasoconstrictor agents. Such decreased vasodilator ability of irradiated blood vessels and their increased responsiveness to external stimuli may be due to, at least, a few main possible reasons: 1) suppression of eNOS-dependent signaling; 2) suppression of BK_{Ca} activity in ECs; 3) PKC-dependent inhibition of BK_{Ca} activity in vascular SMCs; 4) PKC-dependent increase in myofilaments sensitivity to calcium in vascular SMCs. Nevertheless, SMCs are the final common target of malfunctions produced by IR. All these mechanisms are elicited by overproduction of ROS/RNS in excess of endogenous antioxidant activity and oxidative stress development under IR. We believe that a proper regulation of different PKC isoforms in irradiated tissues using novel genetic approaches and others reviewed tools may result in development of new medications for the treating of IR-induced vascular complications.

PKC Involvement in BK_{Ca} Channelopathy

Our research group has shown that in the rat aorta SMCs selective inhibition of PKC effectively reverses the suppression of K^+ currents induced by IR at a dose of 6 Gy from a 60Co source in the post-irradiation period of 9 and 30 days. These data indicate that IR-induced inhibition of the BK_{Ca} current in SMCs is mediated by PKC (Kizub et al. 2010). PKC is a key regulatory enzyme involved in transduction of signals in several cellular functions in vascular SMCs, including VSM growth and contractility (Cosentino-Gomes et al. 2012). PKC is a family of serine/ threonine kinases with 10 isoforms. Based on homology and sensitivity to activators, PKC isoforms are divided into 3 subfamilies: conventional (or classical), novel, and atypical PKC. Classical isozymes include PKC α, PKC-β1, PKC-β2 and PKC-γ. The novel PKC subfamily consists of PKC-δ, PKC-ε, PKC-η, and PKC-θ. The atypical isozymes are represented by PKC-ζ and PKC-ι. PKC-μ and PKC-υ isoforms are now classified as members of the DAG receptor protein kinase D family (Wang, 2006) Expression of different PKC isoforms (α, β1, β2, γ, ε, η, ζ, δ, and ι/λ) in vascular tissues depends on the animal species, as well as on the type and age of vessels (Steinberg, 2008).

PKC is involved in the regulation of vascular SM contractility in various pathways, including changes in myofilaments Ca^{2+}-sensitivity (Soloviev, Bershtein, 1992; Dessy, Matsuda, Hurvelshorn et al, 2000; Somlyo, Somlyo, 2003) and regulation of $[Ca^{2+}]_i$ (Korzic et al, 2004), as well as by reducing endothelium-mediated vasodilatation (Beckman, Goldfine, Gordon et al. 2002). This enzyme is also involved in regulation of the plasmalemmal ion permeability in vascular SMCs. For example, PKC has been shown to regulate the activity of K^+ channels (Boland, Jackson, 1999; Schubrert, Nelson, 2001). PKC can influence vascular tissue function by regulation of the apparent Ca^{2+} - and/or voltage-sensitivity of the BK_{Ca} channels to physiological changes in both Ca^{2+} concentrations and membrane potential (Schubrert, Nelson, 2001). PKC activation has been reported to inhibit the BK_{Ca} channels activity directly in vascular SMCs (Schubrert, Nelson, 2001, Barman et al, 2004; Taguchi, Kaneko, 2004). In addition, it has also been demonstrated that in the vascular

SMCs protein receptor for activated C kinase 1 (RACK1), a scaffolding protein, may bind to the BK_{Ca} channels and directly change its biophysical properties (Isackson et al. 2007).

Importantly, PKC could mediate activity of the other types of K^+ channels in vascular SMCs, delayed rectifier K^+ channels [Aiello et al. 1996], Kv (Shimoda et al. 1998), and KATP (Hayabuchi et al. 2001). There are few studies suggesting that IR activates PKC in various tissues. It has been shown that different doses of γ-radiation from 0.5 to 50 Gy during whole-body and in vitro irradiation caused an increase in expression and activation of PKC in cultured and isolated intestinal SM cells (Claro et al. 2007), fibroblasts (Tachiiri, et al, 2006), skeletal muscle, liver, spleen (Besplug et al, 2005) and ECs (Billis et al. 1998).

In Figure 43, we have summarized and illustrated PKC-mediated involvement of the BK_{Ca} channels in mechanisms of vascular SMCs contractility elevation under IR impact.

The results of the study of the effect of radiation on blood vessels are important not only because radiation, if it is used unwisely, is an extremely serious threat to the very existence of humankind. We found that even a single non-fatal irradiation of rats leads to a persistent increase in blood pressure for up to 6 months (Soloviev, Stefanov, Tishkin et al, 2002; Soloviev, Tishkin, Parshikov et al. 2003).

AH has become widespread among the liquidators of the Chernobyl disaster (Khomazjuk 1998; Klimov, Adziarykha, 2001). In addition, it is certain that this was not a consequence of the emotional stress experienced.

When studying the contractile and electrophysiological characteristics of the vessels of irradiated animals, we found their surprising similarity with similar parameters of the vessels of rats with genetically determined hypertension. The role of reactive oxygen species in the development of AH has long been known, and when exposed to ionizing radiation, it is simply obvious. Maybe, the phenomenon of AH induced by exposure to radiation will help shed light on the causes of essential hypertension.

Considering the important role of reactive oxygen species in the development of such pathological processes, high doses of antioxidants could be recommended for their treatment. For instance, mega-dose sodium ascorbate (NaAscorbate, 30 g over 1 h followed by 30 g over 5 h) appears beneficial in patients with septic shock. However, the mechanisms of this effect remain unknown (Yanase, Spano, Maeda et al, 2023).

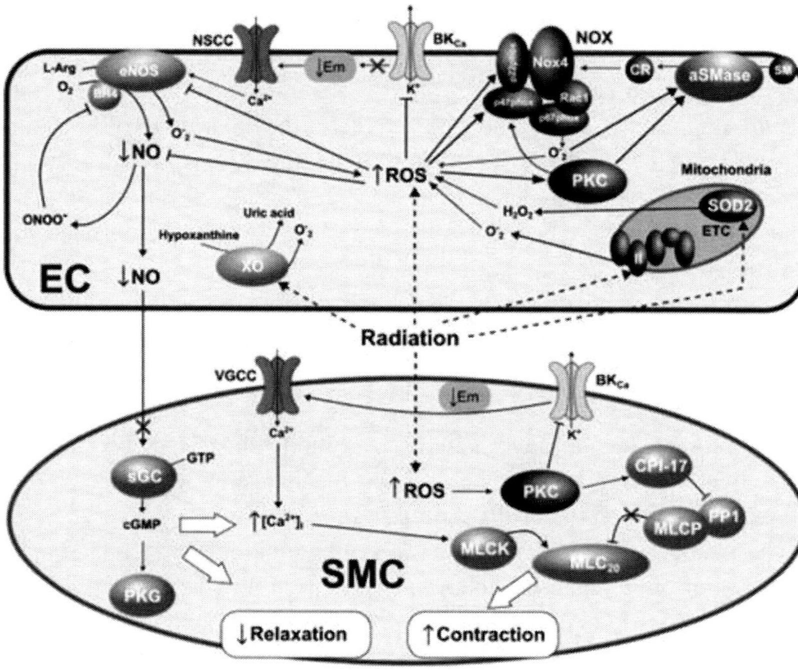

Figure 43. The mechanisms of ionizing radiation effects on endothelial (EC) and smooth muscle cells (SMC) leading to elevation in smooth muscle contractility and vascular tone. Ionizing radiation induces generation of reactive oxygen species (ROS) in ECs. Then, in irradiated cells, ROS are generated secondarily by different biological sources: complex II of mitochondrial electron transport chain (ETC), mitochondrial Mn-superoxide dismutase (SOD2), NADPH oxidase (NOX), xanthine oxidase (XO), and uncoupled endothelial nitric oxide synthase (eNOS). Elevated ROS levels activate NOX and initiate overexpression of Nox4, p22phox, and p47phox NOX subunits to cause additional ROS production. Also, ROS activates NOX via PKC-induced phosphorylation of p47phox. ROS and ROS-activated PKC also activate acidic sphingomyelinase (aSMase) which catalyzes production of ceramide (CR) from sphingomyelin (SM) with the following activation of NOX. Radiation-generated ROS inhibit activity of large conductance Ca^{2+}-activated K^{+} channels (BK_{Ca}) leading to alterations in cell membrane potential and Ca^{2+} entry through non-specific cation channels resulting in decreasing in NO synthesis by eNOS. ROS also inhibits eNOS 38 expression and activity or react with NO forming peroxynitrite (ONOO−) that leads to a decrease in NO production from L-arginine (L-Arg) and NO scavenging. ONOO− in turn may diminish the level of tetrahydrobiopterin (BH4) resulting in eNOS uncoupling and superoxide (O2−) producing instead of NO. Decrease in NO levels leads to inactivation of NO-mediated pathway that involves soluble guanylate cyclase (sGC)/cyclic 3′-5′-guanosine monophosphate (cGMP) protein kinase G (PKG) in vascular SMCs and diminishing relaxation. On the other hand, radiation-induced oxidative stress activates PKC in SMCs. It leads to inhibition of BK_{Ca} channels activity

resulting in membrane depolarization and increase in Ca^{2+} influx through voltage-gated Ca^{2+} channels (VGCC) and elevation in intracellular Ca^{2+} concentration triggering SMCs contraction. ROS-mediated PKC activation in SMCs also results in phosphorylation of PKC-dependent protein phosphatase-1 inhibitor of 17 kDa (CPI-17) which binds to PP1 subunit of myosin light chain phosphatase (MLCP) and inhibits its activity. The inhibition of the MLCP results in elevation in myosin light chain of 20 kDa (MLC20) phosphorylation for any intracellular Ca^{2+} levels and activity of the myosin light chain kinase (MLCK). It leads to an increase in SMCs contraction and vascular tone elevation under ionizing radiation impact.

Chapter 18

miRNAs and Their Possible Role in Myogenic Tone Regulation

How can you embrace the unembraceable? However, among the many other potential modulators of basal tone, and possibly the fundamental mechanisms of its formation, miRNAs occupy a special place. Very briefly about this relatively new direction in the study of vascular tone.

MicroRNAs (miRNAs) are small non-coding RNA molecules 18–25 nucleotides long (on average 22) found in plants, animals, and some viruses that are involved in the transcriptional and post-transcriptional regulation of gene expression by RNA interference. miRNAs are synthesized from DNA during transcription, after which, in turn, it is used during translation as a template for protein synthesis. Thus, mRNAs play an important role in the "manifestation" (expression) of genes.

miRNAs are produced from immature pre-miRNAs, which are processed by the two RNase III endonucleases, Drosha and Dicer (a ribonuclease of the RNase III family that cleaves double-stranded RNA) and pre-miRNA molecules to produce short double-stranded RNA fragments called small interfering RNA (siRNAs) and miRNAs, respectively. These fragments are approximately 20-25 nucleotides long, typically with an overhang of 2-3 nucleotides at the 3' end, and are then incorporated into the RNA-induced silencing complex (RISC). Depending on the complementarity of the miRNA with the 3'-untranslated regions of the target mRNA, the RISC complex will mediate either translational repression/activation or degradation of the target mRNA. Since Dicer is required for processing of almost all mature miRNAs, mutation or disruption of Dicer has been widely used as an approach to investigate the biological significance of miRNAs in various cell types.

There is very little data in the literature on the role of miRNA in the formation of vascular tone, but it already exists. It is likely that phenotypic modulation of smooth muscle cells is known to play a key role in the development of several vascular diseases, including atherosclerosis. Several transcription factors have been proposed to regulate phenotypic modulation of SM cells, but the underlying mechanisms remain unknown.

Recent data Albinsson, Skoura, Yu, DiLorenzo, Fernandez-Hernando, et al. (2011) suggest that certain miRNAs are involved in SMC differentiation and vascular diseases, but the global role of miRNAs in the regulation of postnatal vasculature and, especially, vascular tone has yet to be elucidated. In their study, the role of Dicer-dependent miRNAs in the regulation of blood pressure and contractile function and differentiation of vascular SMCs in vivo was investigated. Tamoxifen-induced SMC-specific deletion of Dicer was achieved by Cre-Lox recombination. It is a site-specific recombinase technology, used to carry out deletions, insertions, translocations, and inversions at specific sites in the DNA of cells. It allows the DNA modification to be targeted to a specific cell type or to be triggered by a specific external stimulus. Dicer deletion resulted in a global loss of miRNAs in aortic SMCs. Furthermore, Dicer-deficient mice exhibited a dramatic decrease in blood pressure due to a significant loss of vascular contractile function and contractile differentiation of SM cells, as well as vascular remodeling. The authors concluded that miRNAs are required for the maintenance of blood pressure and contractile function in resistance vessels.

Below is a more detailed description of their results. Using wire myography, contractile function was examined in the small mesenteric arteries and saphenous arteries of control and Dicer knockout (DK) mice 5 and 10 weeks after tamoxifen. At 10 weeks after tamoxifen, the contractile response to KCl depolarization was almost absent in the small mesenteric arteries of DK mice compared with controls. The level of tonic tension under calcium deprivation conditions was significantly reduced in DK SM, indicating extrinsic remodeling or altered compliance in these vessels. Moreover, the contractile response to the adrenergic a1-agonist phenylephrine was completely lost in DK both when measured as absolute force and when compared to the contraction induced by potassium excess.

Thus, the contractile response to phenylephrine was even further reduced than high potassium -induced contraction in saphenous arteries. Part of this effect may be related to a reduction in phenylephrine-induced calcium influx in DK SM measured in isolated aortic SM. After washout of high potassium-induced contractions, they found that DK SM arteries relaxed significantly more slowly than control arteries. The reason for the reduced relaxation rate in DK is unknown, but it may be related to impaired myosin kinase and myosin phosphatase activity, which regulates the latch state in smooth muscle. Another surprising finding was that the contractile response to 5-HT was not as strongly affected by SM Dicer deletion as were phenylephrine - or high potassium - induced responses, suggesting that Dicer loss may differentiate between these signaling pathways. In support of this theory, the calcium response to 5-HT in isolated SMCs did not differ between control and DK SMC. The reduced ability of DK vascular SM to relax was evident both after washout of high potassium-induced contraction and during sustained contraction in response to 5-HT, which is clearly distinct from contraction in control vessels.

New data on the role of mRNA in the formation of myogenic tone was obtained at the Lund University, Sweden (Bhattachariya, Dahan, Turczynska, Sward, Hellstrand and Albinsson. (2014)). In this study provided at the Department of Experimental Medical Sciences, the novel mechanisms that regulate myogenic tone in resistance arteries, which involves microRNA-dependent control of PI3-kinase/Akt signalling and L-type calcium influx, were identified.

Briefly, they have demonstrated that transient stimulation by Ang II can have long-lasting effects by potentiating myogenic tone. It was suggested that the myogenic response is specifically sensitive to loss of miRNAs in smooth muscle. The mechanism behind this effect involves a reduced voltage gated calcium influx and loss of pressure-induced Akt phosphorylation, possibly due to an increased expression of phosphatase and tensin homologue (PTEN) which triggers a battery of intracellular signaling pathways, especially PI3K/Akt, playing important roles in the cellular function.

In conclusion, the present study provides the first insights into the global, post-natal importance of miRNAs in vascular SMC and it is likely that continual miRNA turnover regulates the levels of key genes in VSM that control contraction, remodeling and phenotypic modulation. The data obtained suggest that the myogenic response is specifically sensitive to loss of miRNAs in smooth muscle. The mechanism responsible for this effect involves a reduced voltage gated calcium influx and loss of pressure-induced Akt phosphorylation, possibly due to an increased expression of PTEN. Their results further emphasize the importance of miRNAs in VSM and demonstrate a novel mechanism participating in the regulation of myogenic tone. Since regulation of myogenic tone is essential for the control of blood pressure and blood flow, the results presented herein can provide a better understanding for the mechanisms underlying vascular diseases, such as hypertension and oedema, and suggest novel targets for therapeutic intervention.

It is known that pressure-induced myogenic tone is involved in autoregulation of local blood flow and confers protection against excessive pressure levels in small arteries and capillaries. Myogenic tone is dependent on smooth muscle miRNAs, but the identity of these miRNAs is unclear.

Holmberg, Bhattachariya, Alajbegovic, et al. (2018) demonstrated that myogenic tone was abolished in miR-143/145 knockout mesenteric arteries, whereas contraction in response to calyculin A and potassium chloride was reduced by ≈30%. Furthermore, myogenic responsiveness was potentiated by angiotensin II in wild-type but not in knockout mice. Angiotensin II administration in vivo elevated systemic blood pressure in both genotypes. Hypertensive knockout mice developed severe vascular lesions characterized by vascular inflammation, adventitial fibrosis, and neointimal hyperplasia in small mesenteric arteries. This was associated with depolymerization of actin filaments and fragmentation of the elastic laminae at the sites of vascular lesions. This study demonstrates that miR-143/145 expression is essential for myogenic responsiveness. In hypertension, the loss of even some of the myogenic basal tone results in an undesirable and potentially dangerous increase in the level of mechanical tension of smooth muscles and a detrimental effect on small arteries. The results presented herein provide novel insights into the pathogenesis of vascular disease and emphasize the importance of controlling mechanical factors to maintain structural integrity of the vascular wall (Figure 44, 45).

Albinsson, Skoura, Yu, DiLorenzo, Fernandez-Hernando et al. (2011) also suppose that phenotypic modulation of smooth muscle cells plays a key role in vascular disease, including atherosclerosis. Several transcription factors have been suggested to regulate phenotypic modulation of SMCs but the decisive mechanisms remain unknown before. Recent reports suggest that specific miRNAs are involved in SMC differentiation and vascular disease, but the global role of miRNAs in postnatal vascular SMC has not been elucidated properly.

Thus, the objective of this study was to identify the role of Dicer-dependent miRNAs for blood pressure regulation and vascular SMC contractile function and differentiation in vivo. Tamoxifen-inducible and SMC specific deletion of Dicer was achieved by Cre-Lox recombination. Deletion of Dicer resulted in a global loss of miRNAs in aortic SMC. Furthermore, Dicer-deficient mice exhibited a dramatic reduction in blood pressure due to significant loss of vascular contractile function and SMC contractile differentiation as well as vascular remodeling. Several of these results are consistent with some previous observations in SM-Dicer deficient embryos.

Therefore, it is possible to conclude that miRNAs are essential for maintaining blood pressure and contractile function in resistance vessels. Although the phenotype of miR-143/145 deficient mice resembles the loss of

Dicer, the phenotypes of SM-Dicer KO mice were far more severe suggesting that additional miRNAs are involved in maintaining postnatal SMC differentiation.

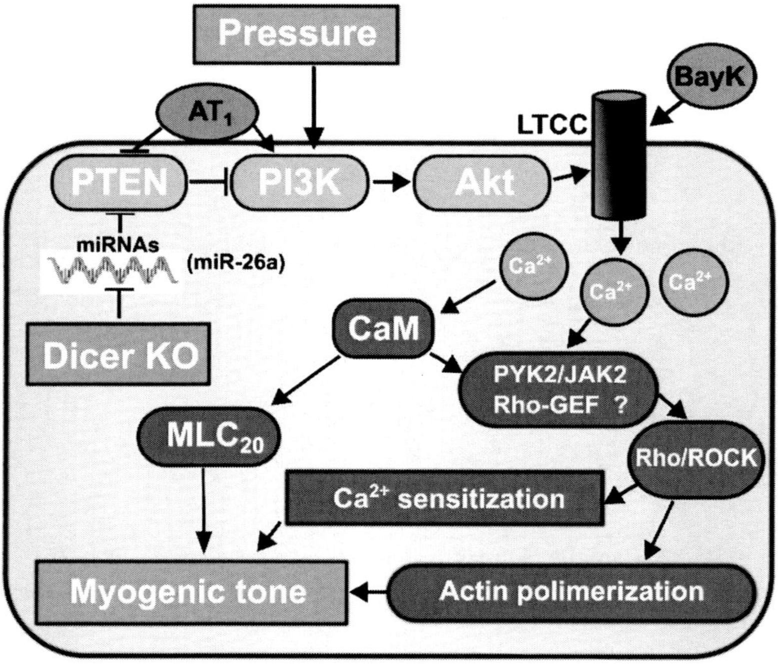

Figure 44. Schematic representation of the chain of events explaining how a decrease in miRNA expression can affect myogenic tone due to an increase in the level of PTEN and inactivation of L-type calcium channels. This model certainly does not exclude any other alternative mechanisms of microRNA participation in the regulation of smooth muscle tone or other alternative signaling pathways also involved in the formation of myogenic tone. The mechanism responsible for calcium-induced Rho-activation is not well clearly understood till this time but may involve PYK2, JAK2, and/or Rho-GEF activation. Symbols in the figure - PTEN, phosphatase and tensin homologue; PI3K, phosphoinositide 3-kinase, AT 1, angiotensin II receptor type 1; LTCC, L-type calcium channel; BayK, Bay K8644; CaM, calmodulin; GEF, guanine nucleotide exchange factor; MLC, myosin light chain. Adapted from Bhattachariya, Dahan, Turczynska, et al. (2014).

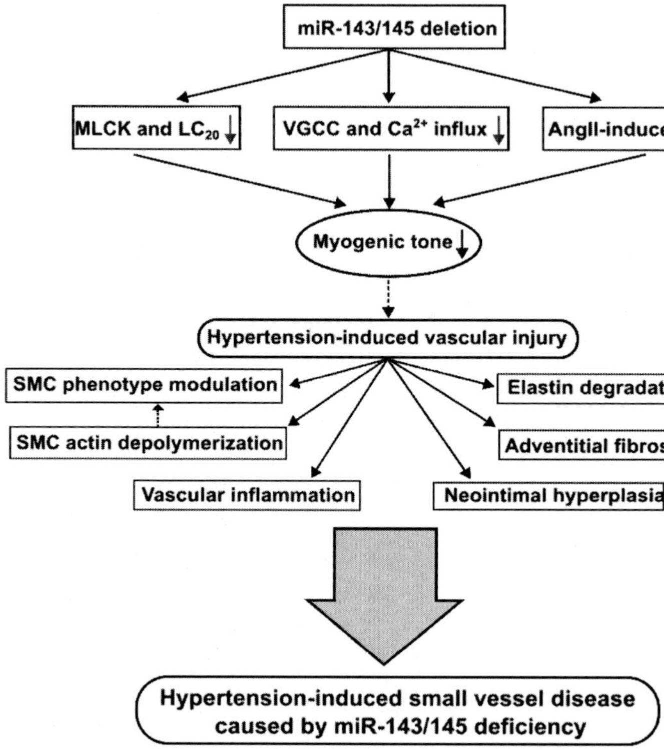

Figure 45. The role of miRNA deficiency in vascular disease.

It is known that the post-transcriptional regulation of genes by RNA-binding proteins, particularly mRNA stability, enables rapid changes in mRNA levels. Dysregulated mRNA stability could contribute to the development of vascular diseases. In recent studies Cui X, Wang Y, Lu H, Wang L, Xie X et al. (2024) established that downregulated RGS proteins (RGS proteins are multi-functional, GTPase-accelerating proteins that promote GTP hydrolysis by the α-subunit of heterotrimeric G proteins) in RNA-binding protein HuR (human antigen is an RNA binding protein in the human antigen protein family) - deficient mice resulted in hypertension. This suggests the important role of RNA-binding proteins in vascular tone development.

Zinc finger protein 36 (ZFP36), encoded by the Zfp36 gene, is another RNA-binding protein containing a tandem Cys-Cys-Cys-His zinc finger domain. The function of ZFP36 is to decay mRNA by binding to adenylate/uridylate-rich-elements in the 3′ untranslated regions of its target mRNAs. Although ZFP36 plays crucial roles in cardiomyocytes and many other cells, its function in vascular SMCs is unclear. ZFP36 is an RNA-binding protein that regulates mRNA stability by binding to adenylate-uridylate-rich elements in the mRNA 3′-untranslated region. This study reveals that ZFP36 expression is highly elevated in the arteries of hypertensive patients and rodents

Cui, Wang, Lu, Wang, Xie et al. (2024) established a functional and mechanistic link between smooth-muscle ZFP36 and blood pressure. Specifically, ZFP36 levels were increased in the arteries of patients and animals with hypertension. According to their in vitro experiments, angiotensin II (AngII) enhanced the transcription of Zfp36 via PARP1. By generating conditional knockout mice, they demonstrated that ZFP36 deletion in VSMCs reduced blood pressure levels and arterial contractility. Mechanistically, ZFP36 reduced GTPase activating protein expression by impairing its mRNA stability and promoting G-protein coupled receptor-mediated intracellular Ca^{2+} increase and subsequent smooth muscle contraction. Moreover, the vascular SM-specific depletion of ZFP36 inhibited AngII-induced hypertension and vascular remodelling in mice, whereas ZFP36 deficiency attenuated hypertension in SHR rats. Thus, these studies suggest that ZFP36 plays a crucial role in smooth muscle contraction and maintaining blood pressure.

Chapter 19

A New View on the Bayliss Concept

The classical point of view on the regulation of vascular tone is that blood flow is constantly regulated by multiple stimuli including the blood flow itself as well as various neural and humoral stimuli. Bayliss (1902), who observed that stretch imposed on the vascular wall by an increase in intraluminal pressure induced a contraction of the vessel, first described the main part of autoregulation, the myogenic response. This ability of VSMCs to respond to mechanical stretch has been observed in a variety of vascular beds. It is assumed that myogenic vasoconstriction is involved in maintaining basal vascular tone to promote constant perfusion despite fluctuations in perfusion pressure and to prevent tissue damage in cases of overperfusion However, experimental evidence for intrinsic mechanisms of this phenomenon until this time is still lacking.

This myogenic response happens through, at least partially, phosphorylation of the myosin light chain (MLC), which allows myosin to interact with actin and to generate contractile force. It is known that MLC phosphorylation can be stimulated by activation of the MLC kinase (MLCK) through a Ca^{2+}- and calmodulin-dependent mechanism or by inhibition of myosin phosphatase via the Rho/Rho-kinase pathway.

The problem is how these two pathways are regulated during myogenic response of VSM. Mederos, Schnitzler, Storch, and Gudermann (2016) postulated that both stretch-activated ion channels and mechanically activated G-protein-coupled receptors (GPCRs) are tightly involved in the initiation of the myogenic response. It is generally accepted that induction of vascular myogenic contraction requires membrane depolarization through activation of mechanically activated ion channels, which would then induce opening of voltage-dependent calcium channels resulting in an increase in intracellular calcium concentration (Jensen et al. 2017).

The data obtained suggest that several type of ion channels have been involved in stretch-induced depolarization, including the transient receptor potential (TRP) channels TRPC6 and TRPM4, the molecular nature of the channel responsible for stretch-induced depolarization of VSMCs has remained poorly understood (Earley and Brayden, 2015).

More recently, it has been demonstrated that some G-protein-coupled receptors (GPCRs) have been involved in the myogenic response of VSMCs to vascular distension (Kauffenstein et al. 2012; Mederos Schnitzler et al. 2016). These receptors include the purinergic P2Y6 receptor, the thromboxane A2 (TR) receptor, sphingosine-1-phosphate receptors as well as the angiotensin AT1 receptor and the cysteinyl leukotriene one receptors (CysLT1Rs). It is likely that stretch-induced activation of P2Y6, TR and S1P receptors is due to the release of agonistic ligands but the data exist that mechanical activation of AT1 and CysLT1 receptors occurs in an agonist-independent manner (Mederos, Schnitzler et al. 2016). The GPCRs involved in vascular myogenic contraction can couple to several G-proteins including Gq/G11 and G12/G13 (Kauffenstein et al. 2012).

Wirth et al. (2008) showed that in VSMCs coupling of receptors to Gq/G11 through stimulation of PLC-β results in the Ca^{2+}- and calmodulin-dependent activation of MLCK, whereas coupling to G12/G13 via activation of the Rho/Rho-kinase pathway results in the inhibition of myosin phosphatase. It is likely that these two pathways can synergize. This conclusion is based on experimental evidence that myogenic contraction can be strongly reduced by pharmacological inhibition of Rho-kinase downstream of G12/G13 as well as of Gq/G11. However, since these pharmacological interventions also affect the function of other vascular cells, including endothelial cells, and this way are not specific, the role of the two major G-protein-mediated signaling transduction pathways inducing VSM contraction in myogenic tone regulation remains unclear.

Chennupati, Wirth, FavreLi, Bonnavion et al. (2019) suppose that G-protein-coupled receptors have been involved in myogenic vasoconstriction, but the downstream signalling mechanisms and the in-vivo-function of this myogenic autoregulation are poorly understood. They demonstrated that small arteries from mice with smooth muscle-specific loss of G12/G13 or the Rho guanine nucleotide exchange factor ARHGEF12 have lost myogenic vasoconstriction. This defect was accompanied by loss of RhoA activation, while vessels showed normal increases in intracellular $[Ca^{2+}]$. In the absence of myogenic vasoconstriction, perfusion of peripheral organs was increased, systemic vascular resistance was reduced, and cardiac output and left ventricular mass were increased. In addition, animals with defective myogenic vasoconstriction showed aggravated hypotension in response to endotoxin. The authors concluded that G12/G13- and Rho-mediated signaling plays a key role in myogenic vasoconstriction and that myogenic tone is required to maintain local and systemic vascular resistance under physiological and pathological conditions.

MLCK-Independent Mechanisms of Smooth Muscle Activation

Once it has been established that smooth muscle can contract in the absence of an increase in intracellular calcium concentration, contraction without the obligatory phosphorylation of the myosin light chain does not seem so shocking.

However, blood vessels from smooth muscle MLCK-null embryos demonstrated contract and showed increased RLC20 phosphorylation in response to both agonists and Ca^{2+} (Somlyo, Wang, Choudhury et al. 2004) as well smooth muscle contracted in response to MLCP inhibitors in the absence of Ca^{2+} (Gong, Cohen, Kitazawa, et al, 1992).

Artamonov, Sonkusare, Good et al. (2019) showed that the p90 ribosomal S6 kinase 2 (RSK2) also possesses the ability to phosphorylated RLC20 to promote smooth muscle contractility. Active, phosphorylated RSK2 in mouse resistance arteries under normal basal tone, and this phosphorylation of RSK2 increased with myogenic vasoconstriction or agonist stimulation. Resistance arteries from Rsk2-deficient mice appeared to be dilated and demonstrated reduced myogenic tone and RLC20 phosphorylation. In addition, RSK2 phosphorylated an activating site in the Na^{+}/H+ exchanger (NHE-1), resulting in cytosolic alkalinization and an increase in intracellular Ca^{2+} that also promotes vasoconstriction. It is important that NHE-1 activity increased upon myogenic constriction, and the increase in intracellular pH was suppressed in Rsk2-deficient mice. Additionally, this ion exchanger is also active on perivascular neurons and could stimulate neurotransmitter release.

In pressured arteries, RSK2-dependent activation of NHE-1 was associated with increased intracellular Ca^{2+} transients, which would be expected to increase MLCK activity, thereby contributing to basal tone and myogenic responses. Accordingly, Rsk2-deficient mice had lower blood pressure than normal littermates. Thus, RSK2 mediates a procontractile signaling pathway that contributes to the regulation of basal vascular tone, myogenic vasoconstriction, and blood pressure and may be a potential therapeutic target in smooth muscle contractility disorders (Artamonov,

Sonkusare, Good, et al, 2019). Of course, this work is a very weighty brick in the overall construction of the future theory of basal vascular tone.

Conclusion

It would be naive to assume that the result of this manuscript will be presented as a final and complete hypothesis of the formation of basal vascular tone. First, it is impossible to grasp the immensity. Second, we focused our attention on the role of glycolysis in the formation of basal smooth muscle tone and some of the associated intrinsic mechanisms. We almost completely excluded from consideration the neurogenic mechanisms of vascular tone control. At best, we wanted to streamline our knowledge in this area and attract the attention of young scientists and specialists from various fields of science - from mathematicians and physics to physiologists, biochemists and pharmacologists - to the problem of basal tone formation and the role of glycolytic oscillator in this matter. This problem certainly deserves close attention and careful study, since its solution can radically change the existing paradigms of the physiology of blood circulation and approaches to pharmacological correction of vascular smooth muscle tone disorders in pathological conditions.

And yet, it would probably be wrong to leave the book without a full conclusion. A number of issues require discussion. How does the complex of intracellular mechanisms, united by the concept of basal tone, function, even hypothetically? What is needed in order for the "backbone" of the vessels to function properly - basal tone? Let us pay tribute to the skeleton of the vascular wall, the structural (connective tissue and elastic component) of the vessels. But first of all, we are interested in the functional system built into smooth muscle cells that reacts to all changes in the external environment and provides a fine adjustment of the blood supply to the organ to the level of its metabolic activity. Moreover, such a system, which solves its tasks at its cellular level on its own, without the intervention of higher control loops.

The main task of any cell is to maintain the level of membrane potential at the appropriate level, i.e., maintenance of the non-equilibrium state and the corresponding ion gradients on the membrane. This task is ensured by the work of the sodium-potassium ATP-ase and the corresponding ion channels.

Alison Gurney and co-authors (Gurney, Osipenko, MacMillan, McFarlane, Tate, Kempsill, 2003) consider that the membrane potential of pulmonary artery smooth muscle cells is determined largely by a non-inactivating K^+ conductance that is sensitive to inhibition by 4-aminopyridine, albeit at relatively high (1 mM) concentrations.

For its normal functioning the sodium-potassium pump, first of all, needs a reliable source of energy, independent (or little dependent) on oxygen supplies. In this regard, let us recall Guyton (Guyton, 1963) – he wrote that the relative oxygen content in the blood is lower than that of other vital ingredients. The so-called safety factor for oxygen is 3, while for glucose it is 30. This means that even a slight decrease in pO_2 in the blood will significantly affect the functional state of tissues. Guyton believed that the coefficient of efficiency of regulation of vascular tone by oxygen deficiency is 2, while the similar parameter of the mechanoreceptor system of the carotid sinus, usually cited as an example of the most effective regulation system, is less than 2 (Scher, Young, 1962).

Thus, based on the principle of the primacy of providing the body with macroergs in conditions of oxygen deficiency, glycolysis is the most acceptable candidate for the role of an energy source to maintain an optimal level of basal tone.

However, this is not the only reason. Glycolysis is a classic example of a self-oscillatory biochemical reaction. Such undamped self-oscillations arise in the absence of external periodic influences due to the internal properties of the system. In this case, an equality of energy loss and energy inflow from an internal source during self-oscillation arises inside the system. Let me remind you that self-oscillations and autowaves, multistability, and non-equilibrium steady-state distributions can exist only in nonlinear systems, which are probabilistic and more aggressive than linear systems. In other words, the choice is small and single - glycolysis.

Thus, there are three main ways of ATP formation: anaerobic creatine phosphokinase (CP) mechanism, spatially localized in the contractile apparatus of muscles; glycolytic (also anaerobic), located in the cytoplasm of muscle cells and the path of oxidative phosphorylation (aerobic), located in mitochondria. The fastest of them is CP (full turn-on time - a few seconds), it is also the most powerful - an average of 1000 cal/min/kg, but it works for a very short time. The second most powerful is the glycolytic pathway - about 800 cal/min/kg. The time to reach full power is 20-30 seconds. Similar parameters for the aerobic pathway are 400 cal/min/kg and 3-4 min, respectively. The highest ATP yield, of course, is in the aerobic pathway - 36 molecules.

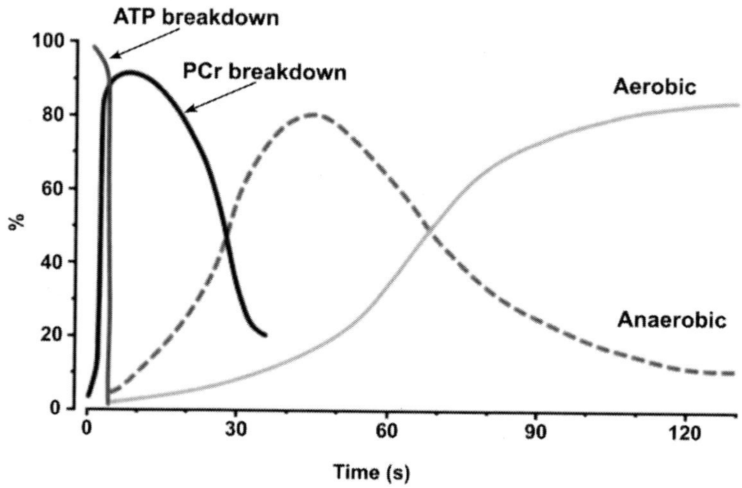

Figure 46. The sequence of inclusion of different pathways of ATP synthesis in skeletal muscle at the beginning of light exercise.

As shown in Figure 46, in the first few seconds, CP and anaerobic pathways provide almost all energy for contraction. The anaerobic process-glycolysis reaches its maximum after about 45 seconds, while due to oxidative reactions, the muscle cannot receive the main part of the energy earlier than after 2 minutes.

All these considerations relate primarily to skeletal muscles. Unfortunately, I do not have such information for smooth muscles. It remains hopeful that the overall picture of the development of events is similar. At the same time, one should not forget that smooth muscles in blood vessels are constantly in a state of tonic tension.

In the field of metabolism, nonlinear effects are especially pronounced in the study of glycolysis. Glycolysis is usually understood as the anaerobic conversion of glucose to lactate, and the biological significance of this process has long been usually explained by the fact that the heat released is used to maintain the heat balance in the body. In fact, as we already understand, everything is much more complicated. During the experimental study of the process of glycolysis, many authors observed chemical oscillations in cells and muscle fibers in which the fermentation process takes place. Glycolytic oscillator, whose oscillation period is from one to 10 minutes, acts due to periodic activation and inhibition of the enzyme phosphofructokinase.

It is interesting that oscillatory reactions in the glycolysis system were first predicted on a mathematical model (Higgins, 1964) and only after that, they were experimentally recorded using the differential spectrophotometry method in the laboratory of Chance et al (1966).

Agree that the mathematical correctness of these harmonic oscillations is somewhat frightening with their seeming mechanistic nature. Harmonic oscillations, as you know, are of two types: free and forced. Free oscillations arise due to the internal forces of the system after it has been brought out of equilibrium. Forced oscillations arise due to an external periodic force. The internal forces that cause glycolysis to periodically change its level of activity can be seen in Figure 48.

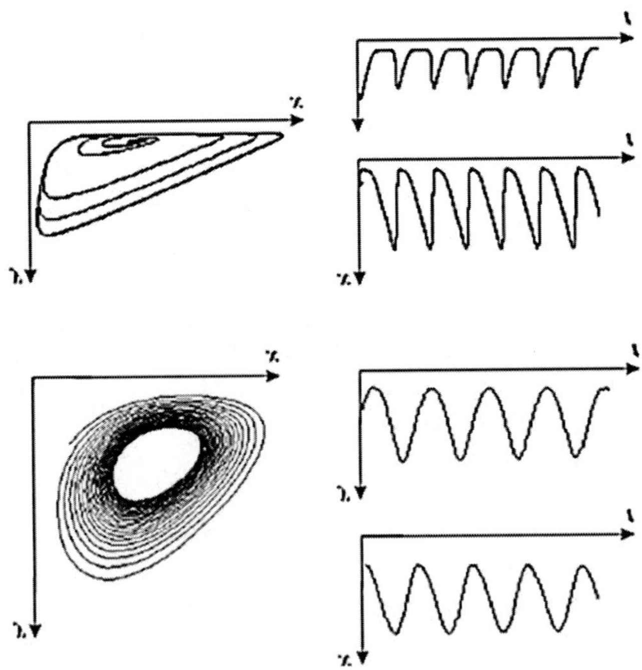

Figure 47. Model of glycolysis. The kinetics of changes in the concentrations of fructose 6 phosphate (x) and fructose diphosphate (yλ) (right) and the phase portrait of the system (left) at different values of the system parameters, c - vibrations with constant amplitude and phase, close to harmonic (limit cycle on the phase plane), $\alpha = 6$; $r = 0.2$. d – relaxation oscillations with constant amplitude and phase, (almost triangular limit cycle on the phase plane) $\alpha = 8$; $r = 0.5$.

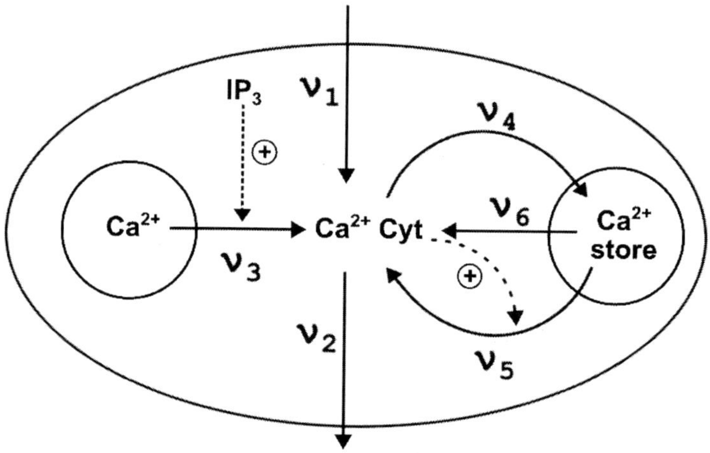

Figure 48. Simple scheme of intracellular calcium oscillation.

Next, you need a reliable signal generation system. Depletion in the cell's energy supply may lead to fluctuations in membrane potential with a crest of depolarization and appearance of action potentials, each of which resulted in a small contraction. Many of the small contractions partially fused to form the major rhythmic contractions (Bose and Bose, 1977). Rhythmic contractile activity is impossible without previous changes in the intracellular concentration of calcium ions. Calcium homeostasis is a sophisticated, multi-pathway process that time-dependently coordinates molecular activity of plasma membrane, cytosolic and store compartments.

In many types of living cells, fluctuations in the intracellular calcium concentration are observed, the period of which can vary from 0.5 to 10 minutes. The simplest scheme of processes leading to harmonically determined calcium fluctuations, which are based on calcium-induced calcium release, is shown in Figure 48. Endo, Tanaka and Ogawa (1970) on skeletal muscle cells, Fabiato A and Fabiato F (1975) on bovine heart sarcoplasmic reticulum cells, and later by many other researchers, first observed such fluctuations.

The scheme and model of the processes proposed and described in the works of Dupont, Goldbeter (1993). They took into account all possible ways of movement of calcium in the cell. Namely, the influx and outflow of calcium into and out of the cell through the plasma membrane (rate constants $\gamma 1$ and $\gamma 2$, respectively). Then, they also did not forget hormone-activated release of calcium from the intracellular pool (rate $\gamma 3$), active transport of cytosolic calcium into the depot (γ4), release of calcium from the depot activated by cytosolic calcium (γ5) and free outflow of calcium from the intracellular storage into the cytosol (γ6).

Below, especially for the advanced reader, are the equations describing this model. This model is relatively simple and consists of two differential equations:

$$dS1/dt = \gamma 1 - \gamma 2 + \gamma 3 - \gamma 4 + \gamma 5 + \gamma 6 \quad (21)$$
$$dS2/dt = \gamma 4 - \gamma 5 - \gamma 6$$

Here, S1 is the calcium concentration in the cytosol; S2 is the calcium concentration in the hormonally sensitive pool. Somogyi and Stuckin (1991) calculated the reaction rates:

$$\gamma 2 = k_2 \cdot S_1;\ \gamma 4 = k_4 \cdot S_1;\ \gamma 5 = k_5 \cdot S_2 \cdot S_1^{nH} / (K_{0.5}^{nH} + S_1^{nH});\ \gamma 6 = k_6 \cdot S_2 \quad (22)$$

The model predicts fluctuations in the calcium concentration over time, which are close in shape to the experimental ones (Figures 49).

Thus, intracellular Ca^{2+} oscillations represent universal signaling mechanisms to control different biological processes including smooth muscle contractility (Parekh, 2011). These oscillations, which carry encoded information for various cellular structures, are encoded by the frequency and amplitude of Ca^{2+} spikes. How the cell extracts all the information it needs from these codes, we still do not fully understand.

Calcium oscillations are triggered either by fluctuations in the membrane potential (due to repeated opening and closing of voltage-gated Ca^{2+} channels) or by activation of membrane receptors mediating the increase in inositol triphosphate levels. The transmission of information in digital form has a number of undoubted advantages in comparison with analog (sustainable) changes in the level of intracellular calcium. First, it is a decrease in the toxic effect of Ca^{2+} on intracellular structures. Secondly, it reduces the effect of possible desensitization of these structures to Ca^{2+}. Thirdly, the oscillatory signal transmits information in the form of frequency and amplitude. Digital oscillations contribute to easier activation of regulatory processes. The fact is that one or two Ca^{2+} spikes are perceived by the corresponding structures more easily than a steady increase in extracellular Ca^{2+} to the same values. Finally, since the oscillatory signal transmits information both in the form of frequency and amplitude, this provides the possibility of selective influence on regulatory structures.

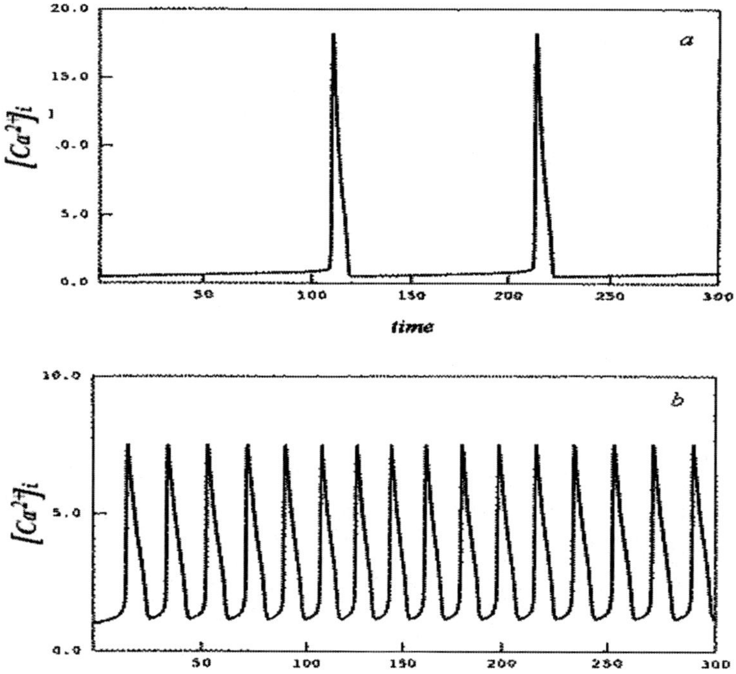

Figure 49. Model behavior of intracellular calcium oscillations (Dupont and Goldbeter, 1993) for various parameters of the equations 22 (rate constants in a and b are equal 1.4 and 3.0, respectively).

A synchronization system is necessary to ensure the synchronous operation of millions of smooth muscle cells. Our understanding of the cellular mechanisms responsible for the synchronized oscillatory activity of the VSM has improved substantially in recent years due to data provided by (Aalkjær & Nilsson, 2005).

Three different types of cellular oscillations have been suggested. One model has suggested that oscillatory release of Ca^{2+} from intracellular stores is important (this type of oscillation is based on a cytosolic oscillator). A second proposed mechanism is an oscillation originating in the sarcolemma (a membrane oscillator). A third mechanism is based on an oscillation of glycolysis (metabolic oscillator). For the two latter mechanisms, only limited experimental evidence is available.

In most situations, a cytosolic oscillator appears to be important because vasomotion, for instance, is very sensitive to interference with release or uptake of Ca^{2+} from intracellular stores.

Furthermore, to achieve synchronization of the cytosolic oscillators in the individual smooth muscle cells, it has been suggested that the cytosolic oscillator interacts with the membrane to establish membrane-potential changes that mediate the synchronization. Other types of oscillations, either based solely on interactions of ion currents in the sarcolemma or based on oscillations of the glycolytic pathway and consequently the Na^+/K^+-pump, have also been suggested and could play a role under some conditions, although these pathways are probably less frequent. The cytosolic oscillator's synchronization may occur via activation of Ca^{2+} -sensitive ion channels by oscillatory Ca^{2+} release. The ensuing membrane potential oscillation feeds back on the intracellular Ca^{2+} stores and causes synchronization of the Ca^{2+} release.

It is well known now that vascular SM metabolism is compartmentalized, such that aerobic glycolysis is associated with membrane energy-dependent functions and oxidative metabolism correlates with vascular contractility (Zhang, Paul, 1994). It is worth dwelling on this work in more detail. The authors of this work investigated the importance of glucose, a primary substrate for glycolysis, in maintenance of resting tension and excitation-contraction coupling in porcine carotid arteries. All arteries were, as generally accepted, precontracted with 80 mM KCl and then exposed to hypoxia in the absence of glucose (6 min) to deplete stored glycogen, an alternative substrate for glycolysis. After such depletion, sensitivity to agonists substantially increased. The concentration of norepinephrine (NE) that induced half-maximal response (EC50) was significantly decreased under glucose-free conditions, and the maximal response was unchanged. The decrease in EC_{50}, or increase in sensitivity, was reversed by glucose, but not by beta-hydroxybutyrate, a substrate for oxidative metabolism.

Similar results were obtained by studying the dose-effect curves for histamine and KCl. Importantly, measurements of high-energy phosphagen content in freeze-clamped arteries indicate that these substrate perturbations were not associated with significant changes in global energy stores. Responses to a single dose of NE or histamine in Ca^{2+}-free medium were significantly lower if intracellular Ca^{2+} stores were loaded in the presence of beta-hydroxybutyrate than in the presence of glucose, suggesting that normal maintenance of intracellular Ca^{2+} stores also depends specifically on glucose. Furthermore, 14 of 26 rings exhibited an increase in resting tension and/or oscillation in the absence of glucose, despite near-normal force responses to KCI. This phenomenon was reversed by nifedipine or glucose.

The main point of this study is that vascular SM cells are glycolysis addicted and characterized by a notable rate of glycolysis with lactate production under fully oxygenated conditions. A similar point of view was previously expressed by Butler, Siegman (1985). The production of lactate in vascular SM cells is comparable with or higher than the oxygen consumption rate on a molar basis; 90% of the glucose utilization could be due to glycolysis, whereas the adenosine triphosphate (ATP) generated from aerobic glycolysis is 30% (Sobue, Hayashi, Nishida, 1999).

Two hypotheses attempt to explain why vascular SM cells rely on glycolysis (generating 2 mol of ATP per molecule of glucose) rather than the mitochondrial glucose oxidation (generating 36 mol of ATP per molecule of glucose) (Michelakis, Weir., 2008). The first one, ATP generated from glycolysis and glucose oxidation provides the energy for different processes; aerobic glycolysis not only reflects a nonspecific defect in vascular metabolism but is also correlated with sodium and potassium transport processes, whereas oxidative metabolism is more highly associated with isometric force and supplies contractile energy (Butler, Siegman, 1985). Second, glycolysis could provide L -lactate, which serves as a substrate that enhances the mitochondrial reserve capacity. Mitochondrial reserve capacity is the difference between mitochondrial maximum respiratory capacity and basal capacity. When energy demand exceeds supply, the reserve capacity is a potent supply source of energy, thereby avoiding the "ATP crisis" and is associated with prolonged cell survival.

It is very important to note that the metabolic and redox signal are closely linked and jointly play a role in the regulation of cellular function due to the fact that pyruvate dehydrogenase acts as an intermediary between these two compartments of energy metabolism.

Thus, these two important metabolic pathways closely interact with each other. Pyruvate dehydrogenase (PDH) could be inhibited by pyruvate dehydrogenase kinase 1 (PDK1), thereby slowing the tricarboxylic acid (TCA) cycle and mediating the glucose metabolic switch from oxidative phosphorylation to glycolysis (Kim, Tchernyshyov, Semenza, Dang, 2006). Currently, the available data on the dominant form of PDK in vascular SM appears to be insufficient and somewhat contradictory. A study reported that both the mRNA and protein of PDK1, PDK2, and PDK3, but not PDK4, were detected in physiological human internal mammary arterial SM cells, and the expression of PDK3 is higher than the other two isoforms, although other studies revealed that all the four PDK isozymes were expressed in both control and damaged human aortic SMCs.

Let us remind also that besides glucose, fatty acids also act as an available source of energy for VSMCs, and fatty acid oxidation (FAO) generates more energy than glucose, although it needs more oxygen per molecule of ATP synthesized (Chen, Austin, Talati, Fessel, Farber-Eger et al. 2017).

Thus, there is strong evidence that glycolysis triggers and maintains oscillatory activity in the smooth muscle. We know many correct and well-identified components of what we call the basal tone. Much more is known about external factors that affect the level of basal tone. However, we still do not see the whole picture. The puzzle does not add up. In addition, not only because there are still empty seats. Something we have not seen yet. In addition, because the individual already known components of the puzzle do not quite exactly match in configuration. We still have a lot to learn and understand in order to put together the correct picture called basal tone.

It is up to the reader to judge how much we managed to get closer to understanding the essence of basal tone and the mechanism of its regulation. It is possible that we are still in the position of the blind men in the Figure 50 below. Nevertheless, this is no reason to give up. The road will be mastered only by going forward, no matter how big the steps are that you need to take. But, as has been said: "The Turtle moves." Moreover, as you know, any road begins with the first step.

Each of us, representatives of various branches of biology (physiologist, biophysicist or biochemist), sees in his own way the problem of the formation of basal tone and its role in the development of pathological processes in the cardiovascular system, in particular arterial hypertension. At the same time, successful treatment of pathological conditions caused by impaired basal tone is impossible without the formation of a holistic and correct picture of pathogenesis.

This picture is not as simple as it seems. Some believe that the crux of the story is that while every blind man proclaims what he thinks is the absolute truth, in reality all their truths are only relative, based on their experience with the elephant. No one has the Truth in its entirety. However, others believe that, of course, the real essence of this story is quite the opposite. For them, the parable of the blind men and the elephant illustrates how our individual perceptions (what Peter Senge calls our "mental models") can lead to misunderstandings and conflicts (Hachinski 2007). However, we leave this problem to philosophers. We have enough urgent special problems of our own waiting to be solved.

And finally, the last drawing of the book and comments on it.

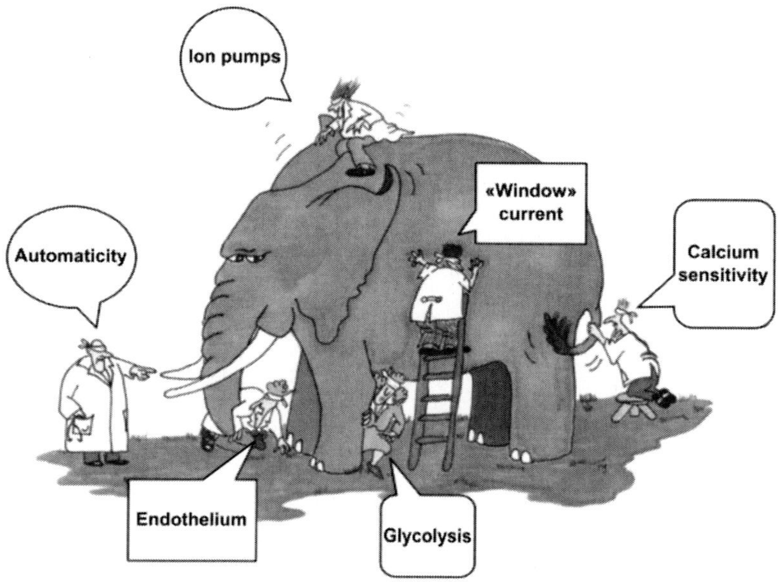

Figure 50. This famous cartoon is based on the story of six blind men from Hindustan who touched different parts of the same elephant and came to completely different conclusions about how this same elephant looks. Agree, the situation in the picture is very similar to what often happens in modern medicine and physiology.

To better understand the essence of the last Figure 51, we should return to Figure 8, which shows the frequency spectrum of a typical radio signal from an AM or FM radio transmitter. This, as you know, consists of a strong signal at the carrier wave frequency, with the modulation information of the signal contained in narrow bands of frequencies, called sidebands, immediately above and below the carrier wave. Thus, in telecommunications there is necessarily a carrier wave, usually sinusoidal, which is modulated in order to convey information in detail. In other words, radio systems use frequency and amplitude modulation to cause the carrier to transmit useful information. It is important to understand that the information transmitted by the radio signal is not at the carrier frequency itself, but is contained in the sidebands (one of the two frequency bands on either side of the carrier wave, containing the modulated signal) on either side of the carrier, i.e. the energy of the carrier component itself is not useful for transmitting information, but without it, signal transmission is impossible.

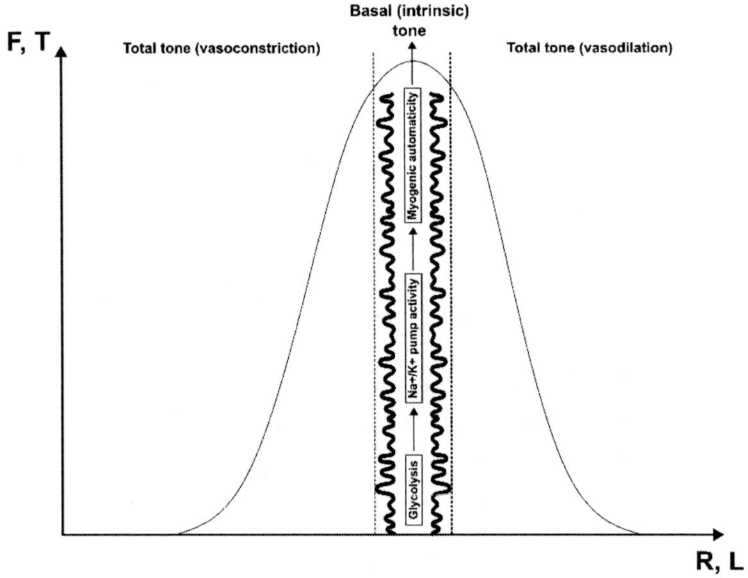

Figure 51. Schematic representation of basal tone as a core factor of the total vascular tone and superimposed on contractile and dilator influences. Abscissa - the length (L), displacement of the contractile element or peripheral resistance (R); ordinate - the level of tonic tension of smooth muscles (T) or the force of contraction developed (F).

We believe that the basal tone is similar to such a carrier frequency with a certain degree of approximation, and external influences (neural and humoral) on it are similar to modulating frequencies. They are the ones that ensure the adjustment of blood flow through the vessel to the metabolic needs of the organ or tissue. However, the presence of a certain basal level of tonic tension of the vascular wall is a prerequisite for normal vascular regulation. There is also a structural part of the basal tone - this is a rigid vascular framework (primarily this concerns large vessels), formed by collagen and elastic fibers, which determines the mechanical resistance of the vessels when the activity of their smooth muscles is completely switched off, but this is a subject for a separate discussion.

The myogenic part of the basal tone is provided by the tension of the smooth muscles of the vessels, which is maintained to a large extent due to the response of the smooth muscles to the force of tension of the vascular wall by intravascular pressure. Consequently, changes in vascular resistance under the influence of nervous or humoral factors change (modulate) the basal tone, which is normally more or less constant for a certain section of the vessel and, by analogy with a radio signal, represents a certain basic "carrier frequency." The level of basal tone can be influenced by a number of different external factors, opening or closing membrane ion channels, activating membrane receptors and their signaling pathways, etc. In the absence of external humoral and nervous influences, the amount of blood flow is determined only by the level of basal tone.

The apparent simplicity and conciseness of Figure 51 may seem excessive to some. Especially when compared to the complexity of the problem we are discussing. But remember Occam's razor - "entities must not be multiple beyond necessity." Indeed, very often a complex problem has a surprisingly simple solution. The solution to the problem of basal tone lies primarily in identifying the source of energy for its initiation and maintenance at a relatively stable level. This is glycolysis and this is the main thing. Next, it is necessary to identify the entire complex of cellular and intercellular communications, ultimately providing the necessary level of isometric contraction of vascular smooth muscle cells. It is important to remember that glycolysis is not only a source of energy, but also a trigger for the entire chain of events leading to autorhythmic activity due to its oscillatory behavior. Moreover, here it is appropriate to recall once again the close connection of the glycolytic and, obviously, the pentose cycle with the mitochondrion as the main suppliers of restored equivalents for the respiratory chain.

In addition, this connection between glycolysis and mitochondrion may be much closer than we imagined.

Deviation 18 and the last. *The glycolytic pathway of eukaryotes, as well as the mitochondrion, apparently have a bacterial origin, and in well-studied model eukaryotes it occurs in the cytosol. There is, however, evidence to suggest that the latter stages of glycolysis may also occur in mitochondria, such as those of stramenopiles, a diverse and ecologically important lineage of eukaryotes (Bartulos CR, Rogers MB, Williams TA, Gentekaki E, Brinkmann H, et al (2018).*

Reference - Stramenopiles are a large and extremely diverse eukaryotic group of organisms, including phototrophic members such as the multicellular algae (brown seaweeds) and unicellular microalgae, including diatoms. They also include the human pathogen Blastocystis

Mitochondria apparently provide the majority of cellular ATP for eukaryotes via oxidative phosphorylation, also known as cellular respiration. Pyruvate, required for cellular respiration, is produced in the cytosol via *glycolysis and imported into the mitochondrion. Pyruvate is then decarboxylated by mitochondrial pyruvate dehydrogenase to acetyl-CoA. This acetyl-CoA enters the citric acid cycle, subsequently producing one GTP (or ATP) and a number of precursors for several anabolic pathways. More importantly, the reduction of NAD^+ to NADH and the formation of succinate fuel the respiratory electron transport chain and hence ATP synthesis via proton gradient-driven ATP synthase, which is responsible for the majority of cellular ATP synthesis.*

Glycolysis is known to depend on the recycling of reducing equivalents that are generated in the reduction of NAD^+ to NADH). How NAD^+ is regenerated depends on the presence of oxygen. Under anoxic conditions, pyruvate is typically reduced by fermentation that regenerates oxidized NAD^+ (most commonly lactic acid or ethanol fermentation). Under aerobic conditions, reducing equivalents are transferred to O2 in the mitochondrial electron transport chain. In organisms that perform glycolysis exclusively in the cytosol, NAD^+/NADH apparently cannot be transported directly into the mitochondria. Instead, two shuttle systems, the glycerol phosphate shuttle and the malate-aspartate shuttle, result in an indirect exchange of reducing equivalents between the cytosol and the mitochondria. The idea of releasing reducing equivalents directly into the mitochondrial matrix, where they can be used by the electron transport chain without the need for a shuttle system, seems to be a very elegant solution. If such a redox shuttle system between the cytosol and the mitochondrial matrix is absent, it is possible that the reaction generating NADPH glucose-6-phosphate dehydrogenase in the Entner-Doudoroff pathway in photosynthetic Stramenopiles occurs in the mitochondria. The end-product of glycolysis, pyruvate, is transported into mitochondria via a specific mitochondrial transporter that has only recently been identified (Herzig, Raemy, Montessuit, Veuthey, Zamboni et al.2012). Taken together, the results of Bartulos, Rogers, Williams, Gentekak, Brinkmann et al. (2018) show that glycolysis, contrary to the textbook view in well-studied model organisms, occurs not only in the cytosol but also in the mitochondria. Reference - The Entner–Doudoroff pathway (ED Pathway) is a metabolic pathway that is most notable in Gram-negative bacteria, certain Gram-positive bacteria and archaea.

Thus, I have depicted my concept of the basal tone of the vascular wall as a basic isometric tension against the background of which all external (constrictor and dilator) metabolic and neurogenic modulating influences are realized. There is no doubt that the basis of the basal tone is myogenic automaticity. The source of energy is probably glycolysis, which ensures the proper performance of the sodium-potassium pump and the corresponding changes in the membrane potential.

The question is how it all works. Folkow very figuratively imagined the smooth muscle cell as a mechanoreceptor with a built-in contractile system. Johnson (1977), in turn, postulated the existence in smooth muscle cells of a sensory element located in series with the contractile element. With an increase in intravascular pressure, the vessel passively stretches, and the tension of the vascular wall increases as a result of both the increase in pressure and the increase in the radius of the vessel. This is accompanied by stretching of the sensory element, which somehow stimulates shortening of the contractile element. If we add to all this the hypothesis of S. Mellander on myogenic reactivity (Mellander, 1978), then the scenario of formation and maintenance of basal tone may look as follows. Let us imagine that the level of basal tone is determined by the sum of spike discharges in smooth muscle cells in response to dynamic and static stimuli. An increase in transmural pressure and the corresponding stretching of the vascular wall under the influence of static and dynamic stimuli leads to an increase in the generation of spike discharges and an increase in the tension of the vascular wall. As a result, the radius of the vessel and the length of the sensory element fall below a certain specified value. This leads to the disconnection of the static stimulus and the appearance of a negative dynamic stimulus for a short time. All this taken together inhibits myogenic activity. As a result, the increased transmural pressure causes passive stretching of the vascular wall and initiates the appearance of a new dynamic stimulus. After which the entire cycle is repeated again. As a result, the vascular tone will fluctuate around a certain value sufficient to maintain a certain perfusion pressure and optimal tissue perfusion.

Obviously, it is time to recall the passive component of the basal vascular tone. The main passive elements are connective tissue proteins. Namely, collagen and elastin. Fibroblasts, due to their insignificant share, obviously do not affect the mechanical characteristics of the vascular wall. It should be noted that the rigidity of collagen is 1000 times greater than that of elastin. It is clear that the larger the vessel, the greater the content of collagen and elastin. Another thing is interesting. In vessels containing these proteins, smooth muscle fibers connect individual layers of elastin. As a result, contraction of muscle fibers leads to an additional increase in the rigidity of the vascular wall. In this case, the diameter of the vessel may not change, but the resistance to stretching pressure and blood flow increases. So, this "passive element" is not so completely passive, but plays the role of a kind of lever system for transforming the mechanical activity of smooth muscles in the vascular wall.

And again, let us return to glycolysis, the main character of the book. Glycolysis is the most ancient and powerful bioenergetic process, occurring uniquely and everywhere in living nature. Particular interest in it is associated with its oscillatory behavior and possible participation in the formation of myogenic autorhythmic activity of smooth muscles (SM) and the formation of basal vascular tone. We assume that glycolysis oscillations play a major role in triggering membrane potential oscillations, initiating automatic myogenic activity in smooth muscle cells, which, in turn, apparently underlies the basal tone in the vascular SM. It is known that the level of glycolysis in vascular SM is extremely high even under aerobic conditions. This clearly indicates a special role of glycolysis in the energetics of vessels.

It is important to emphasize that the ATP produced during oxidative phosphorylation is used by ATPases associated with the contractile process, whereas the ATP produced by glycolysis is specifically used as the main supplier of ATP for the Na^+/K^+-ATPase and the ATP-dependent potassium channels (KATP). Therefore, there is a structuring of metabolism in the vascular SM, which leads to independent metabolic regulation of different SM functions, i.e., contractility and excitability. This compartmentalization of metabolism may be a result of the spatial organization of glycolytic enzymes in the cytoplasm. Glycolytic enzymes are localized not only near the structures of the apparatus, but also in the plasma membrane with a functional connection with membrane ion channels (e.g., the gating properties of KATP depend on ATP obtained from glycolysis) and the outer mitochondrial membrane. It is very important to note that the metabolic and redox signal are closely linked and jointly play a role in the regulation of cellular function due to the fact that pyruvate dehydrogenase acts as an intermediary between these two compartments of energy metabolism.

With respect to the role of calcium, the major source of intracellular calcium oscillations is the sarcoplasmic reticulum, which periodically releases calcium, resulting in regenerative calcium waves through the cell. In the presence of cyclic GMP, this calcium is able to activate a chloride channel in the plasma membrane. If this current is activated in enough cells at once, the cells will depolarize. Cells that are not currently contracting will also depolarize, since all the cells are electrically coupled. Depolarization will cause an influx of calcium through L-type calcium channels, which not only triggers contraction but also releases calcium into resting cells, thereby resetting their intracellular oscillators. Thus, the probability that enough cells will become active together in the next cycle is very high, and the cells will effectively become phase synchronized.

Thus, the basal vascular tone is formed by smooth muscle cells of both the “phasic” and “tonic” types with a high level of aerobic glycolysis and autorhythmic activity. The development of SM contraction is a consequence of the “awakening” of the so-called “silent” cells of the “tonic” type due to a decrease in the outgoing current and their transition to the autorhythmic activity mode. As a result of the summation of these contractions, the level of basal tone. Another possible additional contribution to the formation of basal tone in relatively large blood vessels may be a stable, incoming non-inactivating calcium current that occurs at membrane potential levels when the curves of potential-dependent activation and inactivation overlap (windows current).

Our hypothesis for the formation of basal tone is based on several lines of evidence: i) vascular smooth muscle exhibits abnormally high levels of glycolysis under normal oxygenation; ii) vascular smooth muscle metabolism is functionally compartmentalized, i.e., oxidative phosphorylation appears to be associated with energy-saving contraction, whereas ATP generated by glycolysis may be specifically utilized by ATP-sensitive potassium channels, Na/K-ATPase, and via the Na/Ca exchange calcium pump (i.e., it is involved in electrogenesis); iii) glycolysis may be involved in the generation of slow waves and autorhythmic activity in SM, which in turn underlies the onset and maintenance of basal tone.

In conclusion, BASAL TONE OF RESISTANT VESSELS is the degree of active tension of the vascular wall, which is preserved even after complete elimination of neurogenic and humoral influences. It is based on automatic electrical and contractile activity, inherent in myocytes. The main source of energy for the generation of myogenic automatism is the glycolytic oscillator. Internal myogenic activity is inherent in myocytes of both phasic and tonic types. The contribution of phasic myocytes to the formation of basal tone is determined by the frequency, strength, and duration of spontaneous rhythmic contractions. The contribution of tonic myocytes is determined by their persistent contraction due to the stationary open state of membrane potential-dependent calcium channels or changes in the sensitivity of myofilaments to calcium ions. Basal tone can be modulated by transient receptor potential channels by stimulating calcium entry through voltage-gated calcium channels and subsequent contraction, or by high conductance calcium-activated potassium channels, thereby hyperpolarizing and relaxing vascular smooth muscle cells.

Bibliography

Aalkjær, C., & Nilsson, H. (2005). Vasomotion: Cellular background for the oscillator and for the synchronization of smooth muscle cells. In *British Journal of Pharmacology* (Vol. 144, Issue 5, pp. 605–616). Br J Pharmacol. https://doi.org/10.1038/sj.bjp.0706084.

Abd El-Rahman, R. R., Harraz, O. F., Brett, S. E., Anfinogenova, Y., Mufti, R. E., Goldman, D., & Welsh, D. G. (2013). Identification of L- and T-type Ca^{2+} channels in rat cerebral arteries: role in myogenic tone development. *American Journal of Physiology. Heart and Circulatory Physiology*, *304*(1). https://doi.org/10.1152/AJPHEART.00476.2012.

Abel, H. J., Lee, J. C. F., Callaway, J. C., Foehring, R. C. (2004). Relationships between intracellular calcium and afterhyperpolarizations in neocortical pyramidal neurons. Journal of Neurophysiology, 91: 324–335.

Abernethy, A. D., Stackhouse, K., Hart, S., Devendra, G., Bashore, T. M., Dweik, R., & Krasuski, R. A. (2015). Impact of diabetes in patients with pulmonary hypertension. *Pulmonary Circulation*, *5*(1), 117–123. https://doi.org/10.1086/679705.

Aguilar, H. N., & Mitchell, B. F. (2010). Physiological pathways and molecular mechanisms regulating uterine contractility. *Human Reproduction Update*, *16*(6), 725–744. https://doi.org/10.1093/humupd/dmq016.

Albert, A. P., & Large, W. A. (2003). Store-operated Ca^{2+}-permeable non-selective cation channels in smooth muscle cells. *Cell Calcium*, *33*(5–6), 345–356. http://www.sciencedirect.com/science/article/B6WCC-48F5GHS-1/2/a16e7abb3ab3081cba1e51881dda8881.

Albert, A. P., & Large, W. A. (2006). Signal transduction pathways and gating mechanisms of native TRP-like cation channels in vascular myocytes. *Journal of Physiology*, *570*(1), 45–51. https://doi.org/10.1113/jphysiol.2005.096875.

Albert, A. P., Piper, A. S., & Large, W. A. (2003). Properties of a constitutively active Ca^{2+}-permeable non-selective cation channel in rabbit ear artery myocytes. *Journal of Physiology*, *549*(1), 143–156. http://jp.physoc.org/cgi/content/abstract/549/1/143.

Alonso-Carbajo, L., Kecskes, M., Jacobs, G., Pironet, A., Syam, N., Talavera, K., & Vennekens, R. (2017). Muscling in on TRP channels in vascular smooth muscle cells and cardiomyocytes. In *Cell Calcium* (Vol. 66, pp. 48–61). Elsevier Ltd. https://doi.org/10.1016/j.ceca.2017.06.004.

Álvarez-Miguel, I., Cidad, P., Pérez-García, M. T., & López-López, J. R. (2017). Differences in TRPC3 and TRPC6 channels assembly in mesenteric vascular smooth muscle cells in essential hypertension. *Journal of Physiology*, *595*(5), 1497–1513. https://doi.org/10.1113/JP273327.

Andronov, A. V., Vitt A. A., Khaikin S. E. (1966). Theory of Oscillators. Addison - Wesley Series in Advanced Physics, v .4, Morton Hamermesh, Consulting Editor, Pergamon Press.

Anrep, G. V. (1912). On the part played by the suprarenals in the normal vascular reaction of the body. *The Journal Physiology*, 45, 5, 307-315.

Antoons, G., Volders, P. G. A., Stankovicova, T., Bito, V., Stengl, M., Vos, M. A., & Sipido, K. R. (2007). Window Ca^{2+} current and its modulation by Ca^{2+} release in hypertrophied cardiac myocytes from dogs with chronic atrioventricular block. *Journal of Physiology*, *579*(1), 147–160. https://doi.org/10.1113/jphysiol.2006.124222.

Artamonov, M. V., Sonkusare, S. K., Good, M. E., Momotani, K., Eto, M., Isakson, B. E., Le, T. H, Cope, E. L., Derewenda, Z. S., Derewenda, U., and Somlyo, A. V. (2019). RSK2 contributes to myogenic vasoconstriction of resistance arteries by activating smooth muscle myosin and the Na+/H+ exchanger. *Science Signalling*, 11(554): . doi:10.1126/scisignal.aar3924.

Baguet, J. P., Legallicier, B., Auquier, P., & Robitail, S. (2007). Updated meta-analytical approach to the efficacy of antihypertensive drugs in reducing blood pressure. *Clinical Drug Investigation*, *27*(11), 735–753. https://doi.org/10.2165/00044011-200727110-00001.

Bakhramov, A., Hartley, S. A., Salter, K. J., & Kozlowski, R. Z. (1996). Contractile agonists preferentially activate CL- over K+ currents in arterial myocytes. *Biochemical and Biophysical Research Communications*, *227*(1), 168–175. https://doi.org/10.1006/bbrc.1996.1484.

Barabas, P., Augustine, J., Fernández, J. A., McGeown, J. G., McGahon, M. K., & Curtis, T. M. (2020). Ion channels and myogenic activity in retinal arterioles. In *Current Topics in Membranes* (Vol. 85, pp. 187–226). Academic Press Inc. https://doi.org/10.1016/bs.ctm.2020.01.008.

Barcroft, Joseph. (1934). *Features in the architecture of physiological function: 368 p.* Cambridge University Press.

Barron, E., Bakhai, C., Kar, P., Weaver, A., Bradley, D., Ismail, H., Knighton, P., Holman, N., Khunti, K., Sattar, N., Wareham, N. J., Young, B., & Valabhji, J. (2020). Associations of type 1 and type 2 diabetes with COVID-19-related mortality in England: a whole-population study. *The Lancet Diabetes and Endocrinology*, *8*(10), 813–822. https://doi.org/10.1016/S2213-8587(20)30272-2.

Barron, J. T., Gu, L., & Parrillo, J. E. (2000). NADH/NAD redox state of cytoplasmic glycolytic compartments in vascular smooth muscle. *American Journal of Physiology. Heart and Circulatory Physiology*, *279*(6). https://doi.org/10.1152/AJPHEART.2000.279.6.H2872.

Barajas-López, C., Den Hertog, A., Huizinga, J. D. (1089). Ionic basis of pacemaker generation in dog colonic smooth muscle. *The Journal of Physiology*, Sep; 416:385-402. doi: 10.1113/jphysiol.1989.sp017767. PMID: 2481730; PMCID: PMC1189221.

Bartulos, C. R., Rogers. M. B., Williams, T. A,, Gentekaki, E., Brinkmann, H., Cerff, R., Liaud, M-F., Hehl, A. B., Yarlett, N. R., Gruber, A., Peter, G., Kroth, P. G., and van der Giezen, M. (2018). Mitochondrial Glycolysis in a Major Lineage of Eukaryotes. Genome. Biology and Evolution. 10(9):2310–2325 doi:10.1093/gbe/evy164.

Bayliss, W. M. (1902). On the local reactions of arterial wall to changes of of internal pressurte, *The Journal of Physiology*, 28, 3, 220-237.

Bayliss, W. M. (1923). *The vasomotor system*, London, 123 p.

Bauer, E. S. *Theoretical Biology.* (1935). Moscow-Leningrad, Izd. WIEM, 206 p.

Beech, D. J., Muraki, K., & Flemming, R. (2004). Non-selective cationic channels of smooth muscle and the mammalian homologues of Drosophila TRP. *Journal of Physiology*, *559*(3), 685–706. https://doi.org/10.1113/jphysiol.2004.068734.

Beer, G. (1971). Role of tissue fluid in blood flow regulation. *Circulation Research*, *28*, 154–158.

Benham, C. D., & Bolton, T. B. (1986). Spontaneous transient outward currents in single visceral and vascular smooth muscle cells of the rabbit. *Journal of Physiology*, *381*(1), 385–406. https://doi.org/10.1113/jphysiol.1986.sp016333.

Benham, C. D., Hess, P., & Tsien, R. W. (1987). Two types of calcium channels in single smooth muscle cells from rabbit ear artery studied with whole-cell and single-channel recordings. *Circulation Research*, *61*(4 Pt 2), I10-6.

Benzoni, P., Bertoli, G., Giannetti, F., Piantoni, C., Milanesi, R., Pecchiari, M., Barbuti, A., Baruscotti, M., & Bucchi, A. (2021). The funny current: Even funnier than 40 years ago. Uncanonical expression and roles of HCN/f channels all over the body. *Progress in Biophysics and Molecular Biology*, *166*, 189–204. https://doi.org/10.1016/j.pbiomolbio.2021.08.007.

Berg, J., Yang, H., & Jan, L. Y. (2012). Ca^{2+}-activated Cl-channels at a glance. *Journal of Cell Science*, *125*(6), 1367–1371. https://doi.org/10.1242/jcs.093260.

Bershtein, S., Gurevich, M., Soloviev, A. (1984). *Oxygen deficiency and vascular tone*, Kiev, Naukova dumka.

Biró, S., Kovách, A. G., & Tkatchenko, B. I. (1975). Capillary fluid transfer in the cat hind limb muscles during cardiovascular reflexes. *Bibliotheca Anatomica*, *13*, 84–85.

Blondeau, N., Pétrault, O., Manta, S., Giordanengo, V., Gounon, P., Bordet, R., Lazdunski, M., & Heurteaux, C. (2007). Polyunsaturated fatty acids are cerebral vasodilators via the TREK-1 potassium channel. *Circulation Research*, *101*(2), 176–184. https://doi.org/10.1161/CIRCRESAHA.107.154443.

Boiteux, A., Hess, B. (1974). Oscillations in glycolysis, cellular respiration and communication. *Faraday Symposium of Chemical Society,* 9: 202-214.

Bolton, T. B. (1979). Mechanisms of action of transmitters and other substances on smooth muscle. *Physiological Reviews*, *59*(3), 606–718.

Borda, L. J., Shuchleib, R., & Henry, P. D. (1980). Hypoxic contraction of isolated canine coronary artery. Mediation by potassium-dependent exocytosis of norepinephrine. *Circulation Research*, *46*(6), 870–879. https://doi.org/10.1161/01.RES.46.6.870.

Borysova, L., Dora, K. A., Garland, C. J., & Burdyga, T. (2018). Smooth muscle gap-junctions allow propagation of intercellular Ca^{2+} waves and vasoconstriction due to Ca^{2+} based action potentials in rat mesenteric resistance arteries. *Cell Calcium*, *75*, 21–29. https://doi.org/10.1016/j.ceca.2018.08.001.

Bozler, E. (1962). Initiation of contraction in smooth muscle. *Physiological Reviews*, *5*(Suppl.), 179–192.

Brayden, J. E., Earley, S., Nelson, M. T., & Reading, S. (2008). Transient Receptor Potentila (TRP) channels, vascular tone and autoregulation of cerebral blood flow. *Clinical and Experimental Pharmacology and Physiology*, *35*(9), 1116–1120. https://doi.org/10.1111/j.1440-1681.2007.04855.x.

Bregestovski, P., Zefirov, A. (2019). Optogenetics and photopharmacology — effective tools for managing cell activity using light. *Kazan medical journal*, 100 (1): 158–169. DOI: 10.17816/KMJ2019-158.

Brown, A. C., & Yankowitz, D. (1964). Tooth pulp tissue pressure and hydraulic permeability. *Circulation Research*, *15*, 42–50. https://doi.org/10.1161/01.RES.15.1.42.

Brown, H., & Difrancesco, D. (1980). Voltage-clamp investigations of membrane currents underlying pace-maker activity in rabbit sino-atrial node. *The Journal of Physiology*, *308*(1), 331–351. https://doi.org/10.1113/jphysiol.1980.sp013474..

Brown, H. F., Difrancesco, D., & Noble, S. J. (1979). How does adrenaline accelerate the heart? [13]. In *Nature* (Vol. 280, Issue 5719, pp. 235–236). Nature. https://doi.org/10.1038/280235a0.

Bryan, R. M., Joseph, B. K., Lloyd, E., & Rusch, N. J. (2007). Starring TREK-1: The next generation of vascular K^+ channels. In *Circulation Research* (Vol. 101, Issue 2, pp. 119–121). Lippincott Williams & Wilkins. https://doi.org/10.1161/CIRCRESAHA.107.157412.

Bryan, R. M., You, J., Phillips, S. C., Andresen, J. J., Lloyd, E. E., Rogers, P. A., Dryer, S. E., & Marrelli, S. P. (2006). Evidence for two-pore domain potassium channels in rat cerebral arteries. *American Journal of Physiology - Heart and Circulatory Physiology*, *291*(2). https://doi.org/10.1152/ajpheart.01377.2005.

Byrne, N. G., & Large, W. A. (1988). Membrane ionic mechanisms activated by noradrenaline in cells isolated from the rabbit portal vein. *The Journal of Physiology*, *404*(1), 557–573. http://jp.physoc.org/content/404/1/557.abstract.

Campbell, J. D., & Paul, R. J. (1992). The nature of fuel provision for the Na+,K(+)-ATPase in porcine vascular smooth muscle. *The Journal of Physiology*, *447*(1), 67–82. https://doi.org/10.1113/JPHYSIOL.1992.SP018991.

Casteels, R., & Droogmans, G. (1981). Exchange characteristics of the noradrenaline-sensitive calcium store in vascular smooth muscle cells or rabbit ear artery. *The Journal of Physiology*, *317*(1), 263–279. https://doi.org/10.1113/jphysiol.1981.sp013824.

Chance, B., Estabrook, R. W., & Ghosh, A. (1964). Damped sinusoidal oscillations of cytoplasmic reduced pyridine nucleotide in yeast cells. *Proceedings of the National Academy of Sciences of the United States of America*, *51*(6), 1244–1251. https://doi.org/10.1073/PNAS.51.6.1244.

Chatelain, P., Demol, D., & Roba, J. (1984). Comparison of [3H]nitrendipine binding to heart membranes of normotensive and spontaneously hypertensive rats. *Journal of Cardiovascular Pharmacology*, *6*(2), 220–223. https://doi.org/10.1097/00005344-198403000-00002.

Chen, X., Sooch, G., Demaree, I. S., White, F. A., & Obukhov, A. G. (2020). Transient receptor potential canonical (Trpc) channels: Then and now. In *Cells* (Vol. 9, Issue 9, pp. 1–48). Multidisciplinary Digital Publishing Institute (MDPI). https://doi.org/10.3390/cells9091983.

Clapham, D. E. (2003). TRP channels as cellular sensors. *Nature*, *426*(6966), 517–524–517–524. https://doi.org/10.1038/nature02196.

Cobbold, A. F., Levis, O. L. (1956). The nervous control of joint blood vessels. *The Journal of Physiology*, 28, 133(2), 467-471.

Cohnheim J. (1872). Untersuchungen über die embolischen Processe. Berlin: August Hirschwald.

Connor, J. A., Prosser, C. L., & Weems, W. A. (1974). A study of pace-maker activity in intestinal smooth muscle. *The Journal of Physiology*, *240*(3), 671–701. https://doi.org/10.1113/JPHYSIOL.1974.SP010629.

Crompton, M., Capano, M., Crafolil, E. (1976). The Sodium-Induced Efflux of Calcium from Heart Mitochondria A Possible Mechanism for the Regulation of Mitochondrial Calcium. *European Journal of Biochemistry*, 6: 453- 462.

Devine, C. E., Somlyo, A. V., & Somlyo, A. P. (1972). Sarcoplasmic reticulum and excitation-contraction coupling in mammalian smooth muscles. *Journal of Cell Biology*, *52*(3), 690–718. https://doi.org/10.1083/jcb.52.3.690.

Di, A., & Malik, A. B. (2010). TRP channels and the control of vascular function. *Current Opinion in Pharmacology*, *10*(2), 127–132. http://www.sciencedirect.com/science/article/B6W7F-4Y3SP1S-3/2/5d17e24bb28d337e5695c6da212f38be.

Dietrich, A., Chubanov, V., Kalwa, H., Rost, B. R., & Gudermann, T. (2006). Cation channels of the transient receptor potential superfamily: Their role in physiological and pathophysiological processes of smooth muscle cells. *Pharmacology & Therapeutics*, *112*(3), 744–760. http://www.sciencedirect.com/science/article/B6TBG-4KD5BNN-3/2/e8fec4d0fe8725adb7898359c155d08c.

Dietrich, A., Schnitzler, M., Gollasch, M., Gross, V., Storch, U., Dubrovska, G., Obst, M., Yildirim, E., Salanova, B., Kalwa, H., Essin, K., Pinkenburg, O., Luft, F. C., Gudermann, T., & Birnbaumer, L. (2005). Increased vascular smooth muscle contractility in TRPC6-/- mice. *Molecular and Cellular Biology*, *25*(16), 6980–6989. http://mcb.asm.org/cgi/content/abstract/25/16/6980.

Dryn, D., Melnyk, M., Kizub, I., Hu, H., Soloviev, A. A. I. A., & Zholos, A. (2016). The Role of Trpv4 Cation Channels in the Regulation of Phenylephrine-Induced Contraction of Rat Pulmonary Arter. *Fiziolohichnyi Zhurnal (Kiev, Ukraine : 1994)*, *62*(2), 79–86. https://doi.org/10.1615/intjphyspathophys.v8.i2.30.

Dryn, D. O., Melnyk, M. I., Bon, R. S., Beech, D. J., & Zholos, A. V. (2023). Pico145 inhibits TRPC4-mediated mICAT and postprandial small intestinal motility. *Biomedicine & Pharmacotherapy = Biomedecine & Pharmacotherapie*, *168*. https://doi.org/10.1016/J.BIOPHA.2023.115672.

Dryn, D. O., Melnyk, M. I., Melanaphy, D., Kizub, I. V, Johnson, C. D., & Zholos, A. V. (2023). Bidirectional TRP/L Type Ca^{2+} Channel/RyR/BK<inf>Ca</inf> Molecular and Functional Signaloplex in Vascular Smooth Muscles. *Biomolecules*, *13*(5). https://doi.org/10.3390/biom13050759.

Earley, S., & Brayden, J. E. (2015). Transient receptor potential channels in the vasculature. *Physiological Reviews*, *95*(2), 645–690. https://doi.org/10.1152/physrev.00026.2014.

Ebeigbe, A. B. (1982). Influence of hypoxia on contractility and calcium uptake in rabbit aortas. *Experientia,* 38,8, 935-937.

Eberhard, K. (1973). Krtafte und kraftwwirkungen im Gebiet der Blutkapillaren. *Angiologica,* 10, 5-5, 256-263.

El-Lakany, M. A., Haghbin, N., Arora, N., Hashad, A. M., Mironova, G. Y., Sancho, M., Gros, R., & Welsh, D. G. (2023). CaV3.1 channels facilitate calcium wave generation and myogenic tone development in mouse mesenteric arteries. *Scientific Reports*, *13*(1). https://doi.org/10.1038/S41598-023-47715-3.

Esser, C., Ahmadinejad, N., Wiegand, C., Rotte, C., Sebastiani, F., Gelius-Dietrich, G., Henze, K., Kretschmann, E., Richly, E., Leister, D., Bryant, D., Steel, M. A., Lockhart, P. J., Penny, D., & Martin, W. (2004). A genome phylogeny for mitochondria among α-proteobacteria and a predominantly eubacterial ancestry of yeast nuclear genes. *Molecular Biology and Evolution*, *21*(9), 1643–1660. https://doi.org/10.1093/molbev/msh160.

Evans, A. M., Hardie, D. G., Peers, C., & Mahmoud, A. (2011a). Hypoxic pulmonary vasoconstriction: mechanisms of oxygen-sensing. *Current Opinion in Anaesthesiology*, *24*(1), 13–20. https://doi.org/10.1097/ACO.0B013E3283421201.

Evans, A. M., Hardie, D. G., Peers, C., & Mahmoud, A. (2011b). Hypoxic pulmonary vasoconstriction: mechanisms of oxygen-sensing. *Current Opinion in Anaesthesiology*, *24*(1), 13–20. https://doi.org/10.1097/ACO.0B013E3283421201.

Fabiato, A. (1983). Calcium-induced release of calcium from the cardiac sarcoplasmic reticulum. *American Journal of Physiology - Cell Physiology*, *14*(1). https://doi.org/10.1152/ajpcell.1983.245.1.c1.

Fales, J. T., Heisey, S. R., & Zierler, K. L. (1962). Blood flow from and oxygen uptake by muscle, during and after partial venous occlusion. *The American Journal of Physiology*, *203*, 470–474. https://doi.org/10.1152/ajplegacy.1962.203.3.470.

Fan, G., Cui, Y., Gollasch, M., & Kassmann, M. (2019). Elementary calcium signaling in arterial smooth muscle. In *Channels* (Vol. 13, Issue 1, pp. 505–519). Taylor and Francis Inc. https://doi.org/10.1080/19336950.2019.1688910.

Folkow, B. (1964). Description of the myogenic hypothesis. *Circulation Research*, *15*, 279–287.

Folkow, B. Intravascular pressure as a factor regulating the tone of the small vessels. *Acta Phys. Scand.*, 1949, 17, 4, 239-310.

Franco-Obregon, A., Lopez-Barneo, J. (1996). O-sensing Ca channels in scattered arterial myocytes. *American Journal of Physiology*, 271:H2290–H229.

Freichel, M., Suh, S. H., Pfeifer, A., Schweig, U., Trost, C., Weissgerber, P., Biel, M., Philipp, S., Freise, D., Droogmans, G., Hofmann, F., Flockerzi, V., & Nilius, B. (2001). Lack of an endothelial store-operated Ca^{2+} current impairs agonist-dependent vasorelaxation in TRP4-/- mice. *Nature Cell Biology*, *3*(2), 121–127.

Fretheim, A., Odgaard-Jensen, J., Brørs, O., Madsen, S., Njølstad, I., Norheim, O. F., Svilaas, A., Kristiansen, I. S., Thürmer, H., & Flottorp, S. (2012). Comparative effectiveness of antihypertensive medication for primary prevention of cardiovascular disease: Systematic review and multiple treatments meta-analysis. *BMC Medicine*, *10*, 33. https://doi.org/10.1186/1741-7015-10-33.

Friesen, W. O., & Block, G. D. (1984). What is a biological oscillator? *The American Journal of Physiology*, *246*(6 Pt 2). https://doi.org/10.1152/ajpregu.1984.246.6.R847.

Fuchs, B., Rupp, M., Ghofrani, H. A., Schermuly, R. T., Seeger, W., Grimminger, F., Gudermann, T., Dietrich, A., & Weissmann, N. (2011). Diacylglycerol regulates acute hypoxic pulmonary vasoconstriction via TRPC6. *Respiratory Research*, *12*(1). https://doi.org/10.1186/1465-9921-12-20.

Ganitkevich, V. Y., & Isenberg, G. (1990). Contribution of two types of calcium channels to membrane conductance of single myocytes from guinea-pig coronary artery. *Journal of Physiology*, *426*, 19–42.

Ganitkevich, V. Y., & Isenberg, G. (1995). Efficacy of peak Ca^{2+}currents (ICa) as trigger of sarcoplasmic reticulum Ca^{2+} release in myocytes from the guinea-pig coronary artery. *The Journal of Physiology*, *484*(Pt 2), 287–306. http://jp.physoc.org/content/484/Pt_2/287.abstract.

Ganitkevich, V. Ya., Shuba, M. F., & Smirnov, S. V. (1986). Potential-dependent calcium inward current in a single isolated smooth muscle cell of the guinea-pig taenia caeci. *The Journal of Physiology*, *380*(1), 1–16. https://doi.org/10.1113/jphysiol.1986.sp016268.

Garcia-Elias, A., Mrkonjić, S., Jung, C., Pardo-Pastor, C., Vicente, R., & Valverde, M. A. (2014). The TRPV4 channel. *Handbook of Experimental Pharmacology*, *222*, 293–319. https://doi.org/10.1007/978-3-642-54215-2_12.

Gardener, M. J., Johnson, I. T., Burnham, M. P., Edwards, G., Heagerty, A. M., & Weston, A. H. (2004). Functional evidence of a role for two-pore domain potassium channels in rat mesenteric and pulmonary arteries. *British Journal of Pharmacology*, *142*(1), 192–202. https://doi.org/10.1038/sj.bjp.0705691.

Gaskell W. H. On the tonicity of the heart and blood vessels. *J. Physiol.*, 1880, 3, 48-75.

Gestrelius, S., Borgström, P. (1986). A dynamic model of smooth muscle contraction. *Biophysics Journal,* Jul;50(1):157-69. doi: 10.1016/S0006-3495(86)83448-8. PMID: 3730500; PMCID: PMC1329668.

Ghosh, D., Syed, A. U., Prada, M. P., Nystoriak, M. A., Santana, L. F., Nieves-Cintrón, M., & Navedo, M. F. (2017). Calcium Channels in Vascular Smooth Muscle. In *Advances in Pharmacology* (Vol. 78, pp. 49–87). Academic Press Inc. https://doi.org/10.1016/bs.apha.2016.08.002.

Golenhofen, K. (1976). Theory of P and T systems for calcium activation in smooth muscle. In E. Bülbring & M. F. Shuba (Eds.), *Physiology of Smooth Muscle* (pp. 197–202). New York: Raven Press.

Golovina, V. A., Platoshyn, O., Bailey, C. L., Wang, J., Limsuwan, A., Sweeney, M., Rubin, L. J., & Yuan, J. X. (2001). Upregulated TRP and enhanced capacitative Ca^{2+} entry in human pulmonary artery myocytes during proliferation. *American Journal of Physiology*, *280* (United States PT-Journal Article LG-English NO-HL-54043 (NHLBI), HL-64945 (NHLBI)), H746–H755.

Goltz F. Über den Tonus der Gefäße und seine Bedeutung fur die Blutbewegung. *Arch. Pathol Anat Physiol u fur Klin.* Med, 1864, Neue Folge, 9, 29, 1-2, 394-432).

Gonzales, A. L., Amberg, G. C., & Earley, S. (2010). Ca^{2+} release from the sarcoplasmic reticulum is required for sustained TRPM4 activity in cerebral artery smooth muscle cells. *American Journal of Physiology - Cell Physiology*, *299*(2). https://doi.org/10.1152/ajpcell.00550.2009.

Gonzalez-Cobos, J. C., & Trebak, M. (2010). TRPC channels in smooth muscle cells. *Front Biosci.*, *15:1023-39*, 1023–1039.

Gordienko, D. V, & Bolton, T. B. (2002). Crosstalk between ryanodine receptors and IP3receptors as a factor shaping spontaneous Ca^{2+}-release events in rabbit portal vein myocytes. *Journal of Physiology*, *542*(3), 743–762. http://www.jphysiol.org/cgi/content/abstract/542/3/743.

Gordienko, D. V, & Zholos, A. V. (2004). Regulation of muscarinic cationic current in myocytes from guinea-pig ileum by intracellular Ca^{2+} release: A central role of inositol 1,4,5-trisphosphate receptors. *Cell Calcium*, *36*(5). https://doi.org/10.1016/j.ceca.2004.02.021.

Gordienko, D. V, Zholos, A. V, & Bolton, T. B. (1999). Membrane ion channels as physiological targets for local Ca^{2+} signalling. *Journal of Microscopy*, *196*(3). https://doi.org/10.1046/j.1365-2818.1999.00599.x.

Goulopoulou, S., & Webb, R. C. (2014). Symphony of vascular contraction how smooth muscle cells lose harmony to signal increased vascular resistance in hypertension. *Hypertension*, *63*(3). https://doi.org/10.1161/HYPERTENSIONAHA.113.02444.

Greenidge, E., Keatinge, W. (1983), Reduced K permeability induced by anoxia in sheep carotid arteries. *The Journal of Physiology*, 336: 70-71.

Grimmer, B., & Kuebler, W. M. (2017). The endothelium in hypoxic pulmonary vasoconstriction. *Journal of Applied Physiology (Bethesda, Md. : 1985)*, *123*(6), 1635–1646. https://doi.org/10.1152/JAPPLPHYSIOL.00120.2017.

Guibert, C., Ducret, T., & Savineau, J. P. (2011). Expression and physiological roles of TRP channels in smooth muscle cells. In *Advances in Experimental Medicine and Biology* (Vol. 704, pp. 687–706). https://doi.org/10.1007/978-94-007-0265-3_36.

Gur, S., Alzweri, L., Yilmaz-Oral, D., Kaya-Sezginer, E., Abdel-Mageed, A. B., Sikka, S. C., & Hellstrom, W. J. G. (2021). Ivabradine, the hyperpolarization-activated cyclic nucleotide-gated channel blocker, elicits relaxation of the human corpus cavernosum: a potential option for erectile dysfunction treatment. *Aging Male*, *23*(5), 1088–1097. https://doi.org/10.1080/13685538.2019.1678125.

Gurevich, M. I., Bershtein, S. A., Soloviev, A. I. (1981). Deficiency of oxygen in tissues and their blood supply. *Advances in Physiological Sciences of USSR*, 12, 4: 77-98.

Gurevich, M., Bershtein, S., Evdokimov, I. (1976). The effect of changes in osmolarity and oxygen tension on exicatibility and conduction in vascular smooth muscle. In: *Physiology of Smooth Muscle, New York: Raven Press*, p. 153-161.

Gurney, A. M., Osipenko, O. N., MacMillan, D., McFarlane, K. M., Tate, R. J., & Kempsill, F. E. J. (2003). Two-Pore Domain K Channel, TASK-1, in Pulmonary Artery Smooth Muscle Cells. *Circulation Research*, *93*(10), 957–964. https://doi.org/10.1161/01.RES.0000099883.68414.61.

Gurevich, M. I., Bershtein, S. A., Soloviev, A. I. (1984). *Oxygen deficincy and vascular tone.* Kiev, Naukova dumk, 263 p.

Gurney, A. M., Joshi, S., Manoury, B. (2010). KCNQ potassium channels: new targets for pulmonary vasodilator drugs? *Advances Experimental Medical Biology*, 661:405-17. doi: 10.1007/978-1-60761-500-2_26. PMID: 20204745.

Guyton, A., C. (1963). *Circulatory physiology: cardiac output and its regulation.* Phyladelphia-London: Sounders, 404 p.

Hanson, K. M., & Johnson, P. C. (1962). Evidence for local arteriovenous reflex in intestine. *Journal of Applied Physiology, 17,* 509–513. https://doi.org/10.1152/jappl.1962.17.3.509.

Harhun, M. I., Gordienko, D. V., Povstyan, O. V., Moss, R. F., & Bolton, T. B. (2004). Function of interstitial cells of cajal in the rabbit portal vein. *Circulation Research, 95*(6), 619–626. https://doi.org/10.1161/01.RES.0000143014.04535.a3.

Hartzell, C., Putzier, I., & Arreola, J. (2005). Calcium-activated chloride channels. *Annual Review of Physiology, 67,* 719–758. https://doi.org/10.1146/annurev.physiol.67.032003.154341.

Hellstrand, P., Johansson, B., & Norberg, K. (1977). Mechanical, Electrical, and Biochemical Effects of Hypoxia and Substrate Removal on Spontaneously Active Vascular Smooth Muscle. *Acta Physiologica Scandinavica, 100*(1), 69–83. https://doi.org/10.1111/j.1748-1716.1977.tb05923.x.

Hermsmeyer, K. (1993). Calcium channel function in hypertension. *Journal of Human Hypertension.*

Herzig, S., Raemy, E., Montessuit, S., Veuthey, J. L., Zamboni, N., Westermann, B., Kunji, E. R., Martinou, J. C. (2012). Identification and functional expression of the mitochondrial pyruvate carrier. *Science,* Jul 6;337(6090):93-6. doi: 10.1126/science.1218530. Epub 2012 May 24. PMID: 22628554.

Heyer, C. B., & Lux, H. D. (1976). Properties of a facilitating calcium current in pacemaker neurones of the snail, Helix pomatia. *The Journal of Physiology, 262*(2), 319–348. https://doi.org/10.1113/jphysiol.1976.sp011598.

Hill, A. (1929). Anaerobic survival in muscle. *Proceedings of the Royal Society of London. Series B, Containing Papers of a Biological Character, 105*(737), 298–313. https://doi.org/10.1098/rspb.1929.0044.

Hill, M. A., & Meininger, G. A. (1994). Calcium entry and myogenic phenomena in skeletal muscle arterioles. *The American Journal of Physiology, 267*(3 Pt 2). https://doi.org/10.1152/AJPHEART.1994.267.3.H1085.

Higgins, J., A. (1967). The theory of oscillating reactions, *Industrial & Engineering Chemistry,* v. 59, N5.

Hilzendeger, A. M., Shenoy, V., Raizada, M. K., & Katovich, M. J. (2014). Neuroinflammation in pulmonary hypertension: concept, facts, and relevance. *Current Hypertension Reports, 16*(9), 1–7. https://doi.org/10.1007/S11906-014-0469-1.

Hinshaw, L. (1964). Mechanism of renal autoregulation: role of tissue pressure and description of a multifactor hypothesis. *Circulation Research, Suppl.*, 120–131.

Hinshaw, L. B., Day, S. B., & Carlson, C. H. (1959). Tissue pressure as a causal factor in the autoregulation of blood flow in the isolated perfused kidney. *The American Journal of Physiology, 197,* 309–312. https://doi.org/10.1152/ajplegacy.1959.197.2.309.

House S. J., Potier M, Bisaillon J., Singer H. A., Trebak M. The non-excitable smooth muscle: calcium signaling and phenotypic switching during vascular disease. *Pflugers Arch.* 2008 Aug;456(5):769-85. doi: 10.1007/s00424-008-0491-8. Epub 2008 Mar 26. PMID: 18365243; PMCID: PMC2531252.

Imaizumi, Y., Muraki, K., Takeda, M., & Watanabe, M. (1989). Measurement and simulation of noninactivating Ca current in smooth muscle cells. *American Journal of Physiology - Cell Physiology*, *256*(4). https://doi.org/10.1152/ajpcell.1989.256.4.c880.

Inoue, R., Okada, T., Onoue, H., Hara, Y., Shimizu, S., Naitoh, S., Ito, Y., Mori, Y., Ca, A., & Channel, C. (2001). The Transient Receptor Potential Protein Homologue TRP6 Is the Essential Component of Vascular. *Circulation Research*, *88*(3), 325–332.

Jackson, W. F. (2020). Ion channels and the regulation of myogenic tone in peripheral arterioles. In *Current Topics in Membranes* (Vol. 85, pp. 19–58). Academic Press Inc. https://doi.org/10.1016/bs.ctm.2020.01.002.

Jackson, W. F. (2021). Calcium-Dependent Ion Channels and the Regulation of Arteriolar Myogenic Tone. *Frontiers in Physiology*, *12*. https://doi.org/10.3389/FPHYS.2021.770450.

Jacobsen, J. C. B., Aalkjaer, C., Matchkov, V. V., Nilsson, H., Freiberg, J. J., & Holstein-Rathlou, N. H. (2008). Heterogeneity and weak coupling may explain the synchronization characteristics of cells in the arterial wall. *Philosophical Transactions of the Royal Society A: Mathematical, Physical and Engineering Sciences*, *366*(1880), 3483–3502. https://doi.org/10.1098/rsta.2008.0105.

Jacobsen, J. C. B., Aalkjær, C., Nilsson, H., Matchkov, V. V., Freiberg, J., & Holstein-Rathlou, N. H. (2007). Activation of a cGMP-sensitive calcium-dependent chloride channel may cause transition from calcium waves to whole cell oscillations in smooth muscle cells. *American Journal of Physiology - Heart and Circulatory Physiology*, *293*(1). https://doi.org/10.1152/ajpheart.00726.2006.

Johnson, P.C. (1977). Landis Award Lecture. The myogenic response and the microcirculation. *Microvascular Research*, Jan;13(1):1-18. doi: 10.1016/0026-2862(77)90112-1. PMID: 323643.

Jaggar, J. H., Wellman, G. C., Heppner, T. J., Porter, V. A., Perez, G. J., Gollasch, M., Kleppisch, T., Rubart, M., Stevenson, A. S., Lederer, W. J., Knot, H. J., Bonev, A. D., & Nelson, M. T. (1998). Ca^{2+} channels, ryanodine receptors and $Ca^{(2+)-}$activated K^+ channels: a functional unit for regulating arterial tone. [Review] [69 refs] 243. *Acta Physiologica Scandinavica*, *164*(England PT-Journal Article PT-Review PT-Review, Tutorial LG-English NO-GM14715 (NIGMS), HL-44455 (NHLBI), HL-51728 (NHLBI)), 577–587.

Jiang, Z., Wallner, M., Meera, P., & Toro, L. (1999). Human and rodent MaxiK channel β-subunit genes: Cloning and characterization. *Genomics*, *55*(1), 57–67. https://doi.org/10.1006/geno.1998.5627.

Joyner, M. J. (2013). Physiology and redundancy. In *Physiology* (Vol. 28, Issue 3, pp. 136–137). Physiology (Bethesda). https://doi.org/10.1152/physiol.00015.2013.

Kan, V. N, Levtov, V., A. (1970). Influence of arterial and venous occlusion on hemodynamics and oxygen consumption in skeletal muscle. *Physiological journal of USSR*, 56, 4,618-624.

Kaczorowski, G. J., & Garcia, M. L. (2016). Developing Molecular Pharmacology of BK Channels for Therapeutic Benefit. In *International Review of Neurobiology* (Vol. 128, pp. 439–475). Academic Press Inc. https://doi.org/10.1016/bs.irn.2016.02.013.

Karmazyn, M., Beamish, R. E., & Dhalla, N. S. (1984). Involvement of calcium in coronary vasoconstriction due to prolonged hypoxia. *American Heart Journal*, *107*(2), 293–297. https://doi.org/10.1016/0002-8703(84)90377-6.

Katayama, Y., Coburn, R. F., W. S. Fillers, W.S., C. B. Baron, S. B. (1994). Oxygen sensors in vascular smooth muscle, *Journal of Applied Physiology*,77, 5, 2086-2092. https://doi.org/10.1152/jappl.1994.77.5.2086.

Kaznacheev, V., Dzizinsky, A., A. (1975). *Clinical pathology of transcapillary exchange.* M.: Medicine, 238 p.

Keiser, M. J., Setola, V., Irwin, J. J., Laggner, C., Abbas, A. I., Hufeisen, S. J., Jensen, N. H., Kuijer, M. B., Matos, R. C., Tran, T. B., Whaley, R., Glennon, R. A., Hert, J., Thomas, K. L. H., Edwards, D. D., Shoichet, B. K., & Roth, B. L. (2009). Predicting new molecular targets for known drugs. *Nature*, *462*(7270), 175–181. https://doi.org/10.1038/nature08506.

Khayutin, V., M. (1964). *Vasodomotor reflexes*. Moscow: Science, 376 pp.

Khayutin, V. (1971). Mechanisms controlling the vessels of functional skeletal muscle. Histomechanical hypothesis. In *Problems of Modern Physiological Science* (pp. 123–140).

Khomazjuk, I. (1998). The problem of essential hypertension in survivors after Chernobyl catastrophe, in: *Proceedings of the 2nd Conference on Long-Term Health Consequences of the Chernobyl Disaster, World Health Organization, Geneva, Switzerland,* pp. 398–399.

Kikuchi, Y., & Rodbard, S. (1974). Autoregulatory escape and post-escape hyperaemia in a capillaron model. *Cardiovascular Research*, *8*(3), 395–403. https://doi.org/10.1093/cvr/8.3.395.

Kimrey, J., Vo, T., & Bertram, R. (2020). Canard analysis reveals why a large Ca^{2+} window current promotes early afterdepolarizations in cardiac myocytes. *PLoS Computational Biology*, *16*(11). https://doi.org/10.1371/journal.pcbi.1008341.

Kirk, J. E., Effersøe, P. G., & ChianG, S. P. (1954). The rate of respiration and glycolysis by human and dog aortic tissue. *Journal of Gerontology*, *9*(1), 10–53. https://doi.org/10.1093/geronj/9.1.10.

Kitazawa, T., Semba, S., Huh, Y. H., Kitazawa, K., & Eto, M. (2009). Nitric oxide-induced biphasic mechanism of vascular relaxation via dephosphorylation of CPI-17 and MYPT1. *Journal of Physiology*, *587*(14), 3587–3603. https://doi.org/10.1113/jphysiol.2009.172189.

Kitchin, A. H. (1963). Peripheral blood flow and capillary filtration rates. *British Medical Bulletin*, *19*(2), 155–160. https://doi.org/10.1093/oxfordjournals.bmb.a070036.

Kizub I, Pavlova O, Ivanova I, Soloviev A. Protein kinase C-dependent inhibition of BK_{Ca} current in rat aorta smooth muscle cells following g-irradiation. *Int. J. Radiat. Biol.* 2010; 8: 291-299.

Kizub, I. V., Strielkov, I. V., Shaifta, Y., Becker, S., Prieto-Lloret, J., Snetkov, V. A., Soloviev, A. I., Aaronson, P. I., & Ward, J. P. T. (2013). Gap junctions support the sustained phase of hypoxic pulmonary vasoconstriction by facilitating calcium sensitization. *Cardiovascular Research*, *99*(3), 404–411. https://doi.org/10.1093/CVR/CVT129#.

Klimov, D. V., Adziarykha, K. N. (2001). Risk factors for the development of hypertension in the liquidators of 1986–1987, *International Journal Radiation Medi*cine, 3, 59.

Klymenko, K., Novokhatska, T., Kizub, I., Parshikov, A., Dosenko, V., Soloviev, A. (2014). PKC-δ isozyme gene silencing restores vascular function in diabetic rat. *Journal Basic Clinical Physiology Pharmacology*, 27:1-9.

Kohler R, C. Degenhardt, M. Kuhn, N. Runkel, M. Paul, J. Hoyer, Expression and function of endothelial Ca^{2+}-activated K^+ channels in human mesenteric artery: A single cell reverse transcriptase-polymerase chain reaction and electrophysiological study *in situ*. *Circ. Res.* 87 (2000) 496–503, https://doi.org/10. 1161/01.RES.87.6.496.

Knot, H. J., Standen, N. B., & Nelson, M. T. (1998). Ryanodine receptors regulate arterial diameter and wall $[Ca^{2+}]$ in cerebral arteries of rat via Ca^{2+}-dependent K+ channels. *Journal of Physiology*, *508*(1), 211–221. https://doi.org/10.1111/j.1469-7793. 1998.211br.x.

Komuro, T. (2006). Structure and organization of interstitial cells of Cajal in the gastrointestinal tract. *Journal of Physiology*, *576*(3), 653–658. https://doi.org/10.1113/ jphysiol.2006.116624.

Konradi, G.P. (1944). About peripheral mechanisms for maintaining vascular tone. *Bulletin Experimental Biology and Medicine,* 17, 6, 41-44.

Konradi, G.P. (1973). *Regulation of vascular tone*, Science, Leningrad, 328 pp.

Kotecha, N., & Hill, M. A. (2005). Myogenic contraction in rat skeletal muscle arterioles: smooth muscle membrane potential and Ca^{2+} signaling. *American Journal of Physiology. Heart and Circulatory Physiology*, *289*(4). https://doi.org/10.1152/ AJPHEART.00323.2005.

Kotlikoff, M. I. (2003). Calcium-induced calcium release in smooth muscle: the case for loose coupling. *Progress in Biophysics and Molecular Biology*, *83*(3), 171–191. http://www.sciencedirect.com/science/article/B6TBN-492VMDJ-1/2/a9f8af 43f4f483e626ca137de9b9cb39.

Kuhn, T. S. (1962). *The Structure of Scientific Revolutions*.

Kushmerick, M. J., & Crow, M. (1982). Chemical energy balance in amphibian and mammalian skeletal muscles. *Federation Proceedings*, *41*(2), 163–168.

Kyrychenko, S., Tishkin, S., Dosenko, V., Ivanova, I., Novokhatska, T., Soloviev, A. (201`2). The BKCa channels deficiency as a possible reason for radiation-induced vascular hypercontractility. *Vascular Pharmacology*, 56: 142-149.

Kwan, H. Y., Huang, Y., & Yao, X. (2007). TRP channels in endothelial function and dysfunction. *Biochimica et Biophysica Acta*, *1772*(0006-3002 (Print)), 907–914.

Landis, E. M. (1928). Micro-injection studies of capillary permeability of the capillary wall to fluid and to plasma proteins. *American Journal of Physiology*, 83, 528

Leach, R. M., Hill, H. M., Snetkov, V. A., Robertson, T. P., Ward, J. P. (2001). Divergent roles of glycolysis and the mitochondrial electron transport chain in hypoxic pulmonary vasoconstriction of the rat: identity of the hypoxic sensor. *The Journal of Physiology*, Oct 1;536(Pt 1):211-24. doi: 10.1111/j.1469-7793.2001.00211.x. PMID: 11579170; PMCID: PMC2278857.

Lennon, P. F., & Murray, P. A. (1996). Attenuated hypoxic pulmonary vasoconstriction during isoflurane anesthesia is abolished by cyclooxygenase inhibition in chronically instrumented dogs. *Anesthesiology*, *84*(2), 404–414. https://doi.org/10.1097/00000542-199602000-00020.

Levick. (1991). Capillary filtration-absorption balance reconsidered in light of dynamic extravascular factors. *Experimental Physiology*, *76*(6), 825–857. https://doi.org/10.1113/expphysiol.1991.sp003549.

Levtov, V. A. (1967). *Chemical regulation of local blood circulation*. Nauka, Leningrad, 1967.

Liao, P., Yu, D., Li, G., Tan, F. Y., Jia, L. S., Yeow, L. C., & Tuck, W. S. (2007). A smooth muscle Cav1.2 calcium channel splice variant underlies hyperpolarized window current and enhanced state-dependent inhibition by nifedipine. *Journal of Biological Chemistry*, *282*(48), 35133–35142. https://doi.org/10.1074/jbc.M705478200.

Liao, Y., Erxleben, C., Abramowitz, J., Flockerzi, V., Zhu, M. X., Armstrong, D. L., & Birnbaumer, L. (2008). Functional interactions among Orai1, TRPCs, and STIM1 suggest a STIM-regulated heteromeric Orai/TRPC model for SOCE/Icrac channels. *Proceedings of the National Academy of Sciences of the United States of America*, *105*(8), 2895–2900. https://doi.org/10.1073/pnas.0712288105.

Liu, K. X., Everdell, E., Pal, S., Haas-Kogan, D. A., & Milligan, M. G. (2021). Harnessing Lactate Metabolism for Radiosensitization. *Frontiers in Oncology*, *11*. https://doi.org/10.3389/FONC.2021.672339.

Liu, X., & Pan, Z. (2021). Store-Operated Calcium Entry in the Cardiovascular System. In *Advances in Experimental Medicine and Biology* (Vol. 1349, pp. 303–333). Springer. https://doi.org/10.1007/978-981-16-4254-8_14.

Löfström, B., Pernow, B., & Wahren, J. (1965). Vasodilating Action of Substance P in the Human Forearm. *Acta Physiologica Scandinavica*, *63*(3), 311–324. https://doi.org/10.1111/j.1748-1716.1965.tb04070.x.

Lövgren, B., & Hellstrand, P. (1985). Graded effects of oxygen and respiratory inhibitors on cell metabolism and spontaneous contractions in smooth muscle of the rat portal vein. *Acta Physiologica Scandinavica*, *123*(4), 485–495. https://doi.org/10.1111/j.1748-1716.1985.tb07614.x.

Lumb, C. K. (2017). *Comparative Respiratory Physiology*. In: Nunn's Appl. Respir. Physiol., Elsevier, pp. 357-375.e2. https://doi.org/10.1016/b978-0-7020-6294-0.00025-3).

Lydrup, M. L., Sward, K., & Hellstrand, P. (1994). Effect of glibenclamide on membrane response to metabolic inhibition in smooth muscle of rat oral vein. *Journal of Vascular Research*, *31*(2), 82–91. https://doi.org/10.1159/000159034.

Lyons, T. W., Reinhard, C. T., & Planavsky, N. J. (2014). The rise of oxygen in Earth's early ocean and atmosphere. In *Nature* (Vol. 506, Issue 7488, pp. 307–315). Nature Publishing Group. https://doi.org/10.1038/nature13068.

Madsen, M. F., Danø, S., & Sørensen, P. G. (2005). On the mechanisms of glycolytic oscillations in yeast. *The FEBS Journal*, *272*(11), 2648–2660. https://doi.org/10.1111/J.1742-4658.2005.04639.X.

Majgaard, J., Skov, F. G., Kim, S., Hjortdal, V. E., & Boedtkjer, D. M. B. (2022). Positive chronotropic action of HCN channel antagonism in human collecting lymphatic vessels. *Physiological Reports*, *10*(16). https://doi.org/10.14814/phy2.15401.

Matchkov V. Mechanisms of cellular synchronization in the vascular wall. Mechanisms of vasomotion. *Dan Med Bull* 2010; 57: (10) B4191, 1-50.

Matsuda J. J., Volk K. A., Shibata E. F.: Calcium currents in isolated rabbit coronary arterial smooth muscle myocytes. *J Physiol* 1990, 427:657–680.

Mauban, J. R. H., Zacharia, J., Fairfax, S., & Wier, W. G. (2015). PC-PLC/sphingomyelin synthase activity plays a central role in the development of myogenic tone in murine resistance arteries. *American Journal of Physiology - Heart and Circulatory Physiology*, *308*(12), H1517–H1524. https://doi.org/10.1152/ajpheart.00594.2014.

Maxwell, K. D, Shah, P. T., Shapiro, J. I. (2015). The Plasmalemmal Na/K-ATPase: An Amplifier for Reactive Oxygen Species? *Journal of Hypertension*, 4, 1-7.

McClellan, G., Weisberg, A., & Winegrad, S. (1983). Energy transport from mitochondria to myofibril by a creatine phosphate shuttle in cardiac cells. *American Journal of Physiology - Cell Physiology*, *14*(3). https://doi.org/10.1152/ajpcell.1983.245.5.c423.

McGahon, M. K., Dash, D. P., Arora, A., Wall, N., Dawicki, J., Simpson, D. A., Scholfield, C. N. N., McGeown, J. G. G., & Curtis, T. M. (2007). Diabetes Downregulates Large-Conductance Ca^{2+}-Activated Potassium {beta}1 Channel Subunit in Retinal Arteriolar Smooth Muscle. *Circulation Research*, *100*(5), 703–711. https://doi.org/10.1161/01.RES.0000260182.36481.c9.

McGahon, M. K., Fernández, J. A., Dash, D. P., McKee, J., Simpson, D. A., Zholos, A. V, McGeown, J. G., & Curtis, T. M. (2016). TRPV2 channels contribute to stretch-activated cation currents and myogenic constriction in retinal arterioles. *Investigative Ophthalmology and Visual Science*, *57*(13). https://doi.org/10.1167/iovs.16-20279.

McGregor, A. (2010). JAMES WHYTE BLACK. *British Journal of Pharmacology*, *160*(s1). https://doi.org/10.1111/j.1476-5381.2010.00844.x.

McHale, N., Hollywood, M., Sergeant, G., & Thornbury, K. (2006). Origin of spontaneous rhythmicity in smooth muscle. *The Journal of Physiology Online*, *570*(1), 23–28. http://jp.physoc.org/cgi/content/abstract/570/1/23.

Meech, R. W. (1974). The sensitivity of Helix aspersa neurones to injected calcium ions. *The Journal of Physiology*, *237*(2), 259–277. https://doi.org/10.1113/JPHYSIOL.1974.SP010481.

Mellander, S., Johansson, B. (1968). Control of resistance, exchange, and capacitance functions in the peripheral circulation. *Pharmacological Review*, Sep;20(3):117-96. PMID: 4878307.

Mellander, S. 1978. On the control of capillary fluid transfer by precapillary and postcapillary vascular adjustments. *Microvasc Res* 15, 310–330.

Melanaphy, D., Johnson, C. D., Kustov, M. V, Watson, C. A., Borysova, L., Burdyga, T. V, & Zholos, A. V. (2016). Ion channel mechanisms of rat tail artery contraction-relaxation by menthol involving, respectively, TRPM8 activation and l-type ca^{2+} channel inhibition. *American Journal of Physiology - Heart and Circulatory Physiology*, *311*(6). https://doi.org/10.1152/ajpheart.00222.2015.

Milenkovic, V. M., Langmann, T., Schreiber, R., Kunzelmann, K., & Weber, B. H. F. (2008). Molecular evolution and functional divergence of the bestrophin protein family. *BMC Evolutionary Biology*, *8*(1). https://doi.org/10.1186/1471-2148-8-72.

Minard, A., Bauer, C. C., Wright, D. J., Rubaiy, H. N., Muraki, K., Beech, D. J., & Bon, R. S. (2018). Remarkable progress with small-molecule modulation of TRPC1/4/5 channels: Implications for understanding the channels in health and disease. *Cells*, *7*(6), 1–20. https://doi.org/10.3390/cells7060052.

Minke, B. (2010). The history of the drosophila TRP channel: The birth of a new channel superfamily. *Journal of Neurogenetics*, *24*(4), 216–233. https://doi.org/10.3109/01677063.2010.514369.

Moncada, S., Higgs, A. (1993). The L-arginine-nitric oxide pathway. The New England *Journal of Medicine,* 329, 2002–2012, https://doi.org/10.1056/NEJM1993 12303292706.

Moser, M. (2005). Diuretics should continue to be one of the preferred initial therapies in the management of hypertension: the argument for. In *Journal of clinical hypertension (Greenwich, Conn.)* (Vol. 7, Issue 2, pp. 111–116). J Clin Hypertens (Greenwich). https://doi.org/10.1111/j.1524-6175.2005.03943.x.

Movahed, M. R., Hashemzadeh, M., & Jamal, M. M. (2005). The prevalence of pulmonary embolism and pulmonary hypertension in patients with type II diabetes mellitus. *Chest*, *128*(5), 3568–3571. https://doi.org/10.1378/CHEST.128.5.3568.

Müller, M., & Igamberdiev, A. U. (2024). The emergence of theoretical biology: Two fundamental works of Ervin Bauer (1890–1938) in English translation. *BioSystems*, *241*, 105201. https://doi.org/10.1016/j.biosystems.2024.105201.

Namm, D. H., & Zucker, J. L. (1973). Biochemical alterations caused by hypoxia in the isolated rabbit aorta. Correlation with changes in arterial contractility. *Circulation Research*, *32*(4), 464–470. https://doi.org/10.1161/01.res.32.4.464.

Nelson, M. T., Cheng, H., Rubart, M., Santana, L. F., Bonev, A. D., Knot, H. J., & Lederer, W. J. (1995). Relaxation of arterial smooth muscle by calcium sparks [see comments]. *Science*, *270*(5236), 633–637. https://doi.org/10.1126/science.270.5236.633.

Nelson, M. T., McCarron, J. G., & Quayle, J. M. (1991). Ion Channels in Resistance Arteries. In *The Resistance Vasculature* (pp. 265–279). Humana Press. https://doi.org/10.1007/978-1-4612-0403-9_16.

Nelson, M. T., Patlak, J. B., Worley, J. F., & Standen, N. B. (1990). Calcium channels, potassium channels, and voltage dependence of arterial smooth muscle tone. [Review] [139 refs]. *American Journal of Physiology*, *259*(1 Pt 1), C3–C18. http://ajpcell.physiology.org/content/259/1/C3.abstract.

Nilius, B., & Flockerzi, V. (Eds.). (2014). *Mammalian Transient Receptor Potential (TRP) Cation Channels* (Vol. 222). Springer Berlin Heidelberg. https://doi.org/10.1007/978-3-642-54215-2.

Nosengo, N. (2016). Can you teach old drugs new tricks? *Nature*, *534*(7607), 314–316. https://doi.org/10.1038/534314a.

Novokhatska, T., Tishkin, S., Dosenko, V., Boldyrev, A., Ivanova, I., Strelkov, I,, Soloviev, A (2013). Correction of vascular hypercontractility in spontaneously hypertensive rats using shRNAs-induced delta protein kinase C gene silencing. *European Journal of Pharmacology*, 718, issues 1-3, 401-407.

Numata, T., Kiyonaka, S., Kato, K., Takahashi, N., & Mori, Y. (2016). Activation of TRP channels in mammalian systems. In *TRP Channels* (pp. 43–90). CRC Press. https://doi.org/10.1201/b10896-8.

Ohya, Y., & Sperelakis, N. (1989). Modulation of single slow (L-type) calcium channels by intracellular ATP in vascular smooth muscle cells. *Pflügers Archiv European Journal of Physiology*, *414*(3), 257–264. https://doi.org/10.1007/BF00584624.

Okabe, K., Inoue, Y., Kawarabayashi, T., Kajiya, H., Okamoto, F., & Soeda, H. (1999). Physiological significance of hyperpolarization-activated inward currents (I h) in smooth muscle cells from the circular layers of pregnant rat myometrium. *Pflügers Archiv*, *439*(1), 76–85. https://doi.org/10.1007/s004249900140.

Otto, A. M. (2016). Warburg effect(s) - a biographical sketch of Otto Warburg and his impacts on tumor metabolism. *Cancer & Metabolism*, *4*(1). https://doi.org/10.1186/s40170-016-0145-9.

Ozaki, H., & Karaki, H. (1993). Different Ca^{2+}-sensitivity in phasic and tonic types of smooth muscles. *NeuroSignals*, *2*(5), 253–262. https://doi.org/10.1159/000109506.

Owvsyjannikov, Ph. Die tonishe und reflektorishe Zentren der Gefanervren. Arbeiten aus der physiol. *Anstalt zu Leipzig, mitgeteilt durch C. Ludwig*., 1873, 6, 21-33.

Parekh, A. B. (2011). Decoding cytosolic Ca^{2+} oscillations. In *Trends in Biochemical Sciences* (Vol. 36, Issue 2, pp. 78–87). https://doi.org/10.1016/j.tibs.2010.07.013.

Paul, R. J., Bauer, M., & Pease, W. (1979). Vascular Smooth Muscle: Aerobic Glycolysis Linked to Sodium and Potassium Transport Processes. *Science*, *206*(4425), 1414–1416. https://doi.org/10.1126/Science.505014.

Paul, R., Hellstrand, P., Krisanda, I. (1984). Relations among oxygen consumption, phosphagen and contractility in vascular smooth muscle. In *Stephens, N. (Ed.), Smooth Muscle Contraction. Marcel Dekker, New York,* 245-257.

Pegram, B.,L. (1982). The portal as a model for resistance vessels. *Vascular neuroeffector mechanisms,* New York: Raven, 43-44.

Peppiatt-Wildman, C. M., Albert, A. P., Saleh, S. N., & Large, W. A. (2007). Endothelin-1 activates a Ca^{2+}-permeable cation channel with TRPC3 and TRPC7 properties in rabbit coronary artery myocytes. *Journal of Physiology*, *580*(3), 755–764. https://doi.org/10.1113/jphysiol.2006.126656.

Poms, A. D., Turner, M., Farber, H. W., Meltzer, L. A., & McGoon, M. D. (2013). Comorbid conditions and outcomes in patients with pulmonary arterial hypertension: A reveal registry analysis. *Chest*, *144*(1), 169–176. https://doi.org/10.1378/chest.11-3241.

Potocnik, S. J., Murphy, T. V., Kotecha, N., & Hill, M. A. (2000). Effects of mibefradil and nifedipine on arteriolar myogenic responsiveness and intracellular Ca^{2+}. *British Journal of Pharmacology*, *131*(6), 1065–1072. https://doi.org/10.1038/SJ.BJP.0703650.

Pucovský, V., Moss, R. F., & Bolton, T. B. (2003). Non-contractile cells with thin processes resembling interstitial cells of Cajal found in the wall of guinea-pig mesenteric arteries. *Journal of Physiology*, *552*(1), 119–133. https://doi.org/10.1113/jphysiol.2003.046243.

Putney, J. W. (1986). A model for receptor-regulated calcium entry. *Cell Calcium*, *7*(1), 1–12. https://doi.org/10.1016/0143-4160(86)90026-6.

Putney, J. W. (2009). Capacitative calcium entry: from concept to molecules. *Immunological Reviews*, *231*(1), 10–22. http://dx.doi.org/10.1111/j.1600-065X.2009.00810.x.

Ramsey, I. S. S., Delling, M., & Clapham, D. E. (2006). An introduction to TRP channels. *Annual Review of Physiology*, *68*(2), 619–647. https://doi.org/10.1146/annurev.physiol.68.040204.100431.

Reading, S. A., Earley, S., Waldron, B. J., Welsh, D. G., & Brayden, J. E. (2005). TRPC3 mediates pyrimidine receptor-induced depolarization of cerebral arteries. *American Journal of Physiology - Heart and Circulatory Physiology*, *288*(5 57-5). https://doi.org/10.1152/ajpheart.00861.2004.

Renkin, E. M. (1959). Transport of potassium-42 from blood to tissue in isolated mammalian skeletal muscles. *The American Journal of Physiology*, *197*, 1205–1210. https://doi.org/10.1152/ajplegacy.1959.197.6.1205.

Renkin, E. M, Hudlická, O., Sheehan, R. M. (1966), Influence of metabolic vasodilatation on blood-tissue diffusion in skeletal muscle. *American Journal of Physiology*, 211(1):87-98. doi: 10.1152/ajplegacy.1966.211.1.87. PMID: 5911058.

Rodbard, S. (1971). Capillary control of blood flow and fluid exchange. *Circulation Research*, *28*, 51–58.

Rodbard, S., Takeda, Y., & Takacs, L. (1969). Post-occlusion 'hyperemia': A study on a model. *Quarterly Journal of Experimental Physiology and Cognate Medical Sciences*, *54*(3), 346–365. https://doi.org/10.1113/expphysiol.1969.sp002033.

Rosenberry, R., & Nelson, M. D. (2020). Reactive hyperemia: A review of methods, mechanisms, and considerations. In *American Journal of Physiology - Regulatory Integrative and Comparative Physiology* (Vol. 318, Issue 3, pp. R605–R618). American Physiological Society. https://doi.org/10.1152/AJPREGU.00339.2019.

Rubanyi, G., & Paul, R. J. (1985). Two distinct effects of oxygen on vascular tone in isolated porcine coronary arteries. *Circulation Research*, *56*(1), 1–10. https://doi.org/10.1161/01.RES.56.1.1.

Sadee, W. (2023). Ligand-Free Signaling of G-Protein-Coupled Receptors: Physiology, Pharmacology, and Genetics. In *Molecules* (Vol. 28, Issue 17, p. 6375). Multidisciplinary Digital Publishing Institute (MDPI). https://doi.org/10.3390/molecules28176375.

Saleh, S. N., Albert, A. P., & Large, W. A. (2009a). Activation of native TRPC1/C5/C6 channels by endothelin-1 is mediated by both PIP3 and PIP2 in rabbit coronary artery myocytes. *The Journal of Physiology*, *587*(22), 5361–5375. http://jp.physoc.org/content/587/22/5361.abstract.

Saleh, S. N., Albert, A. P., & Large, W. A. (2009b). Obligatory role for phosphatidylinositol 4,5-bisphosphate in activation of native TRPC1 store-operated channels in vascular myocytes. *The Journal of Physiology*, *587*(3), 531–540. http://jp.physoc.org/content/587/3/531.abstract.

Saleh, S. N., Albert, A. P., Peppiatt, C. M., & Large, W. A. (2006). Angiotensin II activates two cation conductances with distinct TRPC1 and TRPC6 channel properties in rabbit mesenteric artery myocytes. *The Journal of Physiology Online*, *577*(2), 479–495. http://jp.physoc.org/cgi/content/abstract/577/2/479.

Santos, R., Ursu, O., Gaulton, A., Bento, A. P., Donadi, R. S., Bologa, C. G., Karlsson, A., Al-Lazikani, B., Hersey, A., Oprea, T. I., & Overington, J. P. (2016). A comprehensive map of molecular drug targets. *Nature Reviews Drug Discovery*, *16*(1), 19–34. https://doi.org/10.1038/nrd.2016.230.

Sessions, A. L., Doughty, D. M., Welander, P. V., Summons, R. E., & Newman, D. K. (2009). The Continuing Puzzle of the Great Oxidation Event. In *Current Biology* (Vol. 19, Issue 14). Curr Biol. https://doi.org/10.1016/j.cub.2009.05.054.

Shuba, M. F. (1981). Pathways and mechanisms of transmembrane entry of calcium ions into smooth muscle cells, which are involved in the activation of contraction. *Fiziologichnyi Zhurnal*, *27*(4), 533–541.

Siegel G. (1983). Principles of vascular rhythmogenesis. *Progress in Appled Microcirulation,*198; 3: 40-63. https://doi.org/10.1159/isbn.978-3-318-04062-3.

Siegel, G., & Grote, J. (1988). PO2-Induced Changes of Membrane Potential and Tension in Vascular Smooth Musculature. In *Oxygen Sensing in Tissues* (pp. 131–142). Springer Berlin Heidelberg. https://doi.org/10.1007/978-3-642-83444-8_11.

Sigurdsson, S. B., Orlov, R. S., Hellstrand, P., & Johansson, B. (1981). Responses to ions and vasoconstrictor agents and changes of potassium fluxes in vascular smooth muscle during hypoxia. *Acta Physiologica Scandinavica*, *112*(4), 455–462. https://doi.org/ 10.1111/j.1748-1716.1981.tb06844.x.

Smani, T., Hernández, A., Ureña, J., Castellano, A. G., Franco-Obregón, A., Ordoñez, A., & López-Barneo, J. (2002). Reduction of Ca^{2+} channel activity by hypoxia in human and porcine coronary myocytes. *Cardiovascular Research*, *53*(1), 97–104. https://doi.org/10.1016/S0008-6363(01)00422-9.

Smirnov, S. V, Zholos, A. V, & Shuba, M. F. (1992). Potential-dependent inward currents in single isolated smooth muscle cells of the rat ileum. *The Journal of Physiology*, *454*(1). https://doi.org/10.1113/jphysiol.1992.sp019279.

Soloviev, A. (1973). On the mechanisms of regulation of vascular tone of skeletal muscles with short-term and prolonged artery occlusions. *Sechenov Fiziol. Journal of USSR, 59,1: 88-98.*

Soloviev, A., Bazilyuk, O. (1981). Effects of restriction of oxygenation of vascular smooth muscle on contractile effects of direct electrical and mechanical stimulation. *Byull. Eksp. Biol. Med.*, 92: 1469-1471.

Soloviev, A. I. Mechanisms of regulation of vascular smooth muscle tone during changes in the degree of their oxygenation. The dissertation for the degree Doctor of Medical Sciences, Kyiv. 1987.

Soloviev A. I. (1988). The cellular mechanisms of hypoxic coronary spasm. *Sechenov Fiziol. Zh. USSR,* 74: 193-201.

Soloviev, A., Bershtein, S. (1992). The contractile apparatus in vascular smooth muscle cells of spontaneously hypertensive rats possess increased calcium sensitivity: the possible role of protein kinase C. *Journal of Hypertension,* 10: 131-136.

Soloviev, A., Braquet, P. (1992). Platelet-activating factor - a potent endogenous mediator responsible for coronary vasospasm. News in Physiological Science, 10, 166-171.

Soloviev, A., & Basilyuk, O. (1993). Evidence for decrease in myofilament responsiveness to Ca^{2+} during hypoxia in spontaneously active vascular smooth muscle in rats. *Experimental Physiology*, *78*(3), 395–402. https://doi.org/10.1113/expphysiol. 1993.sp003693.

Soloviev, A., Lehen'kyi, V., Zelensky, S., Hellstrand, P. (2004). Nitric oxide relaxes rat tail artery smooth muscle by cyclic GMPindependent decrease in calcium sensitivity of myofilaments. *Cell Calcium*. 2004; 36: 165-173.

Soloviev, A., Parshikov, A., Stefanov, A. (1998). Evidence for the involvement of protein kinase C in development of endothelium-dependent vascular responses in spontaneously rats. *Journal of Vascular Research*, 35: 325-331.

Soloviev, A., Prudnikov, I., Tsyvkin, V., Tishkin S., Kyrychenko, S., Zelensky, S., Ivanova, I. (2010). Electrophysiological and contractile evidence the ability of human mesenchymal stromal stem cells to correct vascular malfunction in rats after ionizing irradiation. *The Journal of Physiological Science, (Japan)*, 60: 161-172.

Soloviev, A. I., Bondarenko, A. I., & Kizub, I. V. (2012). Selective glycolysis blockade in guinea pig pulmonary artery and aorta reverses contractile and electrical responses to acute hypoxia. *Vascular Pharmacology*, *57*(2–4), 119–123. https://doi.org/10.1016/J.VPH.2012.06.001.

Soloviev, A. I., Stefanov, A. V., Baziliyk, O. V., Rekalov, V. V., & Pronchuk, N. F. (1996). Changes in plasma membrane ionic permeability and related contractile responses in vascular smooth muscle at hypoxia. *Pathophysiology*, *3*(1), 11–20. https://doi.org/10.1016/0928-4680(95)00032-1.

Soloviev, A., Stefanov, A., Tishkin, S., Khromov, A, Parshikov, A., Ivanova, I., Gurney, A. (2002). Saline containing phosphatidylcholine liposomes possess the ability to restore endothelial function damaged resulting from gamma-radiation, *Journal Physiology and Pharmacology,* 53, 701–712.

Soloviev, A., Tishkin, S., Parshikov, A., Ivanova, I., Goncharov E., Gurney A. (2003). Mechanisms of endothelial dysfunction after ionized radiation: selective impairment of the nitric oxide component of endothelium-dependent vasodilation. *British Journal of Pharmacology*, 138, 837–844, https://doi.org/10.1038/sj.bjp.0705079.

Soloviev, A., Tishkin, S, Zelensky, S., Ivanova, I., Kizub, I., Pavlova, A., Moreland, R. (2005). Ionizing radiation alter myofilament calcium sensitivity in vascular smooth muscle: potential role of protein kinase C. *American Journal of Physiology. Regul. Integr. Comp. Physiol.*, 289: 755-762.

Soloviev A., Zholos A., Ivanova I., Novokhatska T., Tishkin S., Raevska A., Stroyuk A., Yefanov V. (2015). Plasmonic gold nanoparticles possess the ability to open potassium channels in rat thoracic aorta smooth muscle in a remote control manner. *Vascular Pharmacolology,* 72:190-196.

Soloviev, A., Melnyk, M., Ivanova, I., Dryn, D., Zholos, A. (2016). Non-drug remote control of Maxi-K channels in smooth muscle cells with nano-photonic stimuli using plasmonic gold nanoparticles. *JSM Nanotechnology & Nanomedicine,* 4(1): 1-10.

Soloviev, A., Ivanova, I., Melnyk, M., Dobrelia N., Khromov A. (2019). Hypoxic Pulmonary Vasoconstriction Is Lacking in Rats with Type 1 Diabetes. *Clinical and Experimental Pharmacology and Physiology*, July 2019, 46(5), doi:10.1111/1440-1681.13137.

Somlyo, A. V, & Somlyo, A. P. (1968). Electromechanical and pharmacomechanical coupling in vascular smooth muscle. *Journal of Pharmacology and Experimental Therapeutics*, *159*(1).

Somlyo, A. P., Somlyo, A. V. (1976). Ultrastructural aspects of activation and contraction of vascular smooth muscle. *Federation Proceedings*, 35, p. 1288-1293.

Somlyo, A. P., Somlyo, A. V. (2003). Ca^{2+} sensitivity of smooth muscle and nonmuscle myosin II: modulated by G proteins, kinases, and myosin phosphatase. *Physiological Review*, 83: 1325-1258.

Somlyo, A. V., Wang, H., Choudhury, N., Khromov, A. S., Majesky, M., Owens, G. K., Somlyo, A. P. (2004). Myosin light chain kinase knockout. Journal of Muscle Researches and Cell Motility, 25, 241–242. [PubMed: 15467390].

Sommer, N., Dietrich, A., Schermuly, R. T., Ghofrani, H. A., Gudermann, T., Schulz, R., Seeger, W., Grimminger, F., & Weissmann, N. (2008). Regulation of hypoxic pulmonary vasoconstriction: basic mechanisms. *The European Respiratory Journal*, *32*(6), 1639–1651. https://doi.org/10.1183/09031936.00013908.

Somogyi, R., Stuckin, J. W. (1991). Hormone-induced calcium oscillations in liver cells can be explained by a simple one pool model. *Journal of Biological Chemistrey*, 266 11068-77.

Song, M. Y, Makino, A, Yuan, J., X. J. (2011). Role of Reactive Oxygen Species and Redox in Regulating the Function of Transient Receptor Potential Channels. *Antioxidants & Redox Signaling,* 15, 61549-1565. doi: 10.1089/ars.2010.3648.

Starling, E. H. (1896). On the absorption of fluids from the connective tissue spaces. *The Journal of Physiology,* 19(4):312-26. doi: 10.1113/jphysiol. 1896.sp000596.

Swann, H. G., Montgomery, A. V., Davis, J. C., & Mickle, E. R. (1950). A method for rapid measurement of intrarenal and other tissue pressures. *The Journal of Experimental Medicine*, *92*(6), 625–636. https://doi.org/10.1084/jem.92.6.625.

Swärd, K., Josefsson, M., Lydrup, M. -L, & Hellstrand, P. (1993). Effects of metabolic inhibition on cytoplasmic calcium and contraction in smooth muscle of rat portal vein. *Acta Physiologica Scandinavica*, *148*(3), 265–272. https://doi.org/10.1111/j.1748-1716.1993.tb09557.x.

Sweeney, M., Yu, Y., Platoshyn, O., Zhang, S., McDaniel, S. S., & Yuan, J. X.-J. (2002). Inhibition of endogenous TRP1 decreases capacitative Ca2+ entry and attenuates pulmonary artery smooth muscle cell proliferation. *AJP - Lung Cellular and Molecular Physiology*, *283*(1), L144–L155. http://ajplung.physiology.org/cgi/content/abstract/283/1/L144.

Sylvester, J. T., Shimoda, L. A., Aaronson, P. I., & Ward, J. P. T. (2012). Hypoxic pulmonary vasoconstriction. *Physiological Reviews*, *92*(1), 367–520. https://doi.org/10.1152/PHYSREV.00041.2010.

Szasz, T., Webb, R., C. (2012). Perivascular adipose tissue: more than just structural support. *Clinical Science (Lond)*, 122(1):1-12. doi: 10.1042/CS20110151. PMID: 21910690; PMCID: PMC3966487.

Szymański W., Beierle J. M., Kistemaker H. A., Velema W. A., Feringa B. L. (2013). Reversible photocontrol of biological systems by the incorporation of molecular photoswitches. *Chemical Reviews,* 113 (8): 6114–6178. doi: 10.1021/cr300179f.

Tachiiri, S., Katagiri, T., Tsunoda, T., Oya, N., Hiraoka, M., Nakamura, Y. (2006). Analysis of gene-expression profiles after gamma irradiation of normal human fibroblasts. *International Journal of Radiation Oncology and Biological Physics*. 64 (1), 272–279, https://doi.org/10.1016/j. ijrobp.2005.08.030.

Takahashi, Y., Watanabe, H., Murakami, M., Ono, K., Munehisa, Y., Koyama, T., Nobori, K., Iijima, T., & Ito, H. (2007). Functional role of stromal interaction molecule 1

(STIM1) in vascular smooth muscle cells. *Biochemical and Biophysical Research Communications*, *361*(4), 934–940. https://doi.org/10.1016/j.bbrc.2007.07.096.

Takaki, M. (2003). Gut Pacemaker Cells: The Interstitial Cells of Cajal (ICC). In *Journal of Smooth Muscle Research* (Vol. 39, Issue 5, pp. 137–161). J Smooth Muscle Res. https://doi.org/10.1540/jsmr.39.137.

Tang, J., Lin, Y., Zhang, Z., Tikunova, S., Birnbaumer, L., & Zhu, M. X. (2001). Identification of common binding sites for calmodulin and Inositol 1,4,5-trisphosphate receptors on the carboxyl termini of Trp channels. *Journal of Biological Chemistry*, *276*(24), 21303–21310. http://www.jbc.org/cgi/content/abstract/276/24/21303.

Thakore, P., & Earley, S. (2019). Transient receptor potential channels and endothelial cell calcium signaling. *Comprehensive Physiology*, *9*(3), 1249–1277. https://doi.org/10.1002/cphy.c180034.

Tishkin, S., Rekalov, V., Ivanova, I,, Moreland, R., and Soloviev, A. (2007). Ionizing non-fatal whole-body irradiation inhibits Ca^{2+} -dependent K^{+} channels in endothelial cells of rat coronary artery: Possible contribution to depression of endothelium-dependent vascular relaxation. International Journal of Radiation Biology, 83:3,161-169.

Tomita, K., & Kitahara, K. (1975). A model for oscillating chemical reactions. *Biophysical Chemistry*, *3*(2), 125–141. https://doi.org/10.1016/0301-4622(75)80002-0.

Tykocki, N. R., Boerman, E. M., & Jackson, W. F. (2017). Smooth muscle ion channels and regulation of vascular tone in resistance arteries and arterioles. *Comprehensive Physiology*, *7*(2), 485–581. https://doi.org/10.1002/cphy.c160011.

Tzingounis, A. V., Kobayashi, M., Takamatsu, K., Nicoll, R.A. (2007). Hippocalcin gates the calcium activation of the slow afterhyperpolarization in hippocampal pyramidal cells. *Neuron,* 53:487–493.

Uchida, E., Bohr, D. F., & Hoobler, S. W. (1967). A method for studying isolated resistance vessels from rabbit mesentery and brain and their responses to drugs. *Circulation Research*, *21*(4), 525–536. https://doi.org/10.1161/01.RES.21.4.525.

Ulyanova, A. V., & Shirokov, R. E. (2018). Voltage-dependent inward currents in smooth muscle cells of skeletal muscle arterioles. *PLoS ONE*, *13*(4). https://doi.org/10.1371/journal.pone.0194980.

Vallejo, J., & Hardin, C. D. (2004). Metabolic organization in vascular smooth muscle: distribution and localization of caveolin-1 and phosphofructokinase. *American Journal of Physiology. Cell Physiology*, *286*(1). https://doi.org/10.1152/AJPCELL.00483.2002.

Venkatachalam, K., & Montell, C. (2007). TRP Channels. *Annual Review of Biochemistry*, *76*(1), 387–417. https://doi.org/10.1146/annurev.biochem.75.103004.142819.

Vergara, C., Latorre, R., Marrion, N. V, & Adelman, J. P. (1998). Calcium-activated potassium channels. *Current Opinion in Neurobiology*, *8*(3), 321–329. https://doi.org/10.1016/S0959-4388(98)80056-1.

Wang, H., Cheng, X., Tian, J., Xiao, Y., Tian, T., Xu, F., Hong, X., & Zhu, M. X. (2020). TRPC channels: Structure, function, regulation and recent advances in small molecular probes. In *Pharmacology and Therapeutics* (Vol. 209, p. 107497). Elsevier Inc. https://doi.org/10.1016/j.pharmthera.2020.107497.

Wang, Y., Deng, X., Hewavitharana, T., Soboloff, J., & Gill, D. L. (2008). STIM, ORAI and TRPC channels in the control of calcium entry signals in smooth muscle. *Clinical and Experimental Pharmacology and Physiology*, *35*(9), 1127–1133. https://doi.org/10.1111/j.1440-1681.2008.05018.x.

Watanabe, H., Murakami, M., Ohba, T., Takahashi, Y., & Ito, H. (2008). TRP channel and cardiovascular disease. *Pharmacology & Therapeutics*, *118*(3), 337–351. https://doi.org/10.1016/j.pharmthera.2008.03.008.

Weisbrod, D., Khun, S. H., Bueno, H., Peretz, A., & Attali, B. (2016a). Mechanisms underlying the cardiac pacemaker: The role of SK4 calcium-activated potassium channels. In *Acta Pharmacologica Sinica* (Vol. 37, Issue 1, pp. 82–97). Nature Publishing Group. https://doi.org/10.1038/aps.2015.135.

Weisbrod, D., Khun, S. H., Bueno, H., Peretz, A., & Attali, B. (2016b). Mechanisms underlying the cardiac pacemaker: The role of SK4 calcium-activated potassium channels. In *Acta Pharmacologica Sinica* (Vol. 37, Issue 1, pp. 82–97). Nature Publishing Group. https://doi.org/10.1038/aps.2015.135.

Weissmann, N., Dietrich, A., Fuchs, B., Kalwa, H., Ay, M., Dumitrascu, R., Olschewski, A., Storch, U., Y Schnitzler, M. M., Ghofrani, H. A., Schermuly, R. T., Pinkenburg, O., Seeger, W., Grimminger, F., & Gudermann, T. (2006). Classical transient receptor potential channel 6 (TRPC6) is essential for hypoxic pulmonary vasoconstriction and alveolar gas exchange. *Proceedings of the National Academy of Sciences of the United States of America*, *103*(50), 19093–19098. https://doi.org/10.1073/PNAS.0606728103.

Wenceslau C. F., McCarthy C. G., Earley S., England S. K., Filosa J. A., Goulopoulou S., Gutterman D. D., Isakson B. E., Kanagy N. L., Martinez-Lemus L. A., Sonkusare S. K., Thakore P., Trask A. J., Watts S. W., Webb R. C. (2021). Guidelines for the measurement of vascular function and structure in isolated arteries and veins. *American Journal of Physiology, Heart Circulatory Physiology,* 321(1):H77-H111. doi: 10.1152/ajpheart.01021.2020. Epub 2021 May 14. PMID: 33989082; PMCID: PMC8321813.

Wes, P. D., Chevesich, J., Jeromin, A., Rosenberg, C., Stetten, G., & Montell, C. (1995). TRPC1, a human homolog of a Drosophila store-operated channel. *Proceedings of the National Academy of Sciences of the United States of America*, *92*(21), 9652–9656. https://doi.org/10.1073/pnas.92.21.9652.

Wiedmann, F., Schmidt, C., Lugenbiel, P., Staudacher, I., Rahm, A. K., Seyler, C., Schweizer, P. A., Katus, H. A., & Thomas, D. (2016a). Therapeutic targeting of two-pore-domain potassium (K2P) channels in the cardiovascular system. In *Clinical Science* (Vol. 130, Issue 9, pp. 643–650). Portland Press Ltd. https://doi.org/10.1042/CS20150533.

Wiedmann, F., Schmidt, C., Lugenbiel, P., Staudacher, I., Rahm, A. K., Seyler, C., Schweizer, P. A., Katus, H. A., & Thomas, D. (2016b). Therapeutic targeting of two-pore-domain potassium (K2P) channels in the cardiovascular system. In *Clinical Science* (Vol. 130, Issue 9, pp. 643–650). Portland Press Ltd. https://doi.org/10.1042/CS20150533.

Wong, C. O., & Yao, X. (2011). TRP channels in vascular endothelial cells. *Advances in Experimental Medicine and Biology*, *704*, 759–780. https://doi.org/10.1007/978-94-007-0265-3_40.

Wray, S., & Prendergast, C. (2019). The Myometrium: From Excitation to Contractions and Labour. In *Advances in Experimental Medicine and Biology* (Vol. 1124, pp. 233–263). Springer New York LLC. https://doi.org/10.1007/978-981-13-5895-1_10.

Wu, L. J., Sweet, T. B., & Clapham, D. E. (2010). International Union of Basic and Clinical Pharmacology. LXXVI. Current Progress in the Mammalian TRP Ion Channel Family. *Pharmacological Reviews*, *62*(3), 381–404. https://doi.org/10.1124/pr.110.002725.

Xu, S. Z., & Beech, D. J. (2001). TrpC1 is a membrane-spanning subunit of store-operated $Ca^{(2+)}$ channels in native vascular smooth muscle cells 720. *Circulation Research*, *88*(United States PT-Journal Article LG-English), 84–87.

Yan, S., Sheak, J. R., Walker, B. R., Jernigan, N. L., & Resta, T. C. (2023). Contribution of Mitochondrial Reactive Oxygen Species to Chronic Hypoxia-Induced Pulmonary Hypertension. *Antioxidants (Basel, Switzerland)*, *12*(12). https://doi.org/10.3390/ANTIOX12122060.

Yanagida, H., Inoue, R., Tanaka, M., & Ito, Y. (2000). Temperature-sensitive gating of cation current in guinea pig ileal smooth muscle activated by hyperpolarization. *American Journal of Physiology - Cell Physiology*, *278*(1 47-1). https://doi.org/10.1152/ajpcell.2000.278.1.c40.

Yang, L., Arbona, R. J. R., Smith, C. S., Banks, K. M., Thomas, V. K., Palmer, L., Evans, T., & Hurtado, R. (2023). An evolutionarily conserved pacemaker role for HCN ion channels in smooth muscle. *Journal of Physiology*, *601*(7), 1225–1246. https://doi.org/10.1113/JP283701.

Yang, X. R., Lin, M. J., McIntosh, L. S., & Sham, J. S. K. (2006). Functional expression of transient receptor potential melastatin- and vanilloid-related channels in pulmonary arterial and aortic smooth muscle. *American Journal of Physiology - Lung Cellular and Molecular Physiology*, *290*(6). https://doi.org/10.1152/ajplung.00515.2005.

Yao, X., & Garland, C. J. (2005). Recent developments in vascular endothelial cell transient receptor potential channels. *Circulation Research*, *97*(9), 853–863. http://circres.ahajournals.org/cgi/content/abstract/97/9/853.

Yoshino, M., Someya, T., Nishio, A., Yazawa, K., Usuki, T., & Yabu, H. (1989). Multiple types of voltage-dependent Ca channels in mammalian intestinal smooth muscle cells. *Pflügers Archiv European Journal of Physiology*, *414*(4), 401–409. https://doi.org/10.1007/BF00585049.

Zhang, J., Berra-Romani, R., Sinnegger-Brauns, M. J., Striessnig, J., Blaustein, M. P., & Matteson, D. R. (2007). Role of Cav1.2 L-type Ca^{2+} channels in vascular tone: effects of nifedipine and Mg2+. *American Journal of Physiology. Heart and Circulatory Physiology*, *292*(1). https://doi.org/10.1152/AJPHEART.01214.2005.

Zhang, X., Hu, M., Yang, Y., & Xu, H. (2018). Organellar TRP channels. In *Nature Structural and Molecular Biology* (Vol. 25, Issue 11, pp. 1009–1018). Nature Publishing Group. https://doi.org/10.1038/s41594-018-0148-z.

Zhang, Z., Tang, J., Tikunova, S., Johnson, J. D., Chen, Z., Qin, N., Dietrich, A., Stefani, E., Birnbaumer, L., & Zhu, M. X. (2001). Activation of Trp3 by inositol 1,4,5-trisphosphate receptors through displacement of inhibitory calmodulin from a common binding domain. *Proceedings of the National Academy of Sciences of the United States of America*, *98*(6), 3168–3173. https://doi.org/10.1073/pnas.051632698.

Zhao, Q. Y., Peng, Y. B., Luo, X. J., Luo, X., Xu, H., Wei, M. Y., Jiang, Q. J., Li, W. E., Ma, L. Q., Xu, J. C., Liu, X. C., Zang, D. A., She, Y. S., Zhu, H., Shen, J., Zhao, P., Xue, L., Yu, M. F., Chen, W., Liu, Q. H. (2017). Distinct effects of Ca^{2+} sparks on cerebral artery and airway smooth muscle cell tone in mice and humans. *International Journal of Biological Sciences*, *13*(10), 1242–1253. https://doi.org/10.7150/ijbs.21475.

Zhao, R., & Tsang, S. Y. (2017). Versatile Roles of Intracellularly Located TRPV1 Channel. In *Journal of Cellular Physiology* (Vol. 232, Issue 8, pp. 1957–1965). Wiley-Liss Inc. https://doi.org/10.1002/jcp.25704.

Zholos, A., Johnson, C., Burdyga, T., & Melanaphy, D. (2011). TRPM channels in the vasculature. In *Advances in Experimental Medicine and Biology* (Vol. 704). https://doi.org/10.1007/978-94-007-0265-3_37.

Zholos, A. V. (2006). Regulation of TRP-like muscarinic cation current in gastrointestinal smooth muscle with special reference to PLC/InsP3/Ca^{2+} system. In *Acta Pharmacologica Sinica* (Vol. 27, Issue 7, pp. 833–842). https://doi.org/10.1111/j.1745-7254.2006.00392.x.

Zholos, A. V. (2021). OVERVIEW OF TRP CHANNELS. In *Trips across Epithelial and Endothelial Barriers in Health and Disease.*

Zholos, A. V, Baidan, L. V, & Shuba, M. F. (1991). Properties of the late transient outward current in isolated intestinal smooth muscle cells of the guinea-pig. *The Journal of Physiology*, *443*(1). https://doi.org/10.1113/jphysiol.1991.sp018851.

Zholos, A. V, Baidan, L. V, & Shuba, M. F. (1992). Some properties of Ca^{2+}-induced Ca^{2+} release mechanism in single visceral smooth muscle cell of the guinea-pig. *The Journal of Physiology*, *457*(1). https://doi.org/10.1113/jphysiol.1992.sp019362.

Zholos, A. V, & Curtis, T. M. (2013). TRP channels in vascular disorders. *Current Topics in Medicinal Chemistry*, *13*(3). https://doi.org/10.2174/1568026611313030007.

Zholos, A. V, Komori, S., Ohashi, H., & Bolton, T. B. (1994). Ca^{2+} inhibition of inositol trisphosphate-induced Ca^{2+} release in single smooth muscle cells of guinea-pig small intestine. *The Journal of Physiology*, *481*(1), 97–109. https://doi.org/10.1113/jphysiol.1994.sp020421.

Zholos, A. V, Melnyk, M. I., & Dryn, D. O. (2024). Molecular mechanisms of cholinergic neurotransmission in visceral smooth muscles with a focus on receptor-operated TRPC4 channel and impairment of gastrointestinal motility by general anaesthetics and anxiolytics. In *Neuropharmacology* (Vol. 242). Elsevier Ltd. https://doi.org/10.1016/j.neuropharm.2023.109776.

Zhu, M. X. (2016). TRP channels. *TRP Channels*, 1–464. https://doi.org/10.4324/9781315152837-1.

Zhu, X., Chu, P. B., Peyton, M., & Birnbaumer, L. (1995). Molecular cloning of a widely expressed human homologue for the Drosophila trp gene. *FEBS Letters*, *373*(3), 193–198. https://doi.org/10.1016/0014-5793(95)01038-G.

About the Author

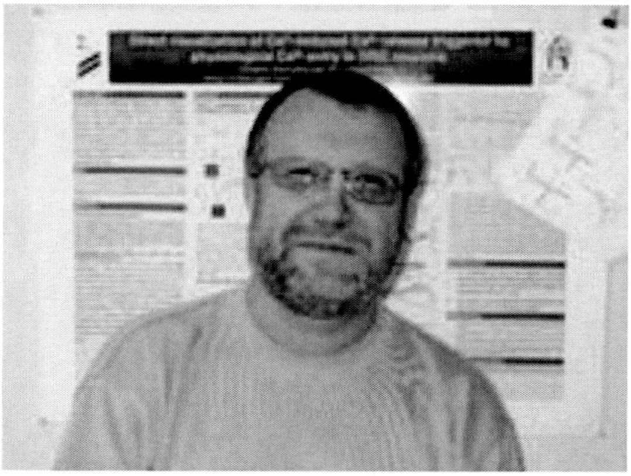

Professor Anatoly I. Soloviev
Institute of Pharmacology and Toxicology,
National Academy of Medical Science of Ukraine, Kyiv, Ukraine

Professor Anatoly I. Soloviev completed a MD in Radiology at Orenburg State Medical University, Russia, in 1972 and a BSc in Biophysics at Academy for Post-Graduate Training, Moscow, Russia, in 1975. He then completed a PhD and DSci in the area of Vascular Physiology, Pharmacology and Biophysics in 1978 and 1987, respectively, at the A. A. Bogomoletz Institute of Physiology, National Academy of Sciences, Kyiv, Ukraine. In 1993, Anatoly joined the Institute of Pharmacology and Toxicology, National Academy of Medical Sciences, Kiev, Ukraine where he is currently a professor (Pharmacology) and a Head of Department for Pharmacology of Cellular Signaling Systems and Experimental Therapeutics. He is also involved in drugs development as a Test Facility Manager of Interagency Laboratory for Non-Clinical Drug Trials. He worked as a visiting professor at the Lund (Sweden) and Strathclyde Glasgow (UK) Universities in 1995-1996 and 1999-2000. He is a Fellow Member of The Physiological Society (UK). Anatoly's research interests focused on the smooth muscle and endothelial function under hypoxia, hypertension, diabetes and ionized irradiation. In these topics, he has authored more than 125 papers in peer-reviewed reputed journals and 9 monographs. His research employed patch-clamp and contractile recording techniques *in vitro*, nitric oxide release and fluorescent calcium measurements, RNA - interference technique, cardiac-hemodynamics in vivo studies, and bioavailability drug studies using the human intestinal Caco-2 cell line. His research was funded by The Wellcome Trust (UK), National Institutes of Health and CRDF (USA), The Royal Society (UK), The Physiological Society (UK), INTAS and CNRS (France). Twice, in 1996 and 2003, he was awarded for these studies the Ukrainian State Prize in Field of Science and Technology. E-mail: tonysolpharm@gmail.com.

Index

A

B

C

D

E

I

K

L

M

N

O

P

R

S

T

U

V

W